# Pediatric neuromuscular diseases

# Pediatric neuromuscular diseases

**KENNETH F. SWAIMAN, M.D.**

Professor and Director, Division of Pediatric Neurology,
University of Minnesota Medical School,
Minneapolis, Minnesota

**FRANCIS S. WRIGHT, M.D.**

Professor, Division of Pediatric Neurology,
University of Minnesota Medical School,
Minneapolis, Minnesota

with 112 illustrations

## The C. V. Mosby Company

ST. LOUIS • TORONTO • LONDON    1979

The C. V. Mosby Company
11830 Westline Industrial Drive, St. Louis, Missouri 63141

**Library of Congress Cataloging in Publication Data**

Swaiman, Kenneth F
    Pediatric neuromuscular diseases.

    Bibliography: p.
    Includes index.
    1.   Neuromuscular diseases in children.   I.   Wright,
Francis S., 1929-         joint author.   II.   Title.   [DNLM:
1.   Neuromuscular diseases—In infancy and childhood.
WS340.3   S971p]
RJ496.N49S94   1979         618.9′27′4         79-20238
ISBN 0-8016-4846-7

GW/CB/B   9  8  7  6  5  4  3  2  1         01/D/071

# Preface

Although technically this text may not be a second edition of our book *Neuromuscular Diseases of Infancy and Childhood*, published in 1970, its ancestry is unmistakable. Very early in our pediatric neurology careers we recognized that among the greatest problems of the practicing physician and physician in training is the formulation of a differential diagnosis. All too often the physician is left without a systematic approach to the patient's difficulties. Enlightenment is further compromised by labels and eponyms that sometimes defy logic and reason. It is our intent that the attempts at anatomic and physiologic correlations in this book will allow a more direct approach to the problems of differential diagnosis. The manner of evaluation is one that has proved valuable through the past two decades in our training of students and house staff.

Although this text is not meant as a definitive textbook of pediatric neuromuscular disease, it is our intention that it provide concise, useful, and current information. We hope that it will in some small way ease the burden of those who undertake the care of children.

**Kenneth F. Swaiman**
**Francis S. Wright**

v

# Acknowledgments

Surely, this book would not have been completed without the care and industry of Mary Currey. It is also appropriate that we acknowledge the expert editorial assistance of Kay Savoie. Laurels are due the Department of Biomedical Graphics of the University of Minnesota, which produced most of the photographs. Line drawings were executed by Martin Finch and demonstrate his special talents.

Year after year, our interchange with colleagues and students helps shape our approaches to teaching pediatric neurology; therefore, they deserve our thanks. Hopefully, they will find this book partial repayment for their efforts.

Parenthetically, we wish to proclaim our survival of this venture in good spirits.

# Contents

# CHAPTER 1

# An approach to the diagnosis of neuromuscular disorders

Neuromuscular diseases of infants and children readily lend themselves to classification in terms of anatomic localization of the disease process.

The motor pathways are divided into a central nervous system or upper motor neuron unit (upper motor unit) and a peripheral or lower motor neuron unit (lower motor unit).

The upper motor unit is comprised of neurons and their axons, which form the corticospinal tract. The neurons that contribute axons to the corticospinal tract come predominantly from the motor cortex, but they also come from other areas of the cerebral cortex and subcortical areas. In effect, the corticospinal tract contains elements of what is classically called the pyramidal tract, as well as fibers from so-called extrapyramidal systems. These anatomic terms are not precise, reflect defects in knowledge about specific anatomic pathways and their relationship to movement and posture, and are not exact enough for many neurophysiologic purposes, but they are useful for purposes of clinical terminology and description.

The lower motor unit consists of the anterior horn cell (lower motor neuron; alpha motor neuron), its axon, neuromuscular junction, and the muscle fibers innervated by this axon (Fig. 1-1). The concept of the lower motor unit as a physiologic entity was developed by Sherrington (1925) and colleagues in work on reflex activity of the spinal cord. Under normal conditions, the lower motor unit responds in an all-or-none manner; the discharge of the anterior horn cell produces a synchronous and full contraction of all its innervated muscle fibers.

Neuromuscular diseases therefore can be classified according to the anatomic site of the pathology and the underlying physiologic disturbance in the lower motor unit. For example, acute anterior poliomyelitis and progressive spinal muscular atrophy are diseases of the anterior horn cell, the former an infectious and the latter a degenerative disease.

The cardinal symptom of diseases of the lower motor unit is weakness, defined as diminished strength in a specific muscle or group of muscles. The patient's history often reveals failure to achieve motor skills or loss of a specific motor skill or ability. The neurologic examination should document the presence of weakness.

Some patients complain of weakness that cannot be demonstrated on examination of individual muscles. This apparent discrepancy is related to lack of stamina and development of fatigue. Fatigue implies loss of ability to perform a repetitive muscular act. Fatigue is a less precise symptom than weakness, and it is important to differentiate fatigue with minimal exercise from fatigue with moderate amounts of exercise. If the patient

1

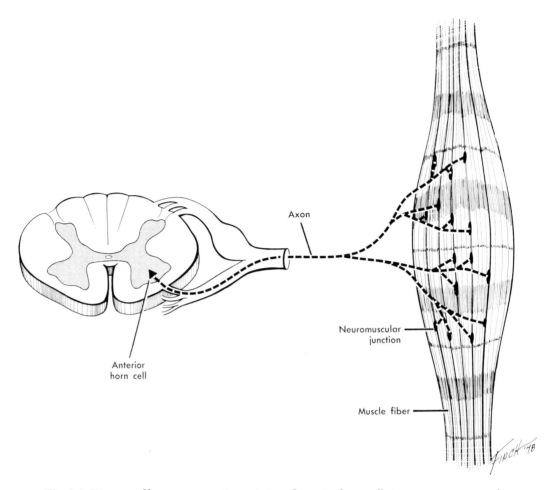

**Fig. 1-1.** Diagram of lower motor unit consisting of anterior horn cell, its axon, neuromuscular junction, and muscle fibers innervated by axon.

experiences difficulty in performing repetitive muscular acts, usually considered to be within the physiologic normal range, fatigue is excessive.

Hypotonia generally accompanies any significant degree of weakness. However, hypotonia also occurs in the absence of weakness. In clinical terms, hypotonia may be described as decreased resistance to passive movement (Holmes, 1939).

Muscle tone normally varies in degree depending on the physiologic demands on the neuromuscular system. It results from the complex interaction of the mechanical properties of joint, tendon, and muscle fiber as well as the dynamic, variable responses of the central and peripheral nervous system (Brooks and Stoney, 1971) that control contraction of muscles that maintain posture.

The mechanism by which disease of the central nervous system alters muscle tone involves the control of tone and posture through the gamma motor system (Leksell, 1945). The gamma system includes the gamma motor neurons, their efferent nerves, the stretch-sensitive muscle spindle located within the muscle, and the primary and secondary gamma afferent nerves coming from the spindle (Boyd et al., 1964; Granit, 1970, 1975; Stein, 1974). The muscle spindle is unique in location. It lies among and parallel to the striated muscle fibers. Therefore,

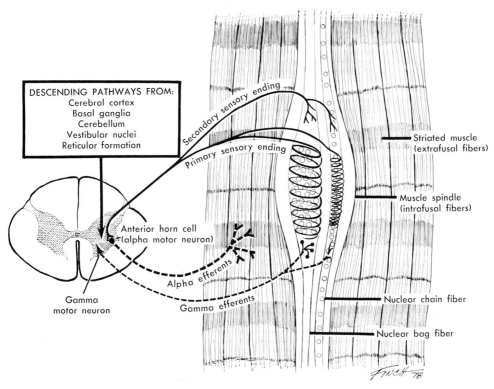

**Fig. 1-2.** Gamma system consists of gamma motor neuron, gamma efferent nerves, muscle spindle, and gamma afferent nerves (that receive impulses from both primary and secondary sensory endings). Gamma motor neuron excitability is affected by several descending pathways from the central nervous system.

when the striated muscle is stretched mechanically, as when a tendon reflex is elicited, the muscle spindle is also stretched, activating its sensory endings. The sensory discharges from the primary and secondary sensory endings travel over the gamma afferent nerves into the spinal cord to alter the excitability of the anterior horn cells, which in turn causes the striated muscle to contract. This sequence of events forms the physiologic basis of the tendon or myotatic reflex.

Several central nervous system structures and their fibers influence the gamma motor neuron activity (Fig. 1-2) (Eldred and Buchwald, 1967). These fibers come from the cerebral cortex, basal ganglia, thalamus, cerebellum, vestibular nuclei, and reticular formation. The gamma motor neurons affect the excitability of the muscle spindle and therefore control the length of the striated

muscle fiber. Thus muscle tone and posture are directly related to gamma motor neuron activity. Motor control is achieved by co-activation of alpha and gamma motor neurons simultaneously to produce a servo-assisted movement, that is, central activation modulated by peripheral feedback information. If the pathologic site of disease is in the central nervous system (cerebellum, cerebral cortex, medullary pyramidal tract), the tonic discharge of gamma motor neurons innervating muscle spindles is depressed producing hypotonia (Gilman, 1973).

Generally, injury to the central nervous system results in spasticity. However, in some areas of the central nervous system injury depresses the tonic discharges of the gamma motor neurons that innervate muscle spindles. This decreased activity results in hypotonia (Gilman, 1973).

### History

An accurate history of weakness should provide a diagnostic impression of the cause and anatomic location of the problem. The manifestation of weakness varies with the patient's age at onset. In the newborn infant, generalized weakness manifests as a weak cry, inadequate suck, respiratory difficulty, lack of body movement, and generalized hypotonia (floppy infant syndrome). After the neonatal period, the most common manifestation of weakness is delayed motor development. During the first year and a half of life, the infant does not attain or belatedly attains the motor landmarks of sitting, crawling, or walking. The older child manifests weakness by an awkward gait when walking or running and by difficulty walking up or down stairs or riding a tricycle. Weakness develops so insidiously sometimes that it is not noticed until the child begins school; as the child attempts to compete with peers, disability may be apparent.

Careful detailed questioning of the parents, and the child when possible, is necessary to determine the temporal characteristics of the weakness. Weakness that comes on within minutes is often vascular or traumatic in origin. Progressive weakness that peaks in a day or several days suggests an exogenous or endogenous toxic process, an electrolyte imbalance, or an infectious process. The physician should determine if there has been exposure to specific toxins such as barbiturates, lead (history of pica), drugs (antibiotics, corticosteroids, diuretics), unusual foods, and insect bites (for example, ticks). Circumstances leading to electrolyte imbalance, such as vomiting, diarrhea, and change in food intake, should be noted, as well as any treatment directed toward correcting the imbalance. Signs of an infectious process, such as fever, headache, rash, and malaise; exposure to a known infectious agent; and history of a recent infection, should be sought.

Weakness that evolves insidiously over many days, weeks, or months is generally associated with degenerative, metabolic, or neoplastic processes. The clinician should determine the time of onset and whether the course is acute, subacute, or chronic. Factors that aggravate the weakness, such as time of day, physical exertion, temperature, and food intake, should be noted. A history of passage of dark brown urine, pain associated with the weakness or exercise, muscle cramps, and muscles that seem to jump spontaneously should be sought.

After the mode of onset of the weakness has been determined, it is necessary to know whether it is static, progressive, or episodic. The examiner should seek objective evidence of progression of the weakness or increase in symptoms as other muscle groups are involved, asking about specific acts that the child can no longer perform. Many progressive diseases are characterized by a period of normal development, followed by loss of previously acquired skills. In addition to the history obtained from the parents, useful information can be gained by reviewing family photographs and motion pictures, as well as from a detailed baby book. Static clinical symptomatology implicates congenital abnormalities, traumatic processes, acute toxicity, or resolved infection.

The presence of progressive disease is documented best by gathering a detailed developmental history that surveys the motor milestones and development of language and adaptive social behavior. Table 1-1 presents pertinent and easily recognized landmarks that most children accomplish within the age periods designated. A thorough developmental history should indicate whether the disease process is confined to the neuromuscular system, with a delay or regression only in motor skills, or is more widespread, with retardation or deterioration in all developmental areas, implicating diffuse involvement of the central nervous system. Obviously, this distinction is more difficult to make in the young infant, whose initial outstanding progress is in the motor area. However, Table 1-1 presents early landmarks suitable for assessing development of both language and adaptive-social behavior.

The neurologic history should indicate

**Table 1-1.** Developmental assessment*

| Age (months) | Motor | Language | Adaptive-social |
|---|---|---|---|
| 0-3 | Prone—lifts head (1)† <br> Follows to midline (1) <br> Follows past midline (3) | Responds to sound (1) <br> Vocalizes—not crying (2) | Regards face (1) <br> Smiles responsively (2) |
| 3-6 | Sit—head steady (4) <br> Rolls over (5) <br> Reaches for object (5) | Laughs (3) <br> Squeals (5) | Smiles spontaneously (5) |
| 6-9 | Pull to sit—no head lag (6) <br> Transfers cube (1″)—hand to hand (7) <br> Sits without support (8) | Turns to voice (8) | Feeds self cracker (8) <br> Works for toy out of reach (9) |
| 9-12 | Pulls self to stand (10) <br> Thumb-finger grasp (11) <br> Gets to sitting (11) | Dada or mama—nonspecific (10) <br> Imitates speech sounds (11) | Plays peek-a-boo (10) <br> Resists toy pull (10) |
| 12-18 | Walks holding on to furniture (13) <br> Walks alone well (14) <br> Neat pincer grasp of object (15) | Dada or mama specific (13) | Plays pat-a-cake (13) <br> Plays ball with examiner (16) |
| 18-24 | Tower of 2 cubes (20) <br> Walks up steps (22) <br> Kicks ball forward (24) <br> Dumps object from bottle — demonstrate (24) | Three words other than mama, dada (21) <br> Points to one named body part (21) | Imitates housework (20) <br> Removes clothes (22) <br> Uses spoon (24) |
| 24-36 | Scribbles spontaneously (25) <br> Tower of 4-6 cubes (26) <br> Jumps in place (36) <br> Pedals trike (36) <br> Imitates vertical line within 30° (36) | Combines 2 different words (28) <br> Names 1 picture (30) <br> Follows 2 or 3 simple directions (32) | Puts on shoes—not tied (36) |

*Modified from several sources (Gesell and Amatruda, 1974; Illingworth, 1972; and Frankenburg and Dodds, 1967).
†Numbers in parenthesis indicate age in months that most normal children will achieve task.

whether the disease process is focal or diffuse. The neurologic examination and appropriate laboratory examinations (Chapter 2) will verify the extent. If the deficit can be produced by a single, discrete anatomic lesion (such as a single peripheral nerve paralysis), the disease is focal. If the deficit implicates two or more discrete anatomic lesions, the process is multifocal or diffuse. Most neuromuscular diseases are diffuse rather than focal, even though the weakness may have a specific distribution.

Toxic, degenerative metabolic, infectious, or dystrophic processes generally cause multifocal or diffuse involvement. Focal diseases are the result of vascular, neoplastic, or traumatic processes.

Familial occurrence of a similar disease or other diseases of the nervous system often suggests the diagnosis. Many neuromuscular diseases are familial or have a predictable hereditary pattern (such as autosomal recessive spinal muscular atrophy and X-linked Duchenne muscular dystrophy).

## Neurologic examination

The general physical examination should focus on detecting evidence of a systemic illness that may be associated with weakness.

The neurologic examination should determine whether the patient's weakness and/or hypotonia results from involvement of the lower motor unit or the upper motor unit. The upper motor unit includes structures in the central nervous system extending from the cerebral cortex to, but not including, the anterior horn cell. Upper motor unit disease is characterized by increased tendon reflexes, Babinski's sign, ankle or knee clonus, persistence of infantile reflexes, and spasticity (increased muscle tone in response to passive stretch). There is no muscular atrophy or muscle fasciculation. In infants, in contrast to older children and adults, hypotonia is a common manifestation of upper motor unit disease. Weakness is occasionally present in upper motor unit disease and typically involves the antigravity muscles of the affected area—the trapezius, deltoid, wrist extensors, hip flexors, and ankle dorsiflexors. The weakness is usually mild except in patients with flaccid hemiplegia.

Lower motor unit disease is characterized by absent or decreased tendon reflexes, significant weakness, hypotonia, atrophy, and muscle fasciculation. Fasciculation is rarely observed in infants because of overlying subcutaneous fat.

Table 1-2 summarizes the differential signs that distinguish between upper and lower motor unit disease.

**INFANT MOTOR EXAMINATION.** The most characteristic features of the neurologic findings on examination of the newborn infant are their variability. Temperature, degree of wakefulness, or feeding pattern may affect the results of the examination. Therefore any suspicious finding on first examination should be reassessed at another time.

It is best to begin the examination with the procedures least disturbing to the infant. Observation of the infant's spontaneous movements will yield information about weakness of the extremities. The specific muscle or muscle groups involved in any weakness, as well as their distribution, whether proximal or distal, should be ascertained.

Examination of the infant may be the only means of detecting hypotonia (Wright, 1971). Decreased resistance to passive flexion and extension of joints of the arms and legs readily gives the impression of hypotonia. The hypotonic infant, when held in vertical suspension, has decreased muscle contraction about the shoulder girdle and slips through the examiner's hands. Placement of the foot to the chin or head and adduction of the elbow past the midline toward the opposite side of the body are maneuvers possible only in the hypotonic infant. Increased extensibility of connective tissues may contribute to the abnormality demonstrated by these tests.

Examination of the cranial nerves provides

**Table 1-2.** Differentiation between upper motor unit and lower motor unit disease

|  | Upper motor unit | Lower motor unit |
|---|---|---|
| Tone | Hypotonia (infants) or spasticity (infants and older children) | Hypotonia |
| Strength | Weakness (normal or minimal) | Weakness (usually profound) |
| Reflexes | Increased tendon reflexes | Decreased or absent tendon reflexes |
|  | Persistence of infantile reflexes | |
|  | Babinski's sign | No Babinski's sign |
|  | Ankle or knee clonus | No clonus |
| Muscle mass | Usually no atrophy | Atrophy (usually not detectable in infants) |
|  |  | Fasciculations (usually not detectable in infants except in tongue) |

several clues. Ptosis, whether unilateral or bilateral, may result from involvement of different parts of the nervous system, such as the sympathetic supply of the levator palpebral muscle (Horner's syndrome), a lesion of the oculomotor nucleus or nerve (cranial nerve III), congenital myasthenia gravis, myotonic dystrophy, congenital muscular dystrophy, centronuclear myopathy, or congenital absence or maldevelopment of the levators of the eyelid.

Careful observation of the eye movements will detect any impairment of the extraocular muscles innervated by the oculomotor nerve (cranial nerve III), the abducens nerve (cranial nerve VI), and the trochlear nerve (cranial nerve IV).

Facial muscle function is most easily determined by observing the symmetry of contraction during crying. A peripheral facial nerve dysfunction (cranial nerve VII) is characterized by complete paralysis of the entire side of the face, especially about the eyes (orbicularis oculi) and mouth. The paralysis is on the side where the lower lip and corner of the mouth are not depressed or turned down during crying. In addition, the strength of the suck reflex is dependent both upon the facial muscles and the muscles innervated by the motor portion of the trigeminal nerve (cranial nerve V).

The gag reflex, movement of the soft palate and pharynx, infant's ability to swallow, and intensity of the infant's cry are used to determine the functions of cranial nerves IX and X.

The tongue should be examined for atrophy or fasciculations. The tongue must be examined at rest in the floor of the mouth. If there are wormlike, rapid contractions visible, fasciculations are present, indicating involvement of cranial nucleus XII or cranial nerve XII.

The tendon reflexes of the newborn infant vary regionally (Critchley, 1968). The Achilles and patellar reflexes are normally always obtainable, while the triceps reflex is difficult to elicit because of the predominant flexor tone in the upper extremities. If all the reflexes are brisk (including the triceps reflex), upper motor unit involvement should be suspected. However, by 6 to 12 weeks the tendon reflexes are normally elicited throughout. Ankle clonus may be present normally (8 to 12 beats). However, unilateral ankle clonus is abnormal. Knee clonus is pathologic.

The plantar response (Babinski's sign) is tested by stroking the lateral aspect of the sole. A systematic study of the plantar reflex of the normal newborn infant (Hogan and Milligan, 1971) emphasizes the value of careful technique when eliciting plantar reflexes. It is important that the infant be awake, supine, and with the head in the midline and the legs either extended spontaneously or held in extension by the examiner. The foot is perpendicular to the leg. Perhaps of most importance, the toes should be in a neutral position when the stimulus is applied to the lateral plantar surface of the foot, beginning at the heel and moving toward the fifth toe. The first movement of the great toe determines the response. If the great toe dorsiflexes, the response is designated extensor (upgoing); if the first movement is plantar flexion, the response is designated flexor (downgoing). In 93% of normal infants, a bilateral flexor-plantar response was obtained. This study demonstrates that the usual response to plantar stimulation in the newborn is flexor. An extensor response is abnormal and constitutes a true Babinski's sign. Babinski's responses in the newborn period are seen most often in the infant with brain stem and spinal cord injuries.

Symmetry is an important factor in the evaluation of the plantar response. The presence of a unilateral extensor response is sufficient evidence for the diagnosis of an upper motor unit lesion. Ankle clonus, which may be normally elicited from the neonate, disappears by 2 months of age. Ankle clonus beyond that time should raise the suspicion of upper motor unit disease; in the presence of overactive tendon reflexes and extensor plantar responses, it is diagnostic of upper motor unit disease.

In addition to the tendon reflexes, there are several useful reflexes unique to infants (Table 1-3). The Moro reflex (Parmelee, 1964) is elicited with the infant in the supine position by lifting the infant's head 30 degrees to 45 degrees and suddenly letting it fall gently on the examiner's hand. This reflex (Fig. 1-3) consists of a sudden symmetric extension and abduction of the arms laterally away from the body accompanied by extension of the fingers and followed by a gradual adduction of the arms over the body with slight shaking movements. The palmar grasp is elicited by stroking the infant's palm or placing a finger on it; a sudden grasping of the examiner's finger comprises a positive response. The plantar grasp consists of toe flexion when the bottom of the toes is stroked. The adductor spread of the knee reflex is a visible contraction of the adductor muscles of the opposite leg after a knee reflex has been elicited on the ipsilateral side.

The Landau reflex, which is observed when the infant is held prone in horizontal suspension, is elicited by flexion of the infant's head by the examiner and characterized by accompanying flexion of the legs on the trunk. The Landau reflex appears at 3 months of age and disappears by 24 months of age. The Landau reflex is used to assess motor maturity (Cupps, Plescia, and Houser, 1976).

The tonic neck reflex is elicited in the supine position by turning the infant's head to one side. If this reflex is present, the infant will extend the arm and leg on the side to which the gaze is directed, while the opposite arm is raised laterally and flexed at the elbow. This position has been referred to as a "fencer's" posture.

**Table 1-3.** Infantile developmental reflexes

| Reflex | Age onset | Age disappears |
|---|---|---|
| Moro | Birth | 6 months |
| Palmar grasp | Birth | 6 months |
| Plantar grasp | Birth | 9-10 months |
| Adductor spread of knee reflex | Birth | 7 months |
| Tonic neck reflex | 2 months | 5 months |
| Landau | 3 months | 24 months |
| Parachute response | 8-9 months | Persists |

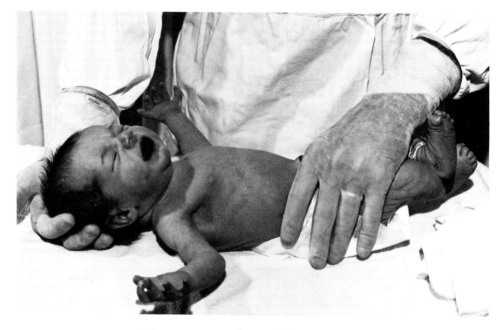

**Fig. 1-3.** Moro reflex in a full-term infant.

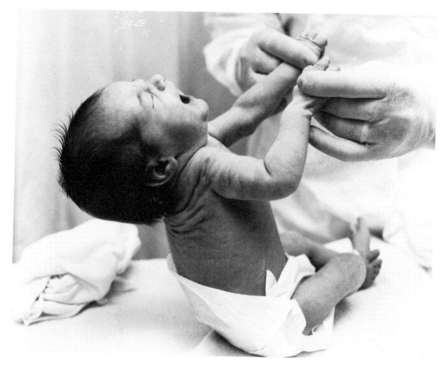

**Fig. 1-4.** Traction response in a full-term infant. Observe normal head lag.

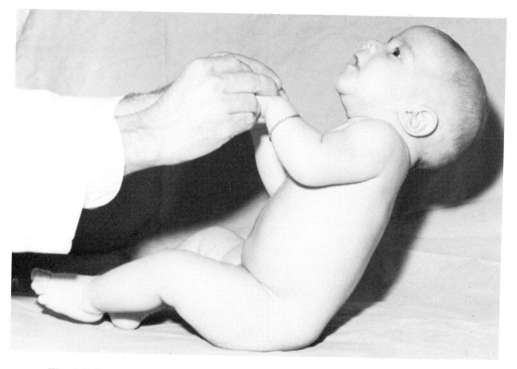

**Fig. 1-5.** Traction response in a 3½-month-old infant. Head is in line with trunk.

The special reflexes of infancy (Table 1-3) are useful in detecting asymmetry of movement. Depression of all the reflexes indicates involvement of the central nervous system due to a toxin, trauma, or anoxia. Asymmetry of the Moro reflex points to involvement of the neuromuscular system, either brachial plexus or single nerve involvement. Involvement of the arm and leg on one side suggests hemiparesis. However, it may also indicate painful limitation of movement from a fracture of the clavicle or humerus without direct involvement of the neuromuscular system. The palmar grasp is well developed in the newborn infant. Any asymmetry indicates weakness of the small muscles (flexors) of the hands, which may be the result of a lower brachial plexus palsy (Klumpke's paralysis).

One test of head and neck control is the traction response. With the infant lying supine, the examiner grasps both hands and pulls the infant gently to a sitting position. In the newborn period, the head lags (Fig. 1-4) while the infant is being pulled up. When in the upright position, the infant's head falls forward and then extends momentarily. By 3 to 5 months of age, the infant is able to keep the head and trunk in a straight line and actively assists in being pulled upright. There is no head lag and the head does not drop forward (Fig. 1-5).

Muscle atrophy in infants is generally not visibly detectable because of the large amount of subcutaneous fat. However, by palpation of the muscle mass beneath the fat, atrophy may be detected. Some experience is needed to assess any variation from normal. The peripheral nerves should be palpated for signs of enlargement.

**OLDER CHILD MOTOR EXAMINATION.** The patient should be examined fully undressed and in a well-lighted area to determine asymmetry of muscle mass. Drooping of a shoulder, pectus excavatum, curvature of the spine, and absence of a specific muscle, such as the pectoralis, are then observed readily. The extent and distribution of muscle atrophy are important. Unusually large muscles, especially deltoid and gastrocnemius, may indicate pseudohypertrophy. Muscle contractures may be obvious, as in arthrogryposis multiplex congenita, or may require examination of range of joint motion for detection. Muscle contractures occur in diverse conditions, such as muscular dystrophies, glycogen storage disease, myositis ossificans, and congenital myopathies.

Observation of the patient's facial expression and standing or sitting position often yields valuable clues in the diagnosis of neuromuscular disease. The facies typical of myopathy is flat and smooth, especially in the areas of the nasolabial folds. The face assumes a bland appearance and lacks spontaneous movement; attempts at smiling produce flattening of the upper lip, minimal elevation of the corners of the mouth, and protrusion of the lips (see Fig. 6-6). The older infant will consistently follow colorful objects with the eyes, allowing assessment of the extraocular muscle function. The symmetry of movement of the face when laughing or crying reveals facial nerve function. If the child will drink from a bottle or cup, the swallowing function can be observed. The young child often can be persuaded to mimic protrusion of the tongue; subsequently, any at-

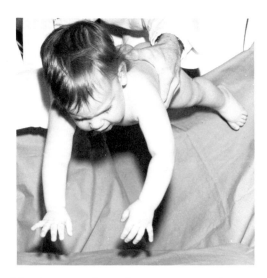

**Fig. 1-6.** Normal parachute response with extension of arms and fingers toward table surface.

rophy or weakness (deviation of the tongue to one side) may be observed.

The tendon reflexes are all elicitable in the older infant and young child. The tendon reflexes in the upper extremities are normally less active than those in the lower extremities. The tendon reflexes generally are depressed or absent in lower motor unit disease; the decrease in reflex activity usually parallels the degree of weakness in anterior horn cell disease but not in peripheral nerve disease or muscle disease. When the tendon reflexes are difficult to obtain, reinforcement techniques should be used. Clonus is not present. The plantar response to stimulation of the sole of the foot is flexor.

Muscle testing in older infants and young children poses unique problems. It is not feasible to test individual muscles. Therefore it is necessary to test gross motor movements. From the history, the development of rolling, sitting, crawling, and walking can be used as indicators of motor strength.

The upper extremities are tested by two means: the parachute response (Fig. 1-6) and the wheelbarrow maneuver (Fig. 1-7). In the parachute response, the infant is held in the prone position by the examiner and then thrust toward a firm surface, for example,

an examining table. The normal response is for the infant to extend both arms toward the table. If the hands are allowed to touch the table, the infant will support its weight largely on the arms. One arm can be slowly pushed aside so that the major portion of the weight is supported on one arm. In this manner, each arm and shoulder girdle is tested individually. From the parachute response the wheelbarrow maneuver may be developed. Once the infant is supporting its weight on the outstretched arms (the body still supported by the examiner), the infant can be induced to crawl by gently pushing the body forward. The 1- to 3-year-old child can be placed on a mat or other protected surface in a crawling position, and the examiner can slowly lift the feet off the mat until the child's weight is supported by the arms. At this point the child is encouraged to crawl using only the arms (wheelbarrow maneuver).

The hip flexors and abdominal muscles are tested by having the child do a sit-up. By the age of 4 years, most children can perform a sit-up without assistance, turning to the side, or using their elbows. However, it may be necessary to hold down the ankles.

The lower extremities are tested by having

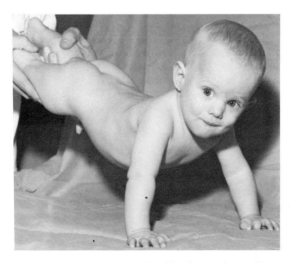

**Fig. 1-7.** Wheelbarrow maneuver in a 7½-month-old infant with excellent strength in arm and shoulder girdle muscles.

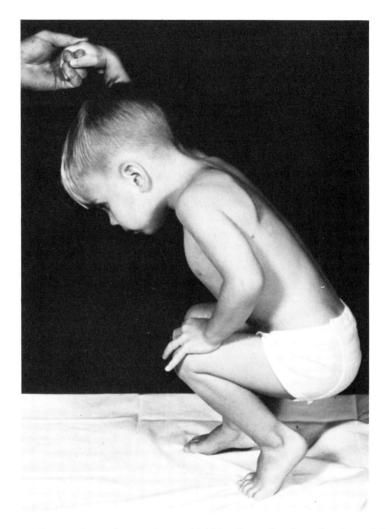

**Fig. 1-8.** Gowers' sign indicates hip weakness. Child has late infantile acid maltase deficiency.

the child walk on toes and heels and perform deep knee bends. Another excellent functional test of hip-girdle and lower extremity strength is to observe the child walking up and down stairs. Children can navigate stairs without assistance, that is, without holding onto a railing or placing a hand on the knee, by 4 years of age.

A similar test of hip function is to have the child rise to a standing position from the prone position on the floor, noting whether a hand is placed on the knee or leg for assistance (Gowers' sign) (Fig. 1-8). Gowers' sign denotes hip weakness from any cause.

In the older child who can cooperate fully, individual muscle testing can be performed, but experience is required to appreciate normal strength at a given age. Individual muscle strength is graded against resistance (Table 1-4). The functional tests just described are generally more satisfactory and more objective in determining the presence and location of weakness.

The muscle response to percussion should be evaluated with a reflex hammer. Normally, percussion should elicit a brisk contraction, visible as a rippling of the overlying skin. This response is often absent in myop-

**Table 1-4.** Strength assessment*

| |
|---|
| 0 = No muscle contraction |
| 1 = Trace of muscle contraction |
| 2 = Active movement at joint—not against gravity |
| 3 = Active movement at joint—against gravity |
| 4 = Active movement against resistance |
| 5 = Normal |

*Modified from Medical Research Council, War Memorandum No. 7: Aids to the investigation of peripheral nerve injuries, ed. 2, London, 1943, His Majesty's Stationery Office, reprinted 1960.

athy and exaggerated in neurogenic disease (Patel and Swami, 1969). If percussion of the deltoid, thenar eminence, or tongue produces a muscle contraction with delayed relaxation, myotonia is present. Muscle percussion may elicit fasciculations that continue for several seconds.

Excessive fatigue is assessed by repetitive muscle contraction. The child is requested to open and close the eyelids several times in rapid succession, repeatedly open and close the hand in a fisting position, or walk up and down several flights of stairs. If the patient is unable to perform these activities without tiring, then an abnormal degree of fatigue is present. Excessive fatigue must be distinguished from the expected fatigue related to mild generalized weakness. Also symptoms resulting from pain, cramps, or stiffness following exercise should be excluded as a cause of excessive fatigue.

Tests of coordination employed to assess cerebellar or posterior column function are generally unreliable in the face of marked muscle weakness. On the other hand, marked incoordination may be perceived by the child as weakness. The neurologic examination should differentiate between incoordination and weakness.

ABNORMALITIES OF GAIT. Normal gait depends on proper function of motor and sensory cortices, basal ganglia, visual receptors, neck proprioceptors, cerebellum, spinal cord centers and tracts, peripheral nerves, neuromuscular junctions, muscles, and muscle spindles. Adequate standing balance is necessary for walking. Patients with profound weakness of the hip may be able to walk, even though they must be assisted to the standing position.

Although the act of walking is almost automatic, it is a highly complex activity. All mechanisms involved in standing must be integrated with the walking sequence. As weight is shifted alternately from leg to leg, the nonsupporting leg is moved forward. The alternating phases of support and forward movement must be evaluated separately and the timing of each phase assessed (Paine and Oppe, 1966; Swaiman, 1975; Aptekar, Ford, and Bleck, 1976a and b).

An abnormal gait is a common symptom in neuromuscular disorders. A critical assessment of gait is necessary for diagnosis. The child should be undressed down to the underwear for examination. The walking and running gait should be observed carefully for the presence of a limp, deviation of the feet, pes planus, genu recurvatum, footdrop, waddling gait, lack of associated movements, and abnormal posturing of the arms or legs.

The examiner should ascertain the presence or absence of curvature of the spine and carefully measure leg lengths from the anterior spine of the ilium to the midpoint of the medial malleolus. The paravertebral area should be scrutinized for skin abnormalities, such as hemangiomas, lipomas, patches of hair, and dimpling, which are often associated with underlying defects of spine and cord. A search should be made for café-au-lait spots. Range of motion of the hip, knee, and ankle joints should be carefully and individually assessed.

The patient should be examined while barefooted, while wearing shoes, and with braces in place if they are worn routinely. The Romberg test should be performed. The child should also be asked to walk down a hallway, turn around, and come back. The examiner should note whether or not the gait is symmetric, whether the child walks normally on the balls of the feet, and whether or not the pelvis remains stable. When the child walks with shoes on, the examiner should listen for scuffing, scraping, and slapping sounds. Split sounds are characteristic of sensory ataxia and steppage gait.

If the patient can cooperate, tandem walking (heel-to-toe) should be executed. At the end of each trial of walking the patient should be asked to reverse direction by turning rapidly.

Abnormalities of associated movements of the arms should be noted. Flexion of the fingers and hands suggests the possibility of upper motor unit abnormality on the same side. Running often potentiates abnormal positioning of the arm and hand.

The child should be asked to walk across the room, initially on the toes and then on the heels. Difficulty with heel-walking suggests weakness of the dorsiflexors of the foot and is also associated with an equinovarus deformity.

The child should also be asked to run and climb steps. It may be necessary to ask the child to run for several minutes in an attempt to induce fatigue.

Specific gait abnormalities found in neuromuscular disorders include sensory ataxia, steppage gait, hip weakness gait, and painful (antalgic) gait.

Sensory ataxia is the result of disruption of input to the cerebellum from peripheral nerves, posterior roots, posterior columns of the spinal cord, or the pathway from posterior columns to the parietal lobes by way of the medial lemnisci.

There is no discrete muscle weakness, but there is great difficulty in standing and walking, and the child has a wide-based gait. The child has little perception of the relation of the feet to the ground and consequently lifts the feet high and stamps them down vigorously with each step. The heel contacts the ground first. The toes then strike the ground, causing a split sound. The child attempts to compensate by watching the ground. The body is flexed slightly forward and the length of the steps varies.

Examination reveals a positive Romberg sign, loss of position sense in the toes, and loss of vibration sense in the feet and legs. Pain, light touch, and temperature sensations are not affected unless a severe peripheral neuropathy is the basis of the difficulty. Sensory ataxia may occur in patients with posterior column degeneration secondary to Friedreich's ataxia, subacute combined degeneration, meningomyelitis, polyneuritis, and demyelinating diseases.

Steppage gait is associated with weakness of dorsiflexion of the feet and toes or permanent contracture in the plantar-flexed position. Paresis is present in the anterior tibial and peroneal muscles. The patient lifts the leg high off the ground with each step. The leg is flexed at the hip and at the knee. The child advances the foot by flinging it forward, and the toe strikes the ground before the heel or the ball of the foot, causing a split sound. The tips of the shoes wear prematurely. The patient's steps are even and rhythmic and no other abnormalities of gait are evident. This difficulty may be confined to one leg and may be the result of a number of conditions, primarily those involving the anterior horn cells of the spinal cord and those leading to severe peripheral neuropathy. Steppage gait occurs in poliomyelitis, progressive muscular atrophy, Charcot-Marie-Tooth disease, and Guillain-Barré syndrome. At times it is also seen in patients with myopathies of predominantly distal distribution.

Profound weakness of the hip, especially of the abductor and extensor muscles, usually leads to an unusual gait. The child waddles and has marked lordosis. He or she cannot stabilize the pelvis and walks with a broad-based gait and exaggerated rotation of the pelvis. The child moves the hips from side to side while shifting the weight with each step. These movements serve to maintain balance and are the result of the weakness of the hip muscles.

In many conditions an associated equinovarus deformity further hampers stability. Among these conditions are various types of muscular dystrophy, myositides, and juvenile proximal hereditary muscular atrophy (Kugelberg-Welander disease).

Painful (antalgic) gait has a multitude of causes, including lesions of the bone, skin, nails, joints, and muscles. It is characterized by a limp comprised of a greatly shortened period of support on the painful leg and prolonged support on the normal leg (Chung, 1974).

**SENSORY EXAMINATION.** Sensory testing in infants is extremely difficult, and, in general, only gross response to pain or touch can be elicited. In injuries of the spinal cord, such as those following a birth traction injury, a sweat level can often be detected merely by running a hand from below upward over the surface of the body and encountering a change from a dry sensation to a moist sensation. Sensory testing in the young child requires a great deal of patience and should be initiated with the least painful stimulus available, that is, touch. In the older child a more detailed examination can be performed that would include the sensory modalities of touch, pain, position, and vibration sense. Gross sensory deficit is found in peripheral nerve, cord, or brain lesions.

**SPECIAL ASPECTS OF THE NEUROLOGIC EXAMINATION OF THE PREMATURE INFANT.** The neurologic status of the prematurely born infant, who is otherwise normal, depends upon gestational age (Table 1-5). The gestational age determines the temporal appearance and disappearance of the special infantile reflexes (Table 1-3).

MUSCLE TONE. The posture that the premature infant assumes when placed in a supine position can be correlated with the gestational age (Robinson, 1966; Amiel-Tison, 1968; and Howard et al., 1976). The premature infant born at 24 weeks gestation rolls onto its side. The premature infant at 32 weeks prefers a posture of total extension with slight increase in tone in the lower extremities.

If an extremity is passively stretched and then released, it will assume its original position. The manner in which this recoil occurs is related to the gestational age. By 34 weeks, there is good recoil in the lower extremities. At 37 weeks, there is slow recoil in the upper extremities and by 40 weeks good recoil in the upper extremities. There are several maneuvers for evaluating muscle tone; these include (1) moving the leg forward and up to touch the big toe to the opposite ear, (2) adducting and flexing the arm across the chin toward the opposite shoulder, and (3) eliciting the traction response. Between 34 and 36 weeks, increased resistance is encountered when attempting these maneuvers.

**Table 1-5.** Neurologic assessment of the prematurely born infant

| | Age | | | | | |
|---|---|---|---|---|---|---|
| | 24 weeks | 28 weeks | 32 weeks | 34 weeks | 36 weeks | 40 weeks |
| Tone | Hypotonic | Hypotonic | Slow recoil in legs | Good recoil in legs | Slow recoil in arms | Good recoil in arms |
| Posture | Limbs extended, rolls onto side | Limbs extended | Flexion of legs | Stronger flexion of legs | Flexion of all limbs | ⟶ |
| Moro | — | Complete but easily exhausted | Complete | ⟶ | | |
| Pupil reaction | — | — | Present (29-31 weeks) | ⟶ | | |
| Suck | Present but weak | Present but weak | Strong | Synchronized with swallowing | ⟶ | |
| Grasp | — | Finger grasp | Fully developed reflex | Stronger | Infant can be lifted off bed | ⟶ |

REFLEXES. Several significant reflexes must be assessed when estimating neurologic maturity. The sucking reflex is present from the twenty-fourth week of gestation. At 32 weeks, the reflex is strong, and at 34 weeks it is usually synchronized with swallowing, which allows the infant to be bottle-fed. The Moro reflex is complete by 28 weeks of gestation but is easily exhausted. The absence of the Moro reflex after 28 weeks indicates serious systemic or primary neurologic dysfunction. The response of the pupil to light is consistently present at 29 to 31 weeks. The grasp reflex is fully developed by 32 weeks, and by 36 weeks some infants can be lifted off the bed by this maneuver. In general, the tendon reflexes are difficult to obtain with the exception of the biceps and ankle reflexes.

POSTNATAL DEVELOPMENT OF THE PREMATURE INFANT. Stages of neurologic development have been used to determine gestational age. Evidence for neuromuscular impairment must take into account the normal neurologic maturation of the premature infant. Knowledge of the circumstances of pregnancy and delivery and of the neonatal course is helpful in determining the origin of retarded motor development in a premature infant.

Studies have shown a lack of influence of extrauterine factors (except injurious ones) on the maturation of the special infantile reflexes. This concept does not necessarily apply to other areas of neurologic maturation.

The same concept applies to the disappearance of the special infantile reflexes as outlined in Table 1-3. Allowance should be made for prematurity. For example, the Moro reflex normally disappears by 6 months of age. In an infant born 1 month prematurely, the Moro reflex may persist normally up to 7 months of age.

### Differential diagnosis in neuromuscular disorders

A list of diseases in the differential diagnosis of lower motor unit disease associated with hypotonia is presented in Table 1-6. If signs of lower motor unit diseases are present, several features are helpful in differentiating disorders of the anterior horn cells, peripheral nerves, and muscles. Fasciculation of the tongue and extremity fasciculations implicate the anterior horn cell. Although fasciculations occur in peripheral nerve disease, they are more common in anterior horn cell disease. Sensory loss indicates involvement of a peripheral nerve. Weakness of the proximal muscles is associated with anterior horn cell disease and muscle disease, while distal weakness is characteristic of peripheral nerve disease. Exceptions are myotonic dystrophy, distal myopathy, and monomelic myopathy, which may be associated with distal weakness.

Localization of muscle weakness to a particular muscle group is often characteristic of some specific disease processes. Ptosis suggests myotonic dystrophy, myasthenia gravis, oculopharyngeal muscular dystrophy, congenital muscular dystrophy, centronuclear myopathy, congenital absence or maldevelopment of the levators of the eyelid, Horner's syndrome, or thiamine deficiency. The extraocular muscles may be involved in myasthenia gravis, oculopharyngeal muscular dystrophy, centronuclear myopathy, and thyroid disease. Hypertrophy of specific muscles, such as the gastrocnemius and deltoid muscles, suggests Duchenne muscular dystrophy, myotonia congenita, hypothyroidism, and late onset X-linked (Becker's) muscular dystrophy. Facial weakness occurs in facioscapulohumeral dystrophy, Möbius syndrome, myotonic dystrophy, centronuclear myopathy, and congenital muscular dystrophy. Weakness, atrophy, and fasciculations of the tongue occur most often in progressive infantile spinal muscular atrophy (Werdnig-Hoffmann disease).

In myasthenia gravis, weakness develops late in the day during periods of activity. Weakness that appears during a rest period following physical activity or after a large carbohydrate meal is typical of periodic paralysis. Aggravation of weakness by cold is common in diseases with associated myotonia but

**Table 1-6.** Diseases associated with hypotonia

| Upper motor unit diseases (central nervous system diseases) | Lower motor unit diseases | Combined upper and lower motor unit diseases |
|---|---|---|
| Acute cerebral insult | Anterior horn cell | Cerebellothalamospinal degeneration |
|   Anoxia |   Arthrogryposis multiplex congenita | Hyperpipecolatemia |
|   Infection—sepsis, meningitis |   Poliomyelitis | Infantile neuroaxonal dystrophy |
|   Intracerebral hemorrhage |   Werdnig-Hoffmann disease | Krabbe's disease |
| Chromosomal abnormality— | Peripheral nerve | Metachromatic leukodystrophy |
|   Down's syndrome |   Familial dysautonomia | Trauma |
| Congenital disease |   Guillain-Barré syndrome | |
|   Ataxia |   Polyneuropathy | |
|   Atonic paraplegia |   Sensory radicular neuropathy | |
|   Choreoathetosis | Neuromuscular junction | |
|   Prader-Willi syndrome |   Myasthenic syndrome—antibiotics, metabolic | |
| Metabolic disease |   Neonatal myasthenia gravis | |
|   Argininosuccinic aciduria | Muscle | |
|   Cerebrohepatorenal syndrome |   Congenital myopathies | |
|   Citrullinemia |   Glycogen storage diseases | |
|   Fucosidosis |   Hypothyroidism | |
|   Hyperammonemia—types I and II |   Myotonic dystrophy | |
|   Hyperlysinemia |   Polymyositis | |
|   Sphingolipidoses—for example, Tay-Sachs and Niemann-Pick diseases | | |
|   Mannosidosis | | |
|   Oculocerebrorenal syndrome (Lowe's syndrome) | | |
| Toxicity | | |
|   Bilirubin | | |
|   Magnesium | | |
|   Phenobarbital | | |

also occurs in Duchenne muscular dystrophy.

Episodic weakness occurs in diseases in which the serum potassium concentration increases or decreases, including classic familial periodic paralysis, aldosteronism, hyperthyroidism, and renal disease. Diseases characterized by episodic weakness without any change in serum potassium concentration are paramyotonia congenita, phosphorylase deficiency (McArdle's disease), and mitochondrial myopathy.

Tenderness or pain in the muscles is associated with breakdown of the muscle cells; severe breakdown produces myoglobinuria, which discolors urine dark brown.

Myositis is often associated with muscle pain. Exercise-related muscle pain may signal impaired glycolysis and energy production, as in deficiency of phosphorylase, phosphofructokinase, or phosphohexoisomerase. Muscle cramps, often painful, are also characteristic of abnormalities in glycolysis (Layzer and Rowland, 1971), and in addition often occur in myotonia, tetanus, and the stiff-man syndrome.

Reflex activity, tone, and strength are interrelated physiologic functions that need to be assessed separately during the neurologic examination. Weakness may be confused with several other conditions. Children with hypotonia, ataxic gait, incoordination of the upper extremities, or vertigo may appear to be weak because they shun activities requiring normal strength. Children with chorea often cannot sustain a muscle contraction and thus appear to be weak.

## REFERENCES

Amiel-Tison, C.: Neurologic evaluation of the maturity of newborn infants, Arch. Dis. Child. **43**:89, 1968.

Aptekar, R. G., Ford, F., and Bleck, E. E.: Light patterns as a means of assessing and recording gait. I: Methods and results in normal children, Dev. Med. Child. Neurol. **18**:31, 1976a.

Aptekar, R. G., Ford, F., and Bleck, E. E.: Light patterns as a means of assessing and recording gait. II: Results in children with cerebral palsy, Dev. Med. Child. Neurol. **18**:37, 1976b.

Boyd, I. A., et al. In Meyers, R., and Swinyard, C. A., editors: The role of the gamma system in movement and posture, New York, 1964, Association for the Aid of Crippled Children.

Brooks, V. B., and Stoney, S. D.: Motor mechanisms: the role of the pyramidal system in motor control, Annu. Rev. Physiol. **33**:337, 1971.

Chung, S. M.: Identifying the cause of acute limp in childhood: some informal comments and observations, Clin. Pediatr. **13**:769, 1974.

Critchley, E. M.: The neurological examination of neonates, J. Neurol. Sci. **7**:427, 1968.

Cupps, C., Plescia, M. G., and Houser, C.: The Landau reaction: a clinical and electromyographic analysis, Dev. Med. Child. Neurol. **18**:41, 1976.

Eldred, E., and Buchwald, J.: Central nervous system: motor mechanisms, Annu. Rev. Physiol. **29**:573, 1967.

Frankenburg, W. K., and Dodds, J. B.: The Denver Developmental Screening Test, Pediatrics **71**:181, 1967.

Gesell, A., and Amatruda, C. S.: Developmental diagnosis, Hagerstown, Md., 1974, Harper & Row, Publishers.

Gilman, S.: Significance of muscle receptor control systems in the pathology of experimental postural abnormalities. In Desmedt, J. E., editor: New developments in electromyography and clinical neurophysiology, vol. 3, Basel, Switzerland, 1973, S. Karger, p. 175.

Granit, R.: The basis of motor control, New York, 1970, Academic Press, Inc., p. 60.

Granit, R.: The functional role of the muscle spindles—facts and hypotheses, Brain **98**:531, 1975.

Hogan, G. R., and Milligan, J. E.: The plantar reflex of the newborn, N. Engl. J. Med. **285**:502, 1971.

Holmes, G.: The cerebellum of man, Brain **62**:1, 1939.

Howard, J., et al.: A neurologic comparison of preterm and full-term infants at term conceptional age, J. Pediatr. **88**:995, 1976.

Illingworth, R. S.: The development of the infant and young child: normal and abnormal, ed. 5, Baltimore, 1972, The Williams & Wilkins Co.

Knobloh, H., and Pasamanick, B.: Gesell and Amatruda Developmental Diagnosis, ed. 3, Hagerstown, Md., 1974, Harper & Row, Publishers.

Layzer, R. B., and Rowland, L. P.: Cramps, N. Engl. J. Med. **285**:31, 1971.

Leksell, L.: The action potential and excitatory effects of the small ventral root fibers to skeletal muscle, Acta Physiol. Scand. **31**(Suppl.):10, 1945.

Medical Research Council, War Memorandum No. 7: Aids to the investigation of peripheral nerve injuries, ed. 2, London, 1943, His Majesty's Stationery Office, reprinted 1960.

Paine, R., and Oppé, T.: Neurological examination of children, London, 1966, William Heinemann Ltd., p. 142.

Parmelee, A. H., Jr.: A critical evaluation of the Moro reflex, Pediatrics **33**:773, 1964.

Patel, A. N., and Swami, R. K.: Muscle percussion and neostigmine test in the clinical evaluation of neuromuscular disorders, N. Engl. J. Med. **281**:523, 1969.

Robinson, R. J.: Assessment of gestational age by neurologic examination, Arch. Dis. Child. **41**:437, 1966.

Sherrington, C. S.: Remarks on some aspects of reflex inhibition, Proc. R. Soc. Biol. **97**:519, 1925.

Stein, R. B.: Peripheral control of movement, Physiol. Rev. **54**:215, 1974.

Swaiman, K. F.: Abnormalities of gait. In Swaiman, K. F., and Wright, F. S., editors: The practice of pediatric neurology, St. Louis, 1975, The C. V. Mosby Co., p. 202.

Wright, F. S.: An approach to hypotonia in children, Postgrad. Med. **50**:116, 1971.

# CHAPTER 2

# Laboratory tests in neuromuscular disease

## Morphology

Laboratory study of neuromuscular disease has advanced substantially in the past several decades. Morphologic study of muscle and nerve continues to be important to the clinician, but concomitant use of biochemical and electrophysiologic studies greatly enhances diagnostic capability. As with all laboratory tests, the technical aspects of these studies must be carefully and reproducibly executed. The results of all of the studies must be correlated, and the physician must realize the importance of the interrelationships between laboratory results and the clinical picture. Only by considering all available information can the physician accurately diagnose neuromuscular disease.

### Histologic findings in muscle

Light and dark fibers are grossly evident in muscle tissue. Muscle is white or red depending on the concentration of myoglobin. Red muscle contracts slowly and maintains a steady tension; white muscle contracts quickly and produces a short-lived twitch. The rapid, brief movement of a bird's wings exemplifies white muscle activity. The ability of a bird to stand for long periods exemplifies red muscle activity. In white muscle fibers the activity of enzymes in the tricarboxylic acid cycle (Krebs cycle) is high. These fibers contain very active oxidative metabolic sys-tems; they have been designated type I fibers. The red muscle fibers, designated type II, manifest high glycolytic metabolic activity. Some fibers possess moderately active glycolytic and oxidative enzyme systems and are classified best as intermediate. (See p. 24.)

A skeletal muscle is encased in a covering of connective tissue called the epimysium (Fig. 2-1) composed of fine fillets that partition the muscles into groups of fibers (fascicles). Such a partition is designated the perimysium. Trabeculae and connective tissue fibers also invest each muscle fiber in a delicate covering of connective tissue known as the endomysium (not to be confused with the sarcolemma, the true cell membrane of the muscle cell). Connective tissue of the epimysium, perimysium, and endomysium forms a continuous fibrous system with the muscle tendon (Fig. 2-1).

The sarcolemma cannot be seen in living muscle fibers unless the fibers are disrupted. Within the sarcolemma are the components characteristic of all living cells as well as some unique to muscle. The cellular protoplasm of muscle cells is called sarcoplasm. Muscle fibers are composed of elongated muscle cells that are multinucleated and therefore constitute a syncytium. Within the fibers are located the contractile elements of muscle, the myofibrils. In a transverse section of muscle

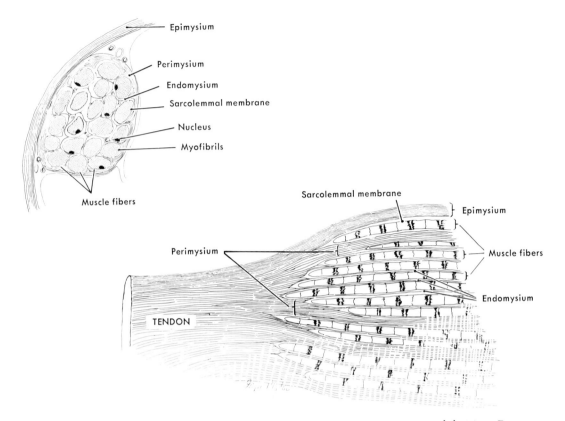

**Fig. 2-1.** Connective tissue of muscle components with a covering at every subdivision. Connective tissue solidly anchors muscle to bone after confluence of connective tissue fibers forms tendon.

fibers (Fig. 2-2) the nuclei are eccentrically located and stain relatively dark with hematoxylin and eosin.

The arrangement of protein filaments in the myofibrils produces the pattern of crossed striation and bands characteristic of voluntary skeletal muscle. The bands change position as the muscle contracts. Although the molecular explanation of the bands and striations is still incomplete, the postulates of Huxley and Hanson (1954) and Huxley (1974) are probably the most correct and form the basis of the explanation that follows.

The myofibrils are divided by dark Z bands of unknown composition that appear regularly along their course. Under the light microscope Z bands in neighboring myofibrils appear to align. They do not change in width as the muscle contracts. The region between the Z bands is the sarcomere. Fig. 2-3 depicts the arrangement of filaments in the myofibril. Thick filaments are composed of myosin and thin filaments of actin. The filament mechanism slides as the muscle shortens or lengthens. Fig. 2-3 explains the microscopic appearance of myofibrillar bands. The Z bands are the basis of reference. The pattern of dark and light in muscle depends on the degree to which the filaments overlap.

The H band is composed entirely of myosin and is apparent because the central portion of the sarcomere does not contain actin filaments. The line down the center of the H band, the M line, may be the result of cross connections between myosin filaments; these connections should not be confused with the cross bridges, discussed later, that project

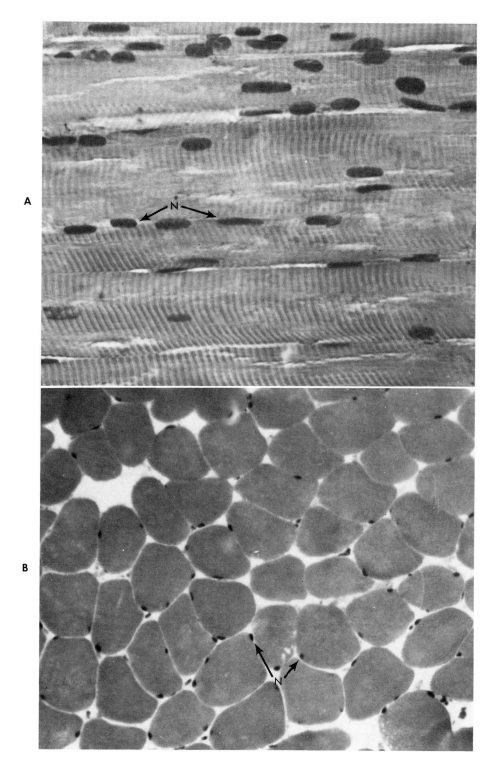

**Fig. 2-2. A,** Normal skeletal muscle showing striations and peripherally placed nuclei *(N).* Note **Z** bands in center of light staining **I** bands and dark **A** bands. (×450.) **B,** Normal skeletal muscle showing peripherally placed nuclei *(N).* (×250.) (Courtesy Dr. Stephen A. Smith.)

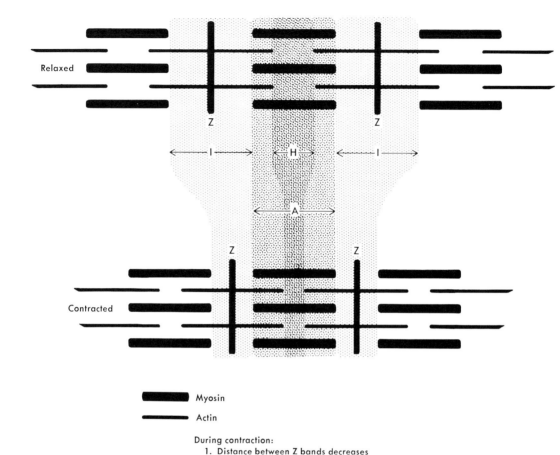

Relaxed

Z          Z

←——I——→  ←H→  ←——I——→

←———A———→

Z          Z

Contracted

████ Myosin

——— Actin

During contraction:
1. Distance between Z bands decreases
2. Widths of H and I bands decrease
3. Width of A band remains unchanged

**Fig. 2-3.** Myosin and actin filaments slide between each other during relaxation and contraction phases. Unique pattern of banding is result of interrelationship of these filaments. One sarcomere extends between two Z bands. The M line is not shown.

from myosin and are important in the sliding process. The cross connections in the H region may be important in stabilizing the hexagonal array of myosin filaments.

The A band is composed of two outer dark segments bisected by the H band. These two dark segments are the result of the overlapping of myosin and actin filaments in this region. The Z band disects the I band. The I band consists primarily of actin and stretches from the stack of myosin filaments in one sarcomere to the beginning of the stack of myosin filaments in the adjacent sarcomere.

As a muscle shortens or lengthens, the re-

lationship of the filaments and the width of the bands change. Shortening of the muscle results in narrower H and I bands and brings the Z bands closer together (Fig. 2-3). Lengthening of the muscle results in wider H bands and I bands and the Z bands move farther apart. In a cross section (Fig. 2-4) each myosin filament is surrounded symmetrically by six actin filaments.

There is a system of cross bridges, which are precisely spaced projections from myosin throughout the length of the myosin filament (Huxley, 1957, 1971), except for a small segment consisting of the M line and abutting portions of the H band.

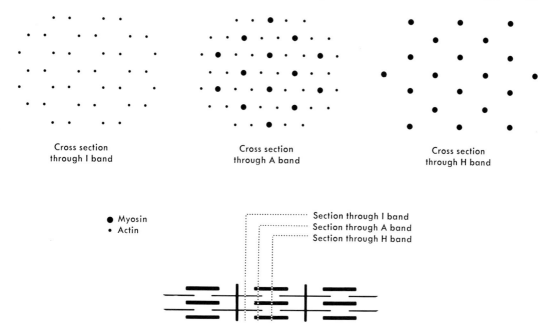

Fig. 2-4. Cross-sectional diagram depicts bands displayed in Fig. 2-3.

The paired myosin projections (cross bridges) are placed at 180 degrees from each other; the next pair of projections is precisely arranged in distance (143 Å) and in angular rotation (120 degrees) from the preceding pair (Huxley, 1971). In the same areas, small knobs composed of complex protein known as troponin-tropomyosin project along the actin filaments (Ebashi and Kodama, 1965) to form a series of catches that the myosin projections may grip transiently.

The muscle cell membrane, the sarcolemma, is composed of a basement membrane and a plasma membrane separated by a poorly characterized cement substance (Price, 1963). The plasma membrane is thinner than the basement membrane, but at the junction of tendon and muscle the plasma membrane thickens where it interdigitates with the endmost Z band of the myofibrils (Mair and Tome, 1972).

There are two systems of tubules that course through muscle and are instrumental in muscle contraction. The transverse tubular system (T-system) membrane is connected directly with the extracellular space. The opening to the sarcolemma is very small and is preceded by a caveola, a membrane-bound structure with a round profile that forms a transition from the sarcolemma to the T-system (Ebashi, 1976). The T-system tubules follow a spiral course around the entire axis of the fiber. The T-system tubules and the "feet" of the terminal cisternae of the sarcoplasmic reticulum provide the structural relationship through which the coupling of the T-system and the sarcoplasmic reticulum occur. (See also p. 135.)

The sarcoplasmic reticulum tubules parallel the myofibrils and encircle them. At the A-I band junction, the terminal cisternae of the sarcoplasmic reticulum and the ramifications of the T-system tubules are adjacent to one another (see Fig. 5-2). It is at this point that the excitation-coupling reaction takes place.

The means by which an electrical potential causes muscle contraction is known as excitation-contraction coupling. Although there are many areas of controversy remaining, the following facts are known (Ebashi, 1976).

1. The action potential of the sarcolemmal membrane is conducted into the interior of the muscle fiber through the T-system.
2. When the T-system membrane is depolarized, calcium ions are released from the terminal cisternae of the sarcoplasmic reticulum (Weber and Murray, 1973; Perry, 1974).
3. The calcium ions form a complex with troponin located in the thin actin filaments and produce contraction through interaction of the thick filament and the thin filament by removing the inhibitory effect of calcium-free troponin located in the thin filament complex (Inesi and Malan, 1976; Endo, 1977).
4. When the depolarization ceases, calcium ions are reaccumulated by the sarcoplasmic reticulum utilizing ATP. There is accompanying reduction of calcium ion concentration, calcium is released from the troponin, and relaxation ensues (Ebashi, 1976; Orentlicher and Gersho, 1977).

### Developing human muscle

There are three constant fiber types and one inconstant type in human muscle that are delineated by differences in their histochemical reaction with myofibrillary ATPase stain (calcium-activated). The three constantly present types are I, IIA, and IIB; on occasion, another fiber type, IIC, is present.

Type I fibers stain predominantly for enzymes associated with the tricarboxylic acid cycle or the electron transport chain. These enzymes are customarily called oxidative enzymes (Dubowitz and Brooke, 1973). Menadione-linked alpha-glycerophosphate dehydrogenase, an oxidative enzyme, is deficient in type I fibers, and thus is an exception.

Type I fibers stain light brownish yellow and type II fibers dark brown with myofibrillary ATPase calcium-activated stain at pH 9.4. Type II fibers may be subdivided by their altered staining properties when incubated for 5 minutes at lower pH. Type IIA fibers are virtually completely inhibited be-

low pH 4.5, type IIB fibers below pH 4.3, and type IIC fibers below pH 3.9 (Brooke and Kaiser, 1970; Tunell and Hart, 1977). Type IIC fibers manifest some inhibition of myofibrillary ATPase activity at pH 4.9, but activity is not completely inhibited until incubation is performed at pH 3.9 or below. Type IIC fibers are often grouped with type IIA fibers in standard reports.

Type I, IIA, and IIB fibers appear in approximately equal proportions in humans. Type I fibers have an average diameter of $58\mu$ in women and $62\mu$ in men. Type II fibers have an average diameter of $50\mu$ in women and $69\mu$ in men.

Other commonly used histochemical stains include nicotinamide-adenine dinucleotide dehydrogenase (NADH), phosphorylase, succinic dehydrogenase, menadione-linked alpha-glycerophosphate dehydrogenase, and lactate dehydrogenase (LDH) (Dubowitz and Brooke, 1973).

In studies of human muscle development from the fifth through the twentieth week of gestation, Fenichel (1966) found that from the fifth to the eighth week most of the cells form a syncytium of myoblasts. Mitochondria concentrate densely just inside the sarcolemma. A few individual myoblasts may be identified, and they are eventually transformed into myotubules by peripheral myofilament formation (Fig. 2-5). Fiber typing by oxidative enzymes or ATPase staining techniques is not feasible at this stage of development.

During the eighth to the tenth week of gestation, myotubules increase greatly in number and become the predominant cellular form. ATPase staining now distinguishes dark myotubules (type II fibers) from a group of smaller, light myotubules (type I fibers). Oxidative enzyme activity is still intense and diffuse, and staining techniques for these enzymes cannot be used for fiber typing at this stage. The nuclei occupy a central position (Fig. 2-5). During the myotubule stage, the motor end-plate is formed in the tenth and eleventh weeks of fetal life (Cuajunco, 1942). A small number of infoldings

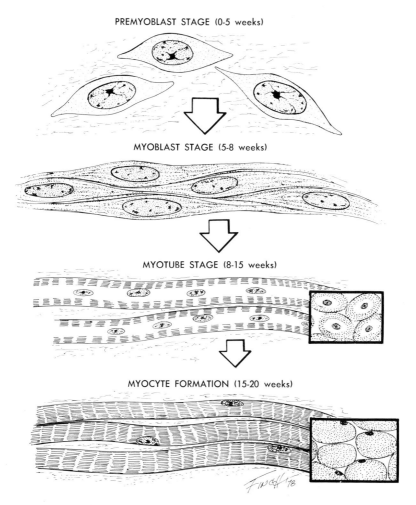

**Fig. 2-5.** Stages of muscle cell development. Pre-myoblast (0-5 weeks). Pre-myoblasts are oval-round primitive cells, indistinguishable from early fibroblasts. Histochemical staining does not distinguish type I from type II fibers. Myoblast stage (5-8 weeks). Pre-myoblasts elongate, and boundaries become indistinct leading to a syncytial pattern typical of myoblast stage. Sarcoplasm becomes granular and vesicular. Staining does not distinguish type I from type II fibers. Myotube stage (8-15 weeks). Myofibrillar formation begins at about fifth week but is not a dominant feature until eighth week. Myofibrils first appear at cell periphery leaving central areas relatively clear and causing myotube appearance. At times central nuclei are seen outlined by clear myotube area. No new myotubes are formed after sixteenth week. When myotubes begin to dominate histologic picture, ATPase histochemical stains can be used to identify dark type II myotubes. Type II fibers are larger than type I fibers at this stage of development. Type II fibers are also more numerous than type I fibers at this time. Myocyte formation (15-20 weeks). Myocytes are formed from myotubes as myofibril formation continues to take place and myofibrils fill in the center of the cell. Oxidative enzyme stains can be employed to identify type I fibers for the first time. Type I fibers overtake and surpass type II fibers in size during this period. The number of type I and type II fibers is about equal by twentieth week. Nuclei tend to become more and more eccentric as development proceeds.

appear in the postsynaptic area, as well as a few synaptic vesicles in the presynaptic area.

From 10 to 20 weeks, myofibrillary development dominates the picture. Type II fibers remain larger in diameter than type I fibers until about the fifteenth week of gestation. Fiber typing by staining for oxidative enzymes can be used now for the first time.

By 20 weeks of gestation, the numbers of type I and type II fibers are about equal, but the type I fibers are larger in diameter. The ratio of type I to type II fibers does not vary thereafter and they are equal in number at birth in humans (Dubowitz, 1963; Dubowitz, 1965).

Suprasegmental factors appear to influence muscle fiber typing. Thus, cordotomy in guinea pigs disrupts the usual shift of predominance of type II fibers to type I fibers in the soleus muscle during the first 6 weeks of postnatal life (Karpati and Engel, 1967). This mechanism is most likely operative in children with brain dysfunction (Fenichel, 1969).

### Muscle biopsy

Failure of muscle biopsy to provide useful diagnostic information in neuromuscular disease all too often reflects improper technique rather than a limitation of the method. The site of biopsy must be carefully chosen. If the disease primarily involves the proximal muscles, the specimen must be taken from an appropriate proximal muscle. The muscle chosen should manifest only moderate clinical involvement. Choosing an uninvolved muscle or one severely destroyed greatly diminishes the value of the biopsy. Although electromyography is valuable in selecting the site, bizarre artifacts may occur if the sample includes the site of needle penetration.

Muscle biopsy must be well planned. All decisions concerning the tests to be conducted must be made before incision. Special biochemical and histochemical studies necessitate immediate preservation of tissue in liquid nitrogen or dry ice at the moment of removal. There is little justification for removing muscle tissue without preparing a portion of the biopsy for electron microscopy

by immersion in 4% glutaraldehyde solution. After 24 hours, the specimen can be placed in 0.1 M phosphate buffer and stored at 4° C (Neville, 1973). Tissue to be examined by light microscopy must be properly preserved in solutions that will not dissolve the accumulations of water-soluble materials in the muscle. At the very least, muscle specimens for light microscopy should be fixed in buffered formalin-saline solution and absolute alcohol.

Biopsy is performed best by the specialist who is responsible for making the diagnosis. This policy assures proper removal, handling, and allocation of the tissue for study.

The patient should be lightly sedated, and adequate local anesthesia should be given without injecting the muscle itself. General anesthesia is rarely needed for muscle biopsy in children. Caution is necessary, because oversedation of an infant with severe intercostal, abdominal, and diaphragmatic muscular weakness may prove catastrophic. Such infants should be sedated minimally and monitored carefully. The value of biopsy in the neonate warrants the extra care (Sarnat, 1978).

Removal of several adjacent superficial strips of muscle (2 to 3 cm long and 0.5 cm wide) is preferable to removal of muscle deep within the muscle bundle (Engel, 1967b). This technique greatly reduces the danger of hematoma formation.

Muscle removed for light microscopic examination must be kept at the same length as the length in situ. This maneuver is one of the most important aspects of the procedure. Muscle tissue can be kept at its original length by tying both ends of the specimen to a piece of tongue blade. Special muscle biopsy clamps allow muscle tissue to be clamped before it is incised and then removed while being held at resting length within the clamp. Failure to hold the muscle tissue properly at its resting length leads to formation of artifact and to unnecessary failures in histologic assessment.

After the muscle tissue is removed and before it is preserved, it should be moistened with saline-soaked gauze for several minutes.

Muscle biopsy is useful only for diagnosis; it cannot be used for purposes of prognosis, evaluation of degree of involvement, or evaluation of therapy. Also, the errors inherent in any sampling technique may, on rare occasions, lead to removal of normal tissue from one area when the neuromuscular disease is histologically detectable only in another area.

### Microscopic picture of disease

The distinguishing histologic picture of the various muscle diseases is described in appropriate sections of this book. However, certain generalizations about the microscopic pathologic patterns can be made. In the late stages of disease, muscle that is severely involved, no matter what the cause, undergoes fatty infiltration and replacement and marked increases in connective tissue. These changes may overshadow all others and make discrete diagnosis impossible.

**NEUROGENIC ATROPHY.** In neurogenic atrophy, fibers are small in cross section. During early stages of disease, bundles of small fibers previously innervated by affected nerves or by anterior horn cells may be interspersed with bundles of fibers of normal size and innervation. The intermingling of normal and atrophied fiber groups is sometimes referred to as the "group" lesion or pattern of neurogenic atrophy resulting from anterior horn cell or motor nerve impairment. The small fibers manifest little change in intracellular structure, and the myofibrillar network is usually intact. Little increase in connective tissue occurs in neurogenic atrophy, but the endomysium appears slightly more prominent (Fig. 3-8, A).

**MYOPATHIC CHANGES.** In myopathic processes, fibers undergo necrosis preceded by swelling and then loss of striations. Rapid phagocytosis is followed by deposition of fat and increase in connective tissue surrounding the fibers. Intense connective tissue proliferation is a dominant sequela of inflammatory muscle (myositic) disease.

In contrast to denervated muscle fibers, those that have been injured or are undergoing dystrophic or myositic change show several types of degeneration, the most common of which are hyaline, granular, and fatty degeneration (Adams, 1975; Adams, Denny-Brown, and Pearson, 1962).

Changes in nuclei are important in pathologic alteration of muscle. In normal tissue, nuclei are eccentrically located in the muscle fiber and usually number five or six, seldom more than eight. A myopathic process or direct trauma leads to changes in portions of the muscle fiber; the nuclei increase in number and tend to migrate centrally. In some processes, notably in myotonic dystrophy, nuclei tend to align in the center of the fiber. They are often enlarged and contain large nucleoli.

**LIGHT MICROSCOPY REPORT.** To be useful, the muscle biopsy report should include the following information whenever possible:
A. Source
B. Description
   1. Presence, absence, or distortion of striations
   2. Evidence of degeneration, necrosis, or phagocytosis
   3. Position, size, and number of sarcolemmal nuclei, nucleolar content of nuclei
   4. Variation of diameter of fiber population
   5. Evidence of basophilia or other signs of regeneration
   6. Positive or negative evidence of storage material within the muscles
   7. Quantity of connective tissue and fat replacement
   8. Blood vessel structure

The microscopist should attempt to differentiate myopathic from neurogenic processes. Specific clinical diagnoses are rarely justified on the basis of biopsy findings alone.

**ELECTRON MICROSCOPIC MORPHOLOGY.** Electron microscopic techniques demonstrate clearly the intricate relationships of the myofibrils and the bands in skeletal muscle. Furthermore, other components of muscle, some poorly seen with light microscopic techniques, others not at all, are clearly demonstrated by use of the electron microscope.

Despite the greater resolution of the electron microscope, the alterations in many disease processes remain nonspecific. Similar changes are found in diseases of such divergent historic and clinical characteristics that it is unlikely they share common pathophysiologic beginnings.

Because of the small sample studied, sampling errors are more likely and more difficult to avoid. The study of muscle that has demonstrable abnormalities on light microscopy with ultramicroscopic techniques is one method of ensuring a higher percentage of detectable abnormalities. However, ultrastructural changes not reflected in light microscopic examination will go unnoticed.

To be sure, the vast majority of muscle diseases do not require ultrastructural studies for identification; nevertheless, there are an increasing number of muscle diseases that

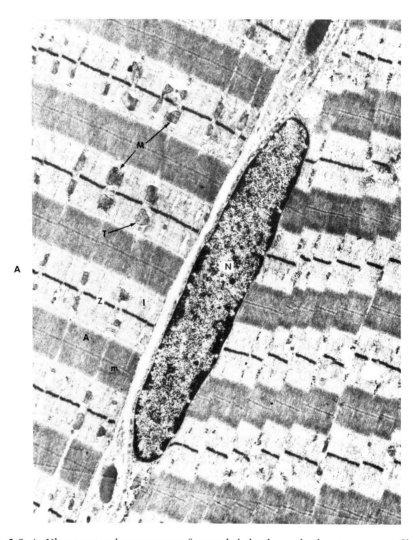

**Fig. 2-6. A,** Ultrastructural appearance of normal skeletal muscle showing a type I fiber with multiple mitochondria *(M)* on left and a type II fiber with a nucleus *(N)* on right. The actin myofibrils meet at Z band *(Z)* and make up I band *(I)*. Myosin myofibrils constitute A band *(A)* meeting at M line *(m)*. The transverse tubular system (T-system) component of a triad is shown. (×8,200.)

can be diagnosed only by electron microscopic study.

The Z band is one of the most prominent landmarks in skeletal muscle. The composition of Z bands is incompletely known, but it is likely that the material is composed primarily of actin filaments that have a predetermined relationship with one another (Kelly, 1967). The Z band is osmiophilic. The pathologic Z band may be blurred, widened, duplicated, or manifest an undulating pattern in a number of myopathies. Nemaline rods likely originate from Z band material and are found in several different conditions. They are not, as once thought, specific for any one myopathy.

Myofilaments, easily seen on electron microscopy, are the result of the interdigitation of actin and myosin in a prescribed pattern (Fig. 2-6). Partial or complete dissolution of this pattern is a common feature of many muscular diseases. The degree of obliteration of the myofilament pattern varies from area to area and from disease to disease.

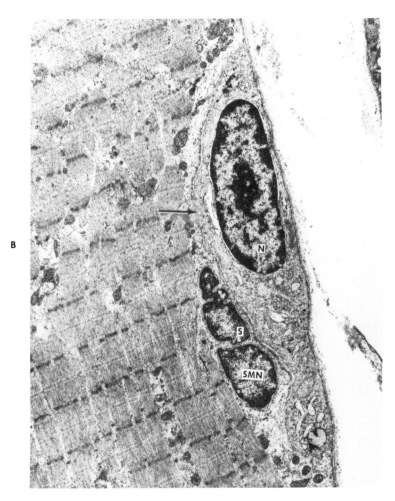

Fig. 2-6 — cont'd. **B**, Muscle biopsy demonstrating ultrastructural appearance of a satellite cell (*S*) with its nucleus (*N*) enclosed within basement membrane of a striated muscle fiber. Note separated striated muscle nucleus (*SMN*) and separate cell walls (*arrow*). (×7,175.) (Courtesy Dr. Stephen A. Smith.)

In the extreme instance, there may be gray smudges of material enclosed in what appears to be normal sarcolemma. Scavenger cells may be embedded in this amorphous material.

The limiting membrane of skeletal muscle cells is the sarcolemma, which consists of a basement membrane and an inner plasma membrane. The latter is homologous to plasma membranes of other cells. Its thickness is approximately 100 Å in width, and it is visualized with more difficulty because it is not as osmiophilic.

In pathologic tissue, there may be random, variable-sized protuberances of both the basement and plasma membranes. These abnormalities have been found in glycogen storage diseases (acid maltase deficiency and McArdle's disease) as well as in polymyositis and neurogenic atrophies. On rare occasion the plasma membrane and basement membrane may separate and reduplicate. This phenomenon has been noted in muscular dystrophies and neurogenic atrophies. Complete dissolution of the plasma membrane may occur leaving only the basement membrane visible.

The internal architecture of the nucleus is rarely changed. The nucleus may become vesicular and grow to an unusually large diameter. Often there is an associated increase in the size of the nucleolus. Nucleolar growth is associated with increased synthesis of ribonucleic acid in the process of regeneration.

Small crystalline inclusions within the nucleus are thought to represent virus particles and have been described in patients with collagen disease (Yunis and Samaha, 1971).

Abnormal location of the nucleus has been described for many years and is readily apparent in light microscopic preparations. The movement from an eccentric position to a central position has been observed in dystrophies (myotonic dystrophy), neurogenic atrophies, and myotubular myopathy (Campbell, Rebetz, and Walton, 1969).

Other abnormalities in muscle are found in the subcellular organelles. Mitochondria are found in large numbers in muscle in close proximity to the I bands. The mitochondria are usually in close association with myofibrils. Mitochondria are sparse in central cores that are devoid of oxidative metabolic activity as well as in neurogenic atrophy in which target fibers appear.

Accurate preservation of mitochondrial morphology is particularly vulnerable to poor technique; therefore decreased number or structural change may not be a reflection of pathology. Mitochondria may be unusually shaped, very large, contain inclusion bodies, or be found in large numbers. Care should be exercised in interpretation of mitochondrial abnormalities.

A T-system tubule flanked by tubules of the sarcoplasmic reticulum constitutes the triad and is found at the abutment of A and I bands. Changes in the triad include: (1) malposition and distortion, (2) reduplication and realignment to form units of five and six components, and (3) dilation, elongation, and reduplication of T-system tubules or sarcoplasmic reticulum tubules (Neville, 1973). Dilatation is usually the result of improper preparation techniques.

Bona fide T-system tubule reduplication and dilation are usually associated with myofilament deterioration; malposition and pathologic rearrangement of triad units are also associated with myofilament degeneration. Although replication of triad components is unusual, it is found in many myopathies and in polymyositis.

In some areas, individual cells with single nuclei are found interposed between the basement and plasma membranes in normal, mature skeletal muscle fibers. It has been postulated that these satellite cells are quiescent myoblasts that have potential for muscle regeneration (Schultz, 1976; Chou, 1977).

At times a convoluted group of flattened tubular structures located in the cytoplasm adjacent to the nuclei is seen; the structures comprise the Golgi complex of the muscle fiber.

There are multiple reports of abnormal

subcellular organelles in various disease conditions. These include myelin bodies, vacuoles that appear to be lysosomal in origin, lipofuscin-like particles, crystalline particles that appear to be virus-like, tubular aggregates, and unusual inclusion bodies including subsarcolemmal inclusions resembling fingerprints and others that contain osmiophilic particles of unexplained composition; the latter structures have been termed "reducing bodies" in the literature. Lipid vacuoles may be evident in some muscle material, usually in type I fibers. Cytoplasmic bodies, thought to represent Z band material, differ widely in shape and mass; the central area is often less dense. They have been associated with collagen disease, mitochondrial myopathies, periodic paralyses, and muscular dystrophies.

### Histochemical technique

Histochemical studies have become more available and are more important than ever in the study of muscle disease. Histochemical techniques lack the precision of quantitative biochemical methods, although they do permit anatomic localization of enzymes and other materials. Histochemical techniques can identify the enzyme, but are not accurate for estimating or comparing enzyme activity.

Enzymes of the Embden-Meyerhof pathway, the tricarboxylic acid cycle, and the electron transport chain are the enzymes usually studied with histochemical techniques; those commonly studied in muscle include the following enzymes of glycogen metabolism and the Embden-Meyerhof pathway: uridine diphosphate glucose-glycogen transferase, phosphorylase, amylo-1, 4→1,6-transglucosidase, and lactate dehydrogenase (Takeuchi and Glenner, 1961; Dubowitz and Pearse, 1960; Takeuchi, 1958; Blanchaer and Van Wijhe, 1962). The enzymes of the tricarboxylic acid cycle frequently studied are isocitric dehydrogenase, malic dehydrogenase, and succinic dehydrogenase (Seligman and Rutenburg, 1951; Hess, Scarpelli, and Pearse, 1958; Dubowitz and Pearse, 1961). An enzyme of the electron transport chain that has been widely studied is cytochrome oxidase (Nachlas et al., 1958).

Histochemical techniques have been used to study a number of other enzymes belonging to other systems and related to these pathways. Most prominent among them are myofibrillar ATPase (calcium-activated), NADH, and NADPH (Farber, Sternberg, and Dunlap, 1956). Certain enzymes thought to be associated with neuromuscular transmission have been studied, including acetylcholinesterase (Cöors and Woolf, 1959).

### Biochemistry
#### Serum enzyme activity

The use of serum enzyme activity in the diagnosis of muscle disease began in 1949, when Sibley and Lehninger reported that serum aldolase activity increases in progressive muscular dystrophy. Since that time, the relationship of numerous other enzymes to muscle diseases has been studied. Prominent among other serum enzyme measurements used clinically are glutamic-oxaloacetic transaminase (GOT), lactic dehydrogenase, glutamic-pyruvic transaminase (GPT), glucose phosphate isomerase, phosphoglucomutase, and creatine phosphokinase (CPK). Of these, the ones most commonly used for clinical purposes are GOT, aldolase, and especially CPK.

The activity of these serum enzymes increases greatly in Duchenne muscular dystrophy and to a lesser extent in limb-girdle dystrophy and facioscapulohumeral dystrophy (Pearce, Pennington, and Walton, 1964; Swaiman and Sandler, 1963). Moderate elevations occur in polymyositis. Elevations are also noted in entities such as severe anoxia and gross muscle trauma (Pearce, Pennington, and Walton, 1964). GOT and LDH are present in almost all known tissues and their elevation in serum may not reflect muscle disease.

**CPK AND ITS ISOENZYMES.** CPK is found primarily in skeletal muscle, smooth muscle, and brain tissue (Dawson and Fine, 1967). Little or no activity is present in liver and red blood cells (Dawson and Fine, 1967; Fujie,

1960). It is likely that serum CPK activity is mildly increased in cerebral disease (Schiavone and Kaldor, 1965), but in practice it is seldom necessary to use this measurement to distinguish between a cerebral vascular accident and muscle disease.

Isoenzymes are enzymes that, while present in one organism, catalyze a specific reaction but differ from one another chemically or physically. Isoenzymes are usually identifiable after electrophoretic separation. Radioimmunoassays are becoming more readily available (Moore, 1978).

CPK is a dimer (82,000 daltons). The two subunits of a specific isoenzyme, which may or may not be similar, have been termed M and B. The MM isoenzyme is virtually the only isoenzyme found in skeletal muscle. The BB isoenzyme predominates in brain tissue. Heart muscle contains MB isoenzyme in addition to MM isoenzyme, a phenomenon that causes MB isoenzyme determinations to be valuable in the diagnosis of myocardial infarction. For practical purposes, the MM isoenzyme is of primary importance in the diagnosis of skeletal muscle disease (Dawson and Fine, 1967; Silverman et al., 1976).

Serum MM isoenzyme activity is usually 20 to 30 times as great as MB activity; therefore major changes of total serum CPK activity virtually always reflect changes in serum MM isoenzyme activity (Roberts and Sobel, 1976). Increased MB isoenzyme activity, probably as a result of cardiac muscle involvement, has been reported in limb-girdle dystrophy, Duchenne dystrophy, congenital muscular dystrophy, and dermatomyositis (Goto, 1974).

Serum CPK activity can be increased up to 48 hours or more by intramuscular injections (Sidell, Culver, and Kaminskis, 1974).

**CLINICAL USES OF SERUM ENZYME STUDIES.** CPK activity is used most often to differentiate myopathic and neurogenic processes. It is particularly useful in distinguishing dystrophies from diseases caused by malfunction of the anterior horn cells. Elevation of the CPK level usually can be interpreted to mean that the process is not neurogenic in origin and that primary myopathic disease is present.

CPK fulfills a number of essential criteria for an enzyme useful in the diagnosis of muscle disease. At present the most sensitive determination of CPK uses the so-called forward reaction, in which ATP is formed (Rosalki, 1967) (Fig. 2-7). Enzymatic activity is assayed in terms of rate of change of nicotinamide-adenine dinucleotide (NAD) as monitored at 340 m$\mu$ on a spectrometer. Studies of CPK activity in newborn infants indicate an unexpected increase that is variable and persists for 4 to 5 weeks (Gilboa and Swanson, 1976).

Shaw and associates (1967) studied GOT, GPT, aldolase, and CPK in Duchenne dystrophy. In their view, a profile of the four enzymes was more valuable diagnostically than evaluation of any of the enzymes separately. In our opinion, CPK study has distinct advantages over study of other enzymes when mild elevation is encountered, because of the unlikelihood that hemolysis or disease of tissue other than muscle significantly contributes to increase in serum CPK activity. In our experience, the elevation of serum CPK activity to three times normal in a patient with neuromuscular disease almost always correlates positively with myositic or myopathic disease. Only rarely is CPK activity elevated in neurogenic muscle disease.

$$\text{ADP} + \text{CP} \xrightarrow{\text{CPK}} \text{ATP} + \text{CREATINE}$$

The symbols refer to the following compounds:

ADP = Adenosine diphosphate
CP = Creatine phosphate
CPK = Creatine phosphokinase
ATP = Adenosine triphosphate

Fig. 2-7. Reaction of creatine phosphokinase.

In the face of elevated serum CPK activity, a diagnosis of neurogenic muscular disease should be considered only in the presence of a characteristic histologic pattern at biopsy.

The method by which muscle enzymes find their way into the circulation is unknown. Pearson (1962) speculated that damage to the sarcolemma allows enzymes to enter the blood. The quantity of enzyme released into the circulation over a period of several years in patients with Duchenne dystrophy exceeds the known amount of enzyme present in the total skeletal muscle mass at any one time (Dreyfus, Schapira, and Schapira, 1954). Thus over a period of years a substantial amount of enzyme must be synthesized.

**ENZYME STUDIES IN THE DETECTION OF THE CARRIER STATE IN MUSCULAR DYSTROPHY.** Serum enzyme activities have been used to detect the carrier state in Duchenne muscular dystrophy (Dennis et al., 1976). CPK has been the enzyme most often used. These studies are not infallible. In fact, only 79% of women who are known to be definite carriers have abnormally increased CPK enzyme activity (Milhorat and Goldstone, 1965). This subject is discussed more completely in Chapter 6.

### Creatine and creatinine

The use of creatine and creatinine determinations to evaluate muscle disease dates back many years. The value of these studies is based on the relatively constant ratio between muscle mass and urinary creatinine excretion. Total muscle mass is estimated from urinary creatinine levels. The estimate will be erroneous if renal disease is present.

Urinary creatinine determinations cannot be used for specific diagnosis. Any disease process that reduces muscle mass also decreases the rate of urinary creatinine excretion. Such varied conditions as disuse atrophy, neurogenic atrophy, and Duchenne dystrophy decrease urinary creatinine excretion.

Creatine is synthesized in the kidneys and liver from three amino acids: glycine, arginine, and methionine (Fig. 2-8). Creatine is then transported through the circulation from the liver to the muscles. In striated muscles, creatine is transformed into the high-energy compound creatine phosphate. During muscle activity, with the aid of CPK the phosphate group of creatine phosphate is transferred to adenosine diphosphate (ADP) to form adenosine triphosphate (ATP). The creatine is released from the muscle cell, transported in the blood to the kidneys, and excreted in the urine. Creatine is not usually present in the urine of adults. The renal threshold in adults is 0.5 mg/dl of blood. Creatinuria is normally present in children, but its presence in adults or children can signify starvation or hyperthyroidism (Tierney and Peters, 1943).

Because urinary excretion of creatinine is relatively constant in adults and parallels

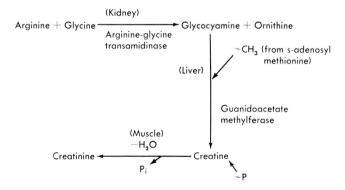

**Fig. 2-8.** Creatine is formed from three amino acids in kidneys and liver. Creatinine is in turn formed from creatine in muscle.

skeletal muscle bulk, its measurement is useful clinically. Creatinine excretion coefficients for children are necessary because the ratios of creatinine to muscle bulk (and body weight) change with age (Clark et al., 1951; Flood and Pinelli, 1949; Harding and Gaebler, 1922; Marples and Levine, 1936; Schwartz et al., 1976). These coefficients must be used accurately to assess the normality of muscle bulk.

In the presence of reduced muscle mass, less muscle tissue is available to convert creatine to creatinine, and an increase in blood creatine ensues. The blood content of creatine then exceeds the renal threshold and is excreted in the urine. At least one exception exists to this mechanism; blood creatine concentration is decreased in myotonic dystrophy, ostensibly because the liver cannot synthesize creatine at a normal rate and there is a subsequent decrease in muscle creatinine synthesis.

## Electrodiagnosis of neuromuscular diseases

Electrodiagnostic studies play a prominent role in the assessment of the complex neuromuscular disorders of childhood. Clinically, the most important facets of electrodiagnosis are electromyography and measurement of nerve conduction velocity. Electrodiagnostic techniques are an extension of the optimal neurologic examination. These techniques can confirm clinical diagnoses and in unusual problems of neuromuscular disease may provide significant diagnostic information. Electrodiagnostic techniques will identify the site and sometimes the pathologic disorder of the lower motor unit, which consists of the anterior horn cell, its axon, the neuromuscular junction, and the muscle fibers innervated by a single anterior horn cell. The muscle fibers of a motor unit are of uniform type (Brandstater and Lambert, 1973) and are diffusely distributed within a given territory, intermingling with fibers of other units.

Electromyography consists of the analysis of the electrical events associated with the contraction of skeletal muscle fibers recorded extracellularly. The electrical activity is analyzed in the form of compound muscle action potentials, which represent the summation of volume-conducted potentials from muscle fibers of a motor unit (Adrian and Bronk, 1929).

### Electromyography

**APPARATUS.** A capacity-coupled amplifier and a cathode-ray oscilloscope are the implements of electrodiagnosis. A needle electrode or surface electrode monitors the electrical potentials extracellularly from the selected muscle and transmits this information to the amplifier. The variation in electrical activity is displayed on the oscilloscope and may be photographed. The impulses are also transformed into sound waves by a high-fidelity loudspeaker. The electrical activity may be simultaneously recorded on a tape recorder or fiberoptic recorder for future evaluation.

**TERMINOLOGY.** Electromyographic terminology is continually modified and revised; some of the terms now in use are defined in Table 2-1. In general, the terms describe the electrical characteristics of the action potentials recorded from muscle. Terms implying a specific diagnostic entity have been discouraged and have been replaced by those that more completely describe electrical events (Simpson, 1969).

**TECHNIQUES.** The electromyographic procedure studies three phases of action potentials: (1) insertion potentials, (2) spontaneous potentials, and (3) motor unit action potentials.

INSERTION POTENTIALS. As the needle is inserted into normal muscle, the mechanical stimulation causes a brief electrical discharge. In normal muscle the activity stimulated by needle insertion persists for less than 300 msec and in normal resting skeletal muscle is followed by electrical silence. If the needle is inserted into the motor end-plate area, brief low-voltage, negative or negative-positive potentials occur irregularly. These irregular potentials have been termed "end-plate noise" or "end-plate potentials."

Abnormal insertion activity, that is, ac-

**Table 2-1.** Electromyographic terminology

| Term | Definition |
| --- | --- |
| Fasciculation potential | Spontaneous contraction of groups of muscle fibers; may be visible |
| Fibrillation potential | Spontaneous discharge of single muscle fiber occurring in absence of voluntary muscle contraction |
| Insertion activity | Electrical activity occurring during insertion or movement of needle electrode |
| Interference pattern | Pattern of overlapping motor unit potentials produced during a maximal muscle contraction |
| Motor unit action potential | Electrical activity recorded extracellularly from the muscle fibers of a motor unit within the recording range of an electrode |
| Polyphasic potential | Motor action potential with five or more phases |
| Positive sharp wave | Diphasic potential initially positive followed by slow negative potential |
| Spontaneous activity | Electrical activity recorded after insertion activity ceases and without voluntary muscle contraction |
| Synchronization | Simultaneous recording of the same action potential from separate electrodes with a greater than normal interelectrode distance |

tivity that persists after the placement of the needle electrode, consists usually of low-voltage (less than 300 mV), short-duration (1 to 5 msec), diphasic or triphasic spikes (usually with an initial positive deflection) and positive sharp waves. These abnormal potentials occur rhythmically at 1 to 10 Hz and indicate denervation.

Prolonged insertion potentials may be followed by fibrillation potentials. The presence of these potentials in combination with prolonged nerve conduction velocity suggests peripheral nerve disease. A moderate number of fibrillation potentials occurring when nerve conduction is normal points to anterior horn cell disease.

A myotonic response may follow insertion of the needle electrode. This is a high-frequency repetitive discharge that waxes and wanes in amplitude and frequency, producing a characteristic "dive bomber" sound. Mechanical stimulation by movement of the needle or by percussion of the muscle may elicit this myotonic response. Voluntary muscle contraction or repetitive electrical stimulation may also evoke this response (Fig. 2-9).

Another abnormal response to insertion is the high-frequency bizarre repetitive discharge, called a pseudomyotonic discharge. It starts and stops abruptly and does not embody the variation in frequency and ampli-

tude characteristic of the true myotonic discharge. Bizarre repetitive potentials are present in chronic neurogenic diseases and dystrophies.

SPONTANEOUS ACTION POTENTIALS. The second phase of electromyography is the study of spontaneous potentials in the muscle at rest (Buchthal and Rosenfalck, 1966). Fibrillation potentials are spontaneous, brief (less than 5 msec), low-amplitude discharges from single muscle fibers. They are diphasic or triphasic in configuration, with an initial positive deflection (Fig. 2-10).

Fibrillation potentials must be differentiated from end-plate potentials. This is best accomplished by recording from areas outside the motor end-plate region. Fibrillation potentials occur in muscle denervated by peripheral nerve disease or anterior horn cell disease. They also occur in polymyositis and late-stage muscular dystrophy. Fibrillation potentials are accompanied by an auditory sound much like rain falling rapidly on a tin roof. When testing for spontaneous activity, the examiner must be certain that the patient is not contracting the muscles. Satisfying this criterion is a problem in the study of a child and may necessitate examination under sedation.

Fasciculations result from spontaneous contraction of groups of muscle fibers and

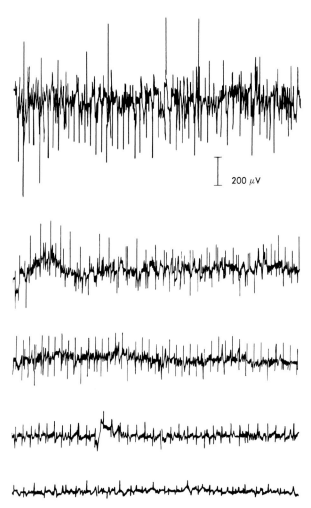

200 μV

**Fig. 2-9.** Myotonic discharge characterized by variation in amplitude and frequency. Traces are continuous from top to bottom. (From Wright, F. S.: Electrodiagnosis of neuromuscular disease. In Swaiman, K. F., and Wright, F. S.: The practice of pediatric neurology, St. Louis, 1975, The C. V. Mosby Co., p. 59.)

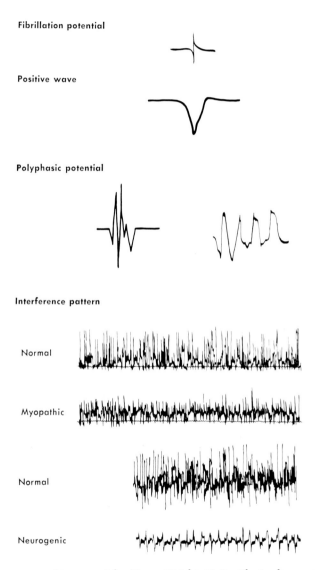

Fibrillation potential

Positive wave

Polyphasic potential

Interference pattern

Normal

Myopathic

Normal

Neurogenic

**Fig. 2-10.** Electromyographic potentials. (From Wright, F. S.: Electrodiagnosis of neuromuscular disease. In Swaiman, K. F., and Wright, F. S.: The practice of pediatric neurology, St. Louis, 1975, The C. V. Mosby Co., p. 59.)

can be monitored electromyographically. Superficial fasciculations are also visible through the skin and often occur normally in the calf muscles and the small muscles of the hands and feet. Pathologic fasciculations occur in diseases of the anterior horn cell, in peripheral neuropathy, and in root compression. They are generally not seen in primary muscular disease.

MUSCLE CONTRACTION POTENTIALS. The third phase of electromyography is the study of motor unit potentials during voluntary contraction of a muscle against varying degrees of resistance. The number, amplitude, and duration of the motor unit potentials are noted. Patience and gentle coaxing may be necessary for proper study of a reticent child.

During a weak contraction, the motor unit potentials discharge with a frequency of 1 to 10 Hz; during maximal contraction, the motor unit potential discharge frequency is 40 to 50 Hz, and many motor units discharge. The combination of an increased frequency of motor unit potential discharges and an increased number of motor units firing (recruitment) obscures the single motor unit potential and forms an interference pattern (Fig. 2-10).

The characteristics of the motor unit potential (configuration, amplitude, and duration) are analyzed best during weak or minimal muscle contraction. The normal action potential has a diphasic or triphasic configuration. If the waveform of the action potential has more than five phases, it is termed a "polyphasic potential." Polyphasic potentials constitute only 10% of the action potentials of normal muscle (Fig. 2-10).

As previously noted, a myotonic response may follow voluntary contraction of the muscle. This type of activity is almost always present in myotonic diseases but occasionally occurs in other myopathies, including progressive muscular dystrophy, glycogen storage disease, hyper- and hypokalemic periodic paralysis, and myotubular myopathy.

Multielectrode recordings can define the extent to which a single motor unit innervates a given muscle (Buchthal and Rosen-falck, 1973; Buchthal, Rosenfalck, and Erminio, 1960). In clinical practice, the electrodes are inserted beyond the established area of activity of a single motor unit; the resulting action potentials recorded by each electrode appear at different times, or nonsynchronously. If the action potentials occur at the same time (synchronously) at widely spaced electrodes, synchronization is abnormal. Abnormal synchronization is a sign of neurogenic disorder, more prevalent in anterior horn cell disease than in peripheral nerve disease.

### Nerve conduction velocity

Muscular contraction evoked by electrical stimulation of peripheral nerves is a useful means of assessing the excitability and function of the peripheral neuromuscular system (Gilliatt, 1966; Hodes, Larabee, and German, 1948; Simpson, 1964).

Measurement of conduction velocity requires a stimulator and stimulating electrodes in addition to the standard electromyographic apparatus. Rectangular or square wave-pulse generators are most commonly used because they allow measurement and predictable alteration of the amplitude and duration of the pulse. In contrast to electromyography, which analyzes spontaneous or volitional motor unit potentials, nerve conduction studies measure potentials evoked by stimulation of either motor or sensory nerves.

MOTOR NERVE CONDUCTION VELOCITY. Certain diseases affect the peripheral nerves, prolonging the conduction time from the point of stimulation of the nerve to the muscle and increasing the duration of the evoked action potential of the muscle. The nerves most often studied by measuring the conduction velocity are the median, ulnar, radial, peroneal, and posterior tibial nerves. Surface or needle electrodes may be used to record the evoked action potentials. In children, surface electrodes placed over the muscle belly are preferred. The nerve is stimulated at two places along its course, and the time (latency) from the application of the stimulus until the onset of the action potential is carefully measured and recorded. To calculate velocity, the measured distance between the two stimulated points is divided by the difference in latency between the two points (Fig. 2-11). This technique measures conduction velocity only in large-diameter fast-conducting nerve fibers.

Conduction velocity of motor and sensory nerves varies with age because of changes in the fiber diameter, degree of myelination, and internodal distance. The normal maturational changes in motor conduction velocity in the ulnar, median, and peroneal nerves are recorded in Table 2-2. Conduction velocity in the ulnar nerve increases rapidly

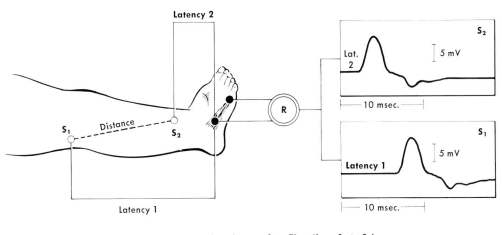

Latency 1 — Latency 2 = Time (from $S_1$ to $S_2$)

$$\frac{\text{Distance}}{\text{Time}} = \text{Velocity}$$

**Fig. 2-11.** Motor nerve conduction velocity is measured by stimulation over two points ($S_1$, $S_2$) along a nerve. Evoked potential is recorded (*R*) with a surface electrode over the muscle and displayed (*inserts*) for analysis. Difference in latency is time required for stimulus to travel distance between the points of stimulation. Distance divided by time yields conduction velocity. (From Wright, F. S.: Electrodiagnosis of neuromuscular disease. In Swaiman, K. F., and Wright, F. S.: The practice of pediatric neurology, St. Louis, 1975, The C. V. Mosby Co., p. 61.)

**Table 2-2.** Maturation of motor nerve conduction velocity*

| | Ulnar | | Median | | Peroneal | |
|---|---|---|---|---|---|---|
| | Mean[†] | S.D.[‡] | Mean | S.D. | Mean | S.D. |
| Newborn[§] | 32 | ± 4 | 29 | ± 8 | 29 | ± 4 |
| 1 to 4 months | 43 | ± 8 | 34 | ± 9 | 37 | ± 7 |
| 4 to 12 months | 50 | ± 7 | 40 | ± 5 | 48 | ± 8 |
| 1 to 3 years | 60 | ± 8 | 50 | ± 6 | 54 | ± 8 |
| 3 to 8 years | 65 | ± 8 | 58 | ± 5 | 58 | ± 7 |
| 8 to 16 years | 68 | ± 6 | 64 | ± 6 | 58 | ± 7 |
| Adult | 63 | ± 6 | 63 | ± 6 | 56 | ± 5 |

*Modified from Gamstorp, I.: Acta Paediatr. Scand. (Suppl.) **146:**68, 1963.
[†]In meters per second.
[‡]Standard deviation.
[§]Full-term infants.

and reaches the lower range of adult normal values by the age of 3 years. Median nerve conduction velocity increases more slowly with maturation; adult values are reached by 8 years of age. Peroneal nerve velocity increases rapidly in the first year of life and achieves adult levels between 1 and 3 years of age (Thomas and Lambert, 1960).

The premature infant exhibits striking maturational changes in motor nerve conduction velocity. Between 30 and 42 weeks' gestation the increase in conduction velocity is two-fold (Table 2-3).

**SENSORY NERVE CONDUCTION VELOCITY.** Sensory nerve function is studied by stimulating the cutaneous nerves, such as the digital (median and ulnar branches), radial, and sural nerves. The evoked action potential, recorded over the course of the nerve, is a small (less than $50\mu V$) triphasic potential that represents the neural activity of large myelinated fibers.

Sensory nerve conduction time, or latency, is most often determined from evoked potentials recorded with surface or needle electrodes over the nerve (Fig. 2-12). The time from onset of stimulation to the beginning of the sensory evoked potential is the latency of response. The true conduction velocity may be determined by recording over two points along the course of the nerve and determining the time required for the impulse to cover the distance between the recording sites (Murai and Sanderson, 1975).

The amplitude of sensory action potentials is small in both normal and pathologic conditions. Amplitudes of less than $5\mu V$ are common. Two techniques improve the detection of small potentials: photographic superimposition (Dawson and Scott, 1949) and electronic averaging (Buchthal and Rosenfalck, 1965). The former involves superimposing a number of oscilloscopic sweeps on film or paper displaying the stimulus and response. The stimulus and response are locked in time and stand out on the film while random potentials are dispersed.

Sensory nerve conduction studies provide useful objective evidence of function, especially in infants, when only gross clinical testing is available. These studies are somewhat more complicated in infants and young children than in adults because of the smaller

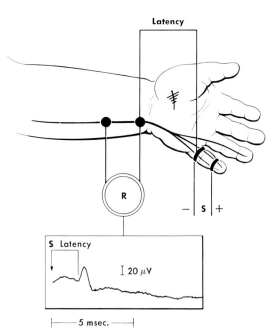

**Fig. 2-12.** Sensory nerve latency is determined by stimulation *(S)* of digital nerves with cathode *(−)* in a proximal location. Potential *(insert)* is recorded *(R)* over nerve at wrist. (From Wright, F. S.: Electrodiagnosis of neuromuscular disease. In Swaiman, K. F., and Wright, F. S.: The practice of pediatric neurology, St. Louis, 1975, The C. V. Mosby Co., p. 62.)

**Table 2-3.** Motor conduction velocity in premature infants*

| Conceptual age† | Ulnar nerve‡ | Peroneal nerve‡ |
|---|---|---|
| 30 | 16 ± 4 | |
| 34 | 20 ± 4 | 15 ± 4 |
| 38 | 26 ± 4 | 20 ± 4 |
| 42 | 30 ± 4 | 27 ± 4 |

*Modified from Wagner, A. L., and Buchtal, F.: Dev. Med. Child. Neurol. **14:**189, 1972.
†Conceptual age equals gestational age plus age from birth in weeks.
‡Mean value ± 2 S.D. in meters per second.

distances involved. Stimulation may be uncomfortable to the patient, but with reassurance most children can be studied without use of sedatives or analgesics.

Data on sensory nerve conduction velocity in infants and children are not extensive. The maximum sensory conduction velocity along median and ulnar nerves in 2- to 4- month-old infants is about 50% of the adult mean value of 62 m/sec. The lower limit of adult conduction velocity is reached by 3 years of age (Minejima, Sato, and Sugiyama, 1971). The distal conduction velocity in the median nerve increases from 55 m/sec at age 2 years to 62 m/sec at age 12 (Wagner and Buchthal, 1972).

Sensory conduction velocity in the peroneal and tibial nerves increases with age. The maximum sensory velocity in 6-month-old infants is 40 m/sec, increasing to 55 m/sec at 3 years of age.

**H-REFLEX.** The H-reflex is a monosynaptic reflex elicited by *submaximal* electrical stimulation of large afferent axons in a mixed nerve. The impulses travel over the sensory nerve to the spinal cord and activate the anterior horn cells, producing an efferent discharge that is recorded from the muscle (Magladery and McDougal, 1950). The H-reflex is readily recorded from the soleus and other muscles of the leg but cannot be recorded in the small muscles of the hand after age 2 years (Thomas and Lambert, 1960). Latency varies with age. In the newborn infant, H-reflex latency is approximately one-half that recorded in adults and increases with age and nerve length until it reaches adult levels (26 to 32 msec) after puberty (Mayer and Mosser, 1973). Persistence of the H-reflex in the hand muscles is an indication of central nervous system dysfunction (Hodes, Gribetz, and Hodes, 1962). H-reflex latency has been used to ascertain sensory nerve conduction velocity (Wager and Buerger, 1974).

**F WAVE RESPONSE.** The F wave is a late response following *supramaximal* stimulation of a mixed peripheral nerve. It results from antidromic activation of a small number of motor neurons. Typically, the F wave is readily recorded from the muscles of the hands and feet. It occurs after the direct motor or M, response. F wave latency represents the summation of centripetal conduction of the stimulus into the spinal cord and centrifugal conduction from the spinal cord, traversing the central segment of the nerve. The advantages of F wave study is that it reflects the latency of the central portion of the nerve in contrast to the usual electrodiagnostic conduction measurements. The F wave response has been useful in diagnosing Charcot-Marie-Tooth disease (Kimura, 1974) and Guillain-Barré syndrome (Kimura and Butzer, 1975). F waves in newborn infants are smaller and more variable than those in children and adults (Mayer and Mosser, 1969).

### Single-fiber electromyography

Motor unit potentials are generated by contraction of a number of muscle fibers distributed randomly over a given area. Ekstedt (1964) recorded from a single muscle fiber using an intramuscular, extracellular needle electrode with a recording surface of $25\mu$. Electrical activity is usually recorded from one or two muscle fibers of the same motor unit. When action potentials from two motor units are recorded, arrival time of the two fiber muscle action potentials at the electrode varies. This variability results from differences in neuromuscular transmission and is termed "action potential jitter."

Single-fiber electromyography, largely a research tool at present, has been used to study myasthenia gravis, myopathy, and neuropathy (Stalberg and Ekstedt, 1973).

### Interpretation of electrodiagnostic studies

Electromyography is most useful in differentiating among diseases affecting the anterior horn cell, peripheral nerve, neuromuscular junction, and muscle. Thus the electromyogram can localize disorders within the lower motor unit and generally can delineate the anatomic level of involvement. Little abnormality is noted on the EMG in the presence of central nervous system disease alone. However, special techniques demonstrate abnormalities of reciprocal innervation in diseases affecting the basal ganglia.

In assessing the results of electrodiagnostic studies, the examiner must remember that these studies are laboratory procedures and most often do not specify a definitive diagnosis; rather they specify the site of involvement and the type of process (neurogenic or myopathic). To arrive at a definitive diagnosis the examiner must combine information from the clinical evaluation with the electrodiagnostic studies.

Electrodiagnostic studies can aid greatly in the differentiation of primary neurogenic and "myopathic" disease processes. No single criterion is sufficient to make this differentiation; a composite of electromyographic findings is necessary. Electromyographic findings are not pathognomonic of a disease process, and the term "myopathic EMG" has been challenged (Drachman et al., 1967; Warmolts and Engel, 1970; Engel, 1975). The electromyographic findings should be interpreted in each case and correlated with the clinical and other laboratory studies to arrive at an appropriate diagnosis. In general, the diagnostic accuracy of electromyographic studies and muscle biopsy concur in more than 90% of cases. The consistency in diagnosis of histologic and electromyographic findings is strong supporting evidence for valid distinction between myopathic and neurogenic disease processes (Black et al., 1974).

Electromyographic analysis is concerned with the duration, amplitude, and shape of the individual motor unit potentials. In addition, the process of recruitment of motor units in relation to strength of force of contraction is compared.

In myopathic processes, the salient features are decreased duration and amplitude of the motor unit potential. The decrease in duration has been hypothesized to result from the loss of muscle fibers within the motor unit. The amplitude of motor unit potential is measured peak to peak. Reduction in amplitude may be seen best on maximal contraction of the muscle during the interference pattern. The shape of the action potential is altered by the appearance of increased polyphasic potentials. Generally, the total duration of a polyphasic unit does not exceed the normal duration and actually may be considerably less. Polyphasic potentials are thought to result from the patchy distribution of fiber loss, with subsequent asynchronization of the contractile process and fragmentation of the motor unit potential. In the normal recruitment process, the increase in muscular output results from the increase in the number of motor units discharging and in the firing rates of the individual units. Normally with maximal contraction of the muscle, the individual motor unit potentials cannot be visualized and a total interference pattern is produced by many potentials occurring at high frequency (Kugelberg, 1947, 1949; Pinelli and Buchthal, 1953).

Neurogenic processes are characterized by

**Table 2-4.** Electrodiagnostic findings in neuromuscular disease

| | Site of disease | | |
| --- | --- | --- | --- |
| | **Anterior horn cell** | **Peripheral nerve** | **Muscle** |
| Denervation potentials (fibrillation, positive sharp wave) | Frequent | Frequent | Rare (except in severe dystrophy, myositis, or periodic paralysis) |
| Unit potential duration | Increased | Increased | Reduced |
| Unit potential amplitude | Increased | Increased | Reduced |
| Interference pattern | Reduced | Reduced | Normal (except with marked weakness) |
| Nerve conduction velocity | Normal | Decreased | Normal |

an increase in the duration and amplitude of the motor unit potential, frequent fibrillation potentials, and a reduced interference pattern (Buchthal and Clemmsen, 1941; Buchthal and Pinelli, 1953; Fuglsang-Frederiksen, Scheel, and Buchthal, 1976).

Neuropathic disease may affect the anterior horn cell, the axon, the myelin covering, or a combination of these sites. In anterior horn cell disease, the mean duration and amplitude of the potentials are increased. In peripheral neuropathy, the mean duration increases while the mean amplitude is normal or decreases. Recruitment in severe neurogenic weakness produces a single motor unit pattern, while in mild to moderate neurogenic weakness only a partial interference pattern is seen with maximal effort. The frequency of unit-discharge firing may be determined easily by visual inspection. Fibrillation potentials, positive sharp waves, and increased insertion activity are common in neurogenic disease. Table 2-4 presents a comparison of electromyographic findings in neurogenic and myopathic disease.

Demyelination of the peripheral nerve is heralded by a decrease in the conduction velocity in both the motor and sensory nerves (Thomas, 1971). Anterior horn cell disease produces an increase in the total volume or territory of the motor unit, with an increase in amplitude and duration of the motor unit potential as the most significant electrodiagnostic feature. In a disease process that affects both the axon and the myelin, a combination of motor unit potential changes and decreased conduction velocity occurs. Electrodiagnostic studies are useful in estimating the prognosis in peripheral nerve or facial nerve injury. Electromyographic study is also helpful in selecting a site for muscle biopsy, although, as previously noted, the tissue should not be taken from a muscle that has recently been subjected to needle electrode examination because an inflammatory reaction occurs at the site of needle electrode penetration (Engel, 1967a) and biopsy specimens of tissue in this area produce a confusing picture of myositis. Consequently the homologous muscle in the opposite body part, if clinically involved, should be selected.

## REFERENCES

Adams, R. D.: General reactions of human muscle to disease. In Adams, R. D.: Diseases of muscle: a study in pathology, ed. 3, Hagerstown, Md., 1975, Harper & Row, Publishers, p. 204.

Adams, R. D., Denny-Brown, D., and Pearson, C. M.: Diseases of muscle, ed. 2, New York, 1962, Harper & Row, Publishers, pp. 15 and 310.

Adrian, E. D., and Bronk, D. W.: The discharge of impulses in motor nerve fibers: II. The frequency of discharge in reflex and voluntary contractions, J. Physiol. **67**:119, 1929.

Becker, P. E.: Generalized non-dystrophic myotonia. In Desmedt, J. E., editor: New developments in electromyography and clinical neurophysiology, Basel, 1973, S. Karger, p. 407, vol. 1.

Black, J. T., et al.: Diagnostic accuracy of clinical data, quantitative electromyography and histochemistry in neuromuscular disease, J. Neurol. Sci. **21**:59, 1974.

Blanchaer, M., and Van Wijhe, M.: Distribution of lactic dehydrogenase in skeletal muscle, Nature **193**:877, 1962.

Brandstater, M. E., and Lambert, E. H.: Motor unit anatomy. In Desmedt, J. E., editor: New developments in electromyography and clinical neurophysiology, Basel, 1973, S. Karger, p. 14, vol. 2.

Brooke, M. H., and Kaiser, K. K.: Some comments on the histochemical characterisation of muscle adenosine triphosphatase, J. Histochem. Cytochem. **17**:431, 1969.

Buchthal, F., and Clemmsen, S.: On the differentiation of muscular atrophy by electromyography, Acta Psychiatr. Neurol. Scand. **16**:143-181, 1941.

Buchthal, F., and Pinelli, P.: Action potentials in muscular atrophy of neurogenic origin, Neurology **3**:591-603, 1953.

Buchthal, F., and Rosenfalck, A.: Action potentials from sensory nerve in man: physiology and clinical applications, Acta Neurol. Scand. (Suppl.) **41**:263, 1965.

Buchthal, F., and Rosenfalch, P.: On the structure of motor units. In Desmedt, J. E., editor: New developments in electromyography and clinical neurophysiology, Basel, 1973, S. Karger, p. 71, vol. 1.

Buchthal, F., Rosenfalch, P., and Erminio, F.: Motor unit territory and fiber density in myopathies, Neurology **10**:398, 1960.

Campbell, M. J., Rebetz, J. J., and Walton, J. N.: Myotubular, centronuclear or peri-centronuclear myopathy? J. Neurol. Sci. **8**:425, 1969.

Chou, S. M.: Satellite cells and muscle regeneration in diseased human skeletal muscle, J. Neurol. Sci. **34**:131, 1977.

Clark, L. C., Jr., et al.: Excretion of creatine and creatinine by children, Am. J. Dis. Child **81**:774, 1951.

Cöors, C., and Woolf, A. L.: The innervation of muscle, Oxford, 1959, Blackwell.

Cuajunco, F.: Development of the human motor endplate, Contrib. Embryol. Carnegie Inst. **30**:127, 1942.

Dawson, D. M., and Fine, I. H.: Creatine kinase in human tissues, Arch. Neurol. **16**:175, 1967.

Dawson, G. D., and Scott, J. W.: The recording of nerve action potentials through the skin in man, J. Neurosurg. & Psychiatr. **12**:259, 1949.

Dennis, N. R., et al.: Use of creatine kinase for detecting severe X-linked muscular dystrophy carriers, Br. Med. J. **2**:577, 1976.

Drachman, D. B., et al.: "Myopathic" changes in chronically denervated muscle, Arch. Neurol. **16**:14-24, 1967.

Dreyfus, J. C., Schapira, G., and Schapira, F.: Biochemical study of muscle in progressive muscular dystrophy, J. Clin. Invest. **33**:794, 1954.

Dubowitz, V.: Enzymatic maturation of skeletal muscle, Nature **197**:1215, 1963.

Dubowitz, V.: Enzyme histochemistry of skeletal muscle: II. Developing human muscle, J. Neurol. Neurosurg. Psychiatry **28**:519, 1965.

Dubowitz, V., and Brooke, M. H.: Histological and histochemical stains and reactions. In Dubowitz, V., and Brooke, M. H., editors: Muscle biopsy: a modern approach, Philadelphia, 1973, W. B. Saunders Co., p. 20.

Dubowitz, V., and Pearse, A. G. E.: Reciprocal relationship of phosphorylase and oxidative enzymes in skeletal muscle, Nature **185**:701, 1960.

Dubowitz, V., and Pearse, A. G. E.: Enzymatic activity of normal and dystrophic human muscle: a histochemical study, J. Path. Bact. **81**:356, 1961.

Ebashi, S.: Excitation-contraction coupling, Annu. Rev. Physiol. **38**:293, 1976.

Ebashi, S., and Kodama, A.: A new protein promoting aggregation of tropomyosin, J. Biochem. (Tokyo) **58**:107, 1965.

Ekstedt, J.: Human single muscle fiber action potentials, Acta Physiol. Scand. (Suppl.) **61**:1-96, 1964.

Endo, M.: Calcium release from the sarcoplasmic reticulum, Physiol. Rev. **57**:71, 1977.

Engel, W. K.: Focal myopathic changes produced by electromyographic and hypodermic needles, Arch. Neurol. **16**:590, 1967a.

Engel, W. K.: Muscle biopsy, Postgrad. Med. **41**:155, 1967b.

Engel, W. K.: Brief, small, abundant motor-unit action potentials: a further critique of electromyographic interpretation, Neurology **25**:173, 1975.

Farber, E., Sternberg, W. H., and Dunlap, C. E.: Histochemical localization of specific oxidative enzymes. I. Tetrazolium stains for diphosphopyridine nucleotide diaphorase and triphosphopyridine nucleotide diaphorase, J. Histochem. Cytochem. **4**:254, 1956.

Fenichel, G. M.: A histochemical study of developing human muscle, Neurology **16**:741, 1966.

Fenichel, G. M.: A cerebral influence on muscle fiber typing: the effect of fetal immobilization, Arch. Neurol. **20**:644, 1969.

Flood, R. G., and Pinelli, R. W.: Urinary glycocyamine, creatine and creatinine. I. Their excretion by normal infants and children, Am. J. Dis. Child. **77**:740, 1949.

Fuglsang-Frederiksen, A., Scheel, U., and Buchthal, F.: Diagnostic yield of analysis of the pattern of electrical activity and of individual motor unit potentials in myopathy, J. Neurol. Neurosurg. Psychiatry **39**:272, 1976.

Fujie, Y.: Distribution of creatine phosphokinase among mammalian tissues, Seitai no Kagaku **11**:207, 1960.

Gilboa, N., and Swanson, J. R.: Serum creatine phosphokinase in normal newborns, Arch. Dis. Child. **51**:283, 1976.

Gilliatt, R. W.: Nerve conduction in human and experimental myopathies, Proc. R. Soc. Med. **59**:989-993, 1966.

Goto, K.: Creatine phosphokinase isoenzymes in neuromuscular disorders, Arch. Neurol. **31**:116, 1974.

Harding, V. J., and Gaebler, O. H.: On the constancy of the creatine-creatinine excretion in children on a high protein diet, J. Biol. Chem. **54**:579, 1922.

Hess, R., Scarpelli, D. G., and Pearse, A. G. E.: The cytochemical localization of oxidative enzymes, J. Cell. Biol. **4**:753, 1958.

Hodes, R., Gribetz, I., and Hodes, H. L.: Abnormal occurrence of the ulnar nerve–hypothenar muscle H-reflex in Sydenham's chorea, Pediatrics **30**:49, 1962.

Hodes, R., Larabee, M. G., and German, W. J.: The human electromyogram in response to nerve stimulation and the conduction velocity of motor axons, Arch. Neurol. Psychiatry **60**:340-365, 1948.

Huxley, A. F.: Review lecture: muscular contraction, J. Physiol. **243**:1, 1974.

Huxley, H. E.: The double array of filaments in cross striated muscle, J. Biophys. Biochem. Cytol. **3**:631, 1957.

Huxley, H. E.: The Croonian Lecture, 1970. The structural basis of muscular contraction, Proc. R. Soc. Lond. **178**:131, 1971.

Huxley, H. E., and Hanson, J.: Changes in the cross striations of muscle during contraction and stretch and their structural interpretation, Nature **173**:973, 1954.

Inesi, G., and Malan, N.: Mechanisms of calcium release in sarcoplasmic reticulum, Life Sci. **18**:773, 1976.

Karpati, G., and Engel, W. K.: A new aspect of the trophic function of the motor nerve: influence of the cytochemical features of the skeletal muscle cell, Neurology **17**:298, 1967.

Kimura, J.: F-wave velocity in the central segment of the median and ulnar nerves. A study in normal subjects and in patients with Charcot-Marie-Tooth disease, Neurology **24**:539, 1974.

Kimura, J., and Butzer, J. F.: F-wave conduction velocity in Guillain-Barré syndrome. Arch. Neurol. **32:** 524, 1975.

Kugelberg, E.: Electromyogram in muscular disorders, J. Neurol. Neurosurg. Psychiatry **10:**122-133, 1947.

Kugelberg, E.: Electromyography in muscular dystrophies with special regard to the differential diagnosis, J. Neurol. Neurosurg. Psychiatry **12:**129-136, 1949.

Magladery, J. V., and McDougal, D. B.: Electrophysiological studies of nerve and reflex activity in normal man, Bull. Johns Hopkins Hosp. **86:**265, 1950.

Mair, W. G. P., and Tome, F. M. S.: The ultrastructure of the adult and developing myotendinous junction, Acta Neuropathol. **21:**239, 1972.

Marples, E., and Levine, S. Z.: Creatinuria of infancy and childhood. I. Normal variations: creatine tolerance tests and the effect of aminoacetic acid in normal infants, Am. J. Dis. Child. **51:**30, 1936.

Mayer, R. F., and Mosser, R. S.: Excitability of motoneurons in infants, Neurology **19:**932, 1969.

Milhorat, A. T., and Goldstone L.: The carrier state in muscular dystrophy of the Duchenne type, J.A.M.A. **194:**130, 1965.

Minejima, T. F., Sato, K., and Sugiyama, S.: Sensory nerve action potentials in infants and children, Abstract IV, Brussels, International Electromyography Congress, 1971, p. 100.

Moore, R. W., and Norris, J. W.: CK-BB isoenzyme detected by radioimmunoassay, Ann. Neurol. **4:**576, 1978.

Murai, Y., and Sanderson, I.: Studies of sensory conduction. Comparison of latencies of orthodromic and antidromic sensory potentials, J. Neurol. Neurosurg. Psychiatry **38:**1187, 1975.

Nachlas, M. M., et al.: The histochemical demonstration of cytochrome oxidase with a new reagent for the Nadi reaction, J. Histochem. Cytochem. **6:**445, 1958.

Neville, H. E.: Ultrastructural changes in muscle disease. In Dubowitz, V., and Brooke, M. H., editors: Muscle biopsy: a modern approach, Philadelphia, 1973, W. B. Saunders Co., p. 383.

Orentlicher, M., and Gersho, A.: A quantitative model of actin-myosin interaction in skeletal muscle, Biophys. J. **18:**141, 1977.

Pearce, J. M. S., Pennington, R. J., and Walton, J. N.: Serum enzyme studies in muscle disease. Part II. Serum creatine kinase activity in muscular dystrophy and in other myopathic and neuropathic disorders, J. Neurol. Neurosurg. Psychiatry **27:**96, 1964.

Pearson, C. M.: Histopathological features in muscle in the preclinical stages of muscular dystrophy, Brain **85:**109, 1962.

Perry, S. V.: Calcium ions and the function of the contractile properties of muscle, Biochem. Soc. Symp. **39:**115, 1974.

Pinelli, P., and Buchthal, F.: Muscle action potentials in myopathies with special regard to progressive muscular dystrophy, Neurology **3:**347-359, 1953.

Price, H. R.: The skeletal muscle fiber in the light of electron microscope studies, Am. J. Med. **35:**589, 1963.

Roberts, R., and Sobel, B. E.: CPK isoenzymes in evaluation of myocardial ischemic injury, Hosp. Pract. **11:**55, 1976.

Rosalki, S. B.: An improved procedure for serum creatine phosphokinase determination, J. Lab. Clin. Med. **69:**696, 1967.

Sarnat, H. B.: Diagnostic value of muscle biopsy in neonatal period, Am. J. Dis. Child. **132:**782, 1978.

Schiavone, D. J., and Kaldor, J.: Creatine phosphokinase levels and cerebral disease, Med. J. Aust. **2:** 790, 1965.

Schultz, E.: Fine structure of satellite cells in growing skeletal muscle, Am. J. Anat. **147:**49, 1976.

Seligman, A. M., and Rutenburg, A. M.: The histochemical demonstration of succinic dehydrogenase, Science **113:**317, 1951.

Shaw, R. F., et al.: Serum enzymes in sex-linked (Duchenne) muscular dystrophy, Arch. Neurol. **16:** 115, 1967.

Sidell, F. R., Culver, D. L., and Kaminskis, A.: Serum creatine phosphokinase activity after intramuscular injection, J.A.M.A. **229:**1894, 1974.

Silverman, L. M., et al.: Significance of creatine phosphokinase isoenzymes in Duchenne dystrophy, Neurology **26:**561, 1976.

Simpson, J. A.: Fact and fallacy in measurement of conduction velocity in motor nerves, J. Neurol. Neurosurg. Psychiatry **27:**381, 1964.

Simpson, J. A.: Terminology of electromyography, Electroencephalogr. Clin. Neurophysiol. **26:**224, 1969.

Stalberg, E., and Ekstedt, J.: Single fiber EMG and microphysiology of the motor unit in normal and diseased human muscle. In Desmedt, J. E., editor: New developments in electromyography and clinical neurophysiology **1:**113, 1973.

Swaiman, K. F., and Sandler, B.: The use of serum enzymes in the diagnosis of progressive muscular dystrophy, J. Pediatr. **63:**116, 1963.

Takeuchi, T.: Histochemical demonstration of branching enzyme (amylo-1, 4→1,6-transglucosidase in animal tissues), J. Histochem. Cytochem. **6:**208, 1958.

Takeuchi, T., and Glenner, G. G.: Histochemical demonstration of uridine diphosphate glucoseglycogen transferase in animal tissues, J. Histochem. Cytochem. **9:**304, 1961.

Thomas, J. E., and Lambert, E. H.: Ulnar nerve conduction velocity and H-reflex in infants and children, J. Appl. Physiol. **15:**1, 1960.

Thomas, P. K.: The morphological basis for alterations in nerve conduction in peripheral neuropathy, Proc. R. Soc. Med. **64:**13, 1971.

Tierney, N. A., and Peters, J. P.: The mode of excretion of creatine and creatine metabolism in thyroid disease, J. Clin. Invest. **22:**595, 1943.

Tosi, C., and Jerusalem, F.: Selective muscle fiber type anomalies in neuro-muscular disorders—analysis of 124 consecutive muscle biopsies, J. Neurol. **214:**13, 1976.

Tunell, G., and Hart, M.: Simultaneous determination of skeletal muscle fiber, types I, IIA and IIB by histochemistry, Arch. Neurol. **34:**171, 1977.

Wager, E. W., Jr., and Buerger, A. A.: A linear relationship between H-reflex latency and sensory conduction velocity in diabetic neuropathy, Neurology **24:**711, 1974.

Wagner, A. L., and Buchthal, F.: Motor and sensory conduction in infancy and childhood: reappraisal, Dev. Med. Child. Neurol. **14:**189, 1972.

Warmolts, J. R., and Engel, W. K.: A critique of the "myopathic" electromyogram, Trans. Am. Neurol. Assoc. **95:**175-177, 1970.

Weber, A., and Murray, J. M.: Molecular control mechanisms in muscle contraction, Physiol. Rev. **53:**612, 1973.

Yunis, E. J., and Samaha, F. J.: Inclusion body myositis, Lab. Invest. **25:**240, 1971.

# CHAPTER 3

# Anterior horn cell and cranial motor neuron disease

## General clinical aspects

The classic clinical pattern of impaired function of the anterior horn cells and cranial motor neurons is profound weakness and atrophy of the muscles, hyporeflexia of the deep tendon reflexes, and fasciculations. Muscles denervated by impairment of the anterior horn cells often are incapable of anti-gravity resistance. Muscle atrophy may not be evident for several months, and in infants with large amounts of subcutaneous fat may not be recognizable at all. The deep tendon reflexes may be difficult to elicit or lost entirely. In normal infants, however, these reflexes are sometimes difficult to obtain in the triceps and biceps muscles and occasionally in the Achilles tendons. Spontaneous contraction of small groups of denervated muscle fibers in a motor unit results in fasciculations that may be stimulated by gentle tapping on the denervated muscle. However, fasciculations, like atrophy, may be masked in infants with abundant subcutaneous fat.

The neurons of the motor nuclei of the cranial nerves are homologous to anterior horn cells. Thus disease processes affecting the cranial motor neurons cause clinical symptoms and signs similar to those found in anterior horn cell impairment. Atrophy, profound weakness, and fasciculations, particularly of the tongue, may be present.

Impairment of the anterior horn cells does not lead to sensory deficit. If a sensory deficit occurs in association with anterior horn cell disease, it indicates damage to adjacent tracts of the spinal cord or to the peripheral nerves.

## Anterior horn cell anatomy

Anterior horn cells are motor neurons distributed throughout the length of the spinal cord in the anterior gray masses (Fig. 3-1). They are most prominent in the cervical and lumbosacral enlargements. The anterior horn cell masses may be divided into medial cell and lateral cell groups. The medial cell group contains dorsomedial and ventromedial components. The dorsomedial cells supply the small, deep muscles of the spine; the ventromedial cells supply the superficial, larger muscles. The lateral cell group comprises centrodorsal and ventrolateral components. The centrodorsal cells innervate flexor muscles; the ventrolateral cells innervate extensor muscles (Romanes, 1951). Because of the proximity of these groups to one another, damage to the anterior horn cells usually affects many types of muscle. Differentiation of the anterior horn cells is most pronounced around 12 to 14 weeks of gestation (Vassilopoulos and Emery, 1977).

## Congenital defects
### Diastematomyelia

CLINICAL FEATURES. Because the mesodermal septum usually disrupts the anterior horn cell column, there are resulting muscle

**47**

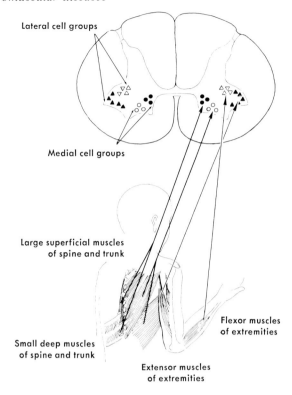

Lateral cell groups

Medial cell groups

Large superficial muscles
of spine and trunk

Small deep muscles
of spine and trunk

Flexor muscles
of extremities

Extensor muscles
of extremities

**Fig. 3-1.** Anterior horn cells are grouped in systematic pattern forming central spinal gray matter. Lateral cell groups are connected with muscles of extremities and medial cell groups with muscles of spine and trunk.

atrophy, reduction or loss of deep tendon reflexes, and profound weakness of the muscles of the lower legs and feet. Involvement is usually bilateral. Patients with diastematomyelia usually have deformities of the feet, particularly talipes equinovarus. Atony of the bladder and weakness of the lower legs are common presenting signs. Skin lesions over the spine are a frequent finding and include lipoma, hypertrichosis, sacrococcygeal sinus, soft-tissue swelling, and myelomeningocele; rarely, pigmented nevi or hemangiomas are seen over the lower spine (James and Lassman, 1964).

Pain and temperature sensations are often diminished, since the septum interferes with the fibers that transmit these sensations as they cross from one side of the spinal cord to the other. Occasionally, light touch sensation (superficial sensation) is also impaired. Corticospinal tract involvement with resulting upper motor neuron symptoms and signs are uncommon but have been reported.

The presence of a septum can be determined by x-ray study, but because calcification is delayed, the septum may not be detectable until the child is several years old (Fig. 3-2). The septum is usually in the lower thoracic and lumbar areas, but it has been reported as high as the second thoracic vertebra (Cowie, 1951). Other associated skeletal changes include spina bifida occulta, often present, and scoliosis or kyphoscoliosis, less frequently present. Diastematomyelia should be suspected in the presence of intersegmental laminar fusion with spina bifida at or adjacent to the level of fusion (Hilal, Marton, and Pollack, 1974).

In diastematomyelia a septum of variable length divides the spinal cord laterally into more or less equal portions (Fig. 3-3). Originating from mesoderm, the septum is com-

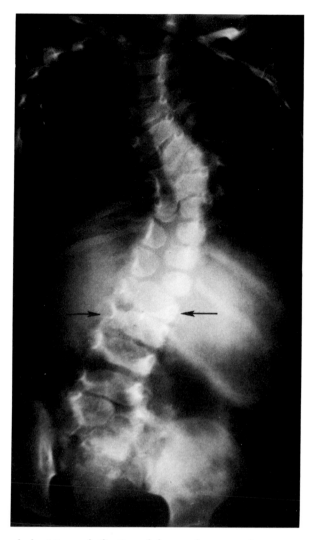

**Fig. 3-2.** Radiograph depicting calcification of abnormal septum. Arrows point to a small area of calcification.

posed of cartilage, fibrous tissue, bone, or a combination of these tissues. The septum is attached to the posterior aspect of the vertebral bodies and passes through the neural canal, where it divides the spinal cord and is often affixed posteriorly to the bony neural arch or dura mater (Moes and Hendrick, 1963).

### PATHOPHYSIOLOGY

EMBRYOLOGY. When development is normal, the neural tube forms a closed cavity during the first month of gestation. The tube then distends, the roof becomes permeable, and fluid escapes into the space above, which eventually becomes the subarachnoid space. The developmental abnormality that results in diastematomyelia has not been precisely defined, but at least two theories are widely entertained.

One theory proposes that in diastematomyelia the roof of the neural tube does not become permeable but is split by the increasing pressure, resulting in lateral displacement of the neural tissues. The distention of

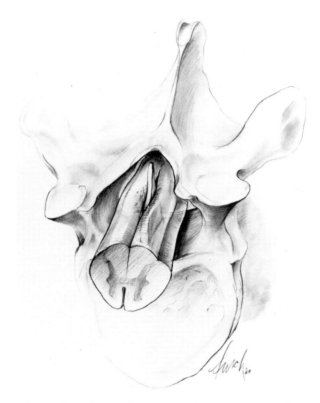

**Fig. 3-3.** Abnormal mesodermal central septum in diastematomyelia disrupts gray matter of cord. (From Swaiman, K. F., and Wright, F. S. In Baker, A. B., and Baker, L. H., editors: Clinical neurology, Hagerstown, Md., 1977, Harper & Row, Publishers, vol. 3, chap. 40.)

the tube also ruptures the floor plate (Gardner, 1960) and displaces other structures, which results in development of hemivertebrae and spina bifida.

The second theory is based on the probability of persistence of the early developing neurenteric canal, which traverses a path from the primitive intestinal canal (yolk sac cavity) to the amniotic cavity. The connection between the intestinal tract and the dorsal surface of the embryo quickly disappears, and during normal development the canal migrates to the tip of the coccyx. According to this theory, an accessory neurenteric canal is present that does not migrate caudally, and a rent develops in midline structures with resultant diastematomyelia. The accessory canal may later disappear and the medial bony processes may fuse to form the characteristic fibrous or bony spur (Ford, 1966).

The term "myelodysplasia" is used to denote congenital malformations of the spinal cord. These malformations are almost always associated with mesodermal abnormalities or abnormalities of the overlying skin or soft tissue. Use of the term in the absence of these associated abnormalities is rarely justified.

**TREATMENT.** Surgery often prevents or greatly retards progression of symptoms. If the septum is not removed, scoliosis is almost inevitable. Laminectomy and removal of the mesodermal septum, including all portions attached to the anterior dural surface, are indicated. A detailed discussion of the surgical technique is available (Meacham, 1967).

### Syringomyelia

**CLINICAL FEATURES.** Patients with syringomyelia frequently have difficulty in per-

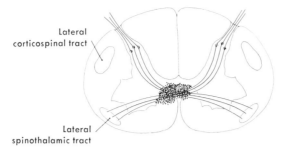

**Fig. 3-4.** Syringomyelia involves anterior white commissure. There is bilateral loss of pain and temperature sensation because crossing fibers of lateral spinothalamic tracts are involved. As lesion enlarges, gray matter of anterior horn is compromised.

ceiving pain and temperature and often have trophic ulcers of the fingers. Because the areas of the cord usually involved are those of the cervical and lumbosacral enlargements, the associated weakness is often severe. Muscle wasting is obvious, usually appearing first in the small muscles of the hand. Deep tendon reflexes are depressed or absent and fasciculations are present in the elbow, shoulder, and hip. Papilledema has been described in association with cervical syringomyelia. Intracranial pressure may be increased and associated with hydrocephalus, neoplasm, or obstruction of the foramina of Luschka and Magendie (Alpers and Comroe, 1931).

Syringomyelia occasionally occurs secondary to trauma or infections that damage the spinal cord, but this acquired type is very unusual in children. In patients with hydrocephalus, syringomyelia has been implicated as a complication of lumboureteral shunting (Fischer, Welch, and Shillito, 1977).

During early growth, intramedullary tumors can cause symptoms similar to those of syringomyelia (Williams and Timperley, 1977). Differentiation between syringomyelia and intramedullary tumors may be impossible even after extensive neurologic and radiologic examinations and may require surgical exploration of the spinal cord.

Composition and dynamics of cerebrospinal fluid are usually normal in syringomyelia. Occasionally, however, the fluid is xan-thochromic and its flow is obstructed. Diagnosis is best approached by myelography or computed tomography (DiChiro et al., 1975), which confirms widening of the spinal cord.

The symptoms caused by cysts in the cord may be grossly exaggerated by coughing, straining, and postural changes that affect hydrodynamics. The transient increase in intracranial pressure brought on by these actions may hasten the development of syringomyelia and syringobulbia (Bertrand, 1973).

**LABORATORY FINDINGS**

PATHOLOGY. Syringomyelia is a slowly progressive, degenerative disease involving the spinal cord, the medulla, or both. A cavity forms within the spinal cord and gliosis ensues. Similar involvement of the medulla is known as syringobulbia. Cavitation usually occurs in the cervical and lumbar segments of the cord, primarily in the anterior white commissure. As the cavity enlarges, the anterior horn cells are involved. There is bilateral loss of temperature and pain sensations because the crossed fibers of the lateral spinothalamic tracts are disrupted (Fig. 3-4). Light touch sensation remains intact, however, because the tracts subserving this function run dorsally and do not cross. Simultaneous preservation of light touch sensation and loss of pain and temperature sensations are known as "dissociation of sensation."

Asymmetric, bilateral involvement is usual in the early stages. The long tracts, including the corticospinal tracts, may be compromised if the process of cavitation becomes greatly extended. Horner's syndrome may be present if sympathetic cells in the cervical cord are compromised. In syringobulbia, the motor neurons in the medulla may be involved.

Only rarely has syringomyelia been diagnosed before age 15. It may be associated with other congenital malformations, including cervical ribs, scoliosis, basilar impression, and Klippel-Feil syndrome (Berke and Magee, 1976). On rare occasions it appears to be the result of a hereditary factor (Jackson, 1949).

### PATHOPHYSIOLOGY

EMBRYOLOGY. Syringomyelia has been attributed to incompetent closing of the neural tube in the fourth week of gestation. Normally, the differentiation of cells results in an inner grouping of spongioblastic cells that later form glial tissue and an outer grouping of neuroblastic cells that later form nerve cells and nerve processes. In congenital syringomyelia, differentiation of the spongioblastic cells may be delayed, causing cavitation and gliosis (Leyden, 1876).

Another explanation is that there is a congenital abnormality of the hindbrain similar to the one present when myelomeningocele is associated with Arnold-Chiari malformation. Gardner (1965) found that in many cases the foramen of Magendie is closed by a membrane. Clear fluid was removed, possibly the result of an accumulation between the syrinx and the fourth ventricle. Distention of the syrinx and fourth ventricle may result from failure of the foramina to open sufficiently in prenatal life.

Some of these cases may represent hydromyelia, but more likely the underlying pathophysiologic defect is an anomaly of the intramedullary vascular supply. The vessels appear to be susceptible to infarction or hemorrhage, and inadequate circulation leads to cavity formation (Netsky, 1953).

Williams (1977) has advanced still another explanation for syringomyelia. Using a questionnaire to determine if mothers of syringomyelia patients had had a high incidence of difficult labor, he found that a high proportion had experienced forceps delivery. Furthermore, he found that in a high proportion of the cases the syringomyelia patient was the firstborn child. Williams postulated that as a result of birth injury the tonsils descend through the foramen magnum, causing arachnoiditis. The difference in fluid pressure between cranial and spinal cavities may lead to continued insidious descent of the tonsils, resulting in communicating syringomyelia.

*Hydromyelia* is another congenital abnormality arising from distention of the central canal that compromises the surrounding structures in the spinal cord, including the anterior horn cells. Symptoms are similar to those of syringomyelia. Hydromyelia, like syringomyelia, occurs most often in the cervical and lumbar enlargements. The abnormally distended cavity may traverse the length of the cord and is lined with ependyma, in contrast with the glial cell lining of the syrinx.

The cause of hydromyelia is unknown. It is possible that at least in the cervical region the dilation of the central canal results from failure of the foramina of the fourth ventricle to form (Gardner, 1965; Lassman, Michael, and Foster, 1968).

## Degenerative conditions
### Progressive infantile spinal muscular atrophy (Werdnig-Hoffman disease)

Progressive infantile spinal muscular atrophy is an inherited degenerative disease of the anterior horn cells and the cranial nerve motor nuclei that becomes clinically apparent in the first 2 years of life.

The term "amyotonia congenita" is a modification of one originally used by Oppenheim (1900) to describe infants who were born with weakness, hypotonia, and areflexia but who improved in time. Oppenheim's brief report did not present pathologic details or long-term clinical assessment of the infants. The term has been used to designate a number of conditions in which weakness and hypotonia are the principal symptoms. Because the term is so vague that it engenders confusion,

**Table 3-1.** Hereditary degenerative anterior horn cell diseases of infancy and early childhood: general characteristics

| Type of muscular atrophy | Age of onset | Pattern of weakness | Sit | Stand | Walk | Tendon reflexes | Prognosis |
|---|---|---|---|---|---|---|---|
| Progressive infantile spinal (Werdnig-Hoffmann) | | | | | | | |
| Group 1 | Before 2 months | Frog-leg position; hands at head level; active movement of fingers and toes | No | No | No | Absent | Most die by age 3 |
| Group 2 | 2-12 months | Thigh and hip muscle | Yes | Yes | No | May be present early; patellar reflex absent | Most die in first decade, some live through teens |
| Group 3 | 12-24 months | Thigh and hip muscle | Yes | Yes | May walk early; in wheelchair by teens | Usually present early; patellar reflexes lost first | May live through second decade and beyond |
| Juvenile proximal hereditary (Kugelberg-Welander) | 2-17 years (mean: 9 years) | Normal early development followed by atrophy of shoulder and hip (Gowers' sign often present) | Yes | Yes | May walk for 20-40 years after onset | Present early; patellar reflexes lost first | Most live through fourth decade and beyond |

it should be avoided. It should never be used as a synonym for progressive infantile spinal muscular atrophy.

The earlier the manifestations of the disease are found, the more fulminating is the course and the more disseminated and catastrophic is the motor weakness. Onset occurs from infancy to age 2 years, and severity ranges from extreme proximal weakness of the limbs and bulbar weakness to gradually progressive proximal weakness of the hip and shoulder girdle.

**CLINICAL FEATURES AND CLASSIFICATION.** Because of the need for clarification, several authors have divided progressive infantile spinal muscular atrophy into clinical groups on the basis of age of onset (Byers and Banker, 1961). As the disease process shows an almost continuous spectrum, however, no classification is entirely satisfactory.

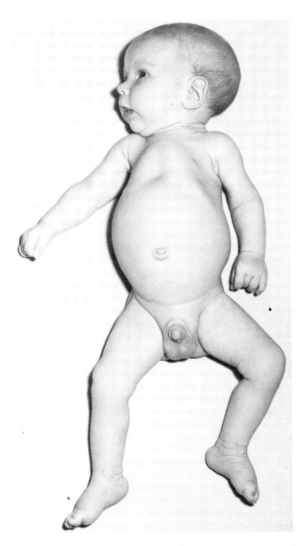

**Fig. 3-5.** Patients with group 1 Werdnig-Hoffmann disease maintain typical posture of abduction of legs at hips and flexion of knees. There is slight flexion of arms at elbow with little movement of shoulders. Movements of fingers and toes occur frequently. Pectus excavatum deformity of chest is common and is result of unopposed diaphragmatic breathing.

Nevertheless, some guidelines are helpful in establishing the diagnosis and prognosis. The categories recommended by Byers and Banker are summarized here (Table 3-1).

GROUP 1. Group 1 comprises infants who acquire the disease in utero or during the first 2 months of life. If the symptoms are present at birth, the history often shows that there was relatively little movement in utero. In about one third of all pregnancies resulting in birth of infants with the disease, there is history of reduced fetal movement. Some movement is almost always noted, however, and the time of fetal quickening is not delayed (Pearn, 1973).

Children in this group display marked weakness of the proximal muscles of the extremities and of the thoracic muscles. There is little movement of the arms and legs proximally but some movement of the hands and feet. The infant remains in a frog-leg position with the legs externally rotated, abducted, and flexed at the hips and knees (Fig. 3-5). The arms are usually slightly flexed at the elbows; the hands are held at the level of the head. Active movement of the limbs is often confined to the fingers and toes.

The chest is narrow, with pectus excavatum deformity and flaring of the lower ribs. The abdomen protrudes and the infant depends on diaphragmatic respiration. Involvement of the upper cranial nerve nuclei, including those subserving extraocular muscle function, is rare. However, weakness of the tongue and fasciculations are almost always obvious; the latter must be differentiated from normal tongue movements.

The features characteristic of anterior horn cell disease are usually present. Weakness is profound and usually the deep tendon reflexes are absent. The cry is weak and short. Sensations of pain, temperature, or light touch do not appear to be impaired.

Generally these infants do not progress sufficiently to sit alone, roll over, or walk. They have progressive weakness, increasing problems with oropharyngeal secretions, and recurrent pneumonia. Progressive difficulty in swallowing may ultimately necessitate feeding by nasogastric or gastrostomy tube. The clinical pattern varies somewhat, but almost all of the children in this group die by age 3.

GROUP 2. Group 2 includes infants who manifest the disease between 2 and 12 months of age. The symptoms are less devastating and the course less fulminating than in group 1 (Fig. 3-6). At first the weakness is limited to the arms and legs and only later becomes generalized. The legs are usually more severely involved than the arms. Deep tendon reflexes of the biceps, triceps, and gastrocnemius muscles are sometimes obtainable, but those of the quadriceps muscles are absent. Pectus excavatum is prominent, and diaphragmatic respiration becomes more evident as the disease progresses. Fasciculations are almost always present in the tongue and occasionally in the extremities.

An unusual tremor, called minipolymyoclonus, has been described in patients with slowly progressive disease. It is characterized by barely visible intermittent, irregular movements that involve primarily the distal joints and head and sometimes the proximal joints. The tremor ceases during complete relaxation or sleep, but stress, fatigue, and self-consciousness increase the amplitude. Formerly these movements were often attributed to weakness or fasciculations. They are not noted in myopathic processes (Spiro, 1970). Respiratory distress becomes evident after an initial asymptomatic period of 1 to 2 months. Two cases have been reported in which bilateral eventration of the diaphragm preceded loss of the deep tendon reflexes or other manifestations of muscle weakness (Mellins et al., 1974).

Some of the children in group 2 can sit if placed in position, and on rare occasions some can stand by holding onto furniture. In one study, the age of death ranged from 7 to 84 months (Byers and Banker, 1961). Rare cases of survival into the third decade have been reported in group 2 (Guinter, Hernried, and Kaplan, 1977).

GROUP 3. Patients in the third group experience onset of difficulty between the first

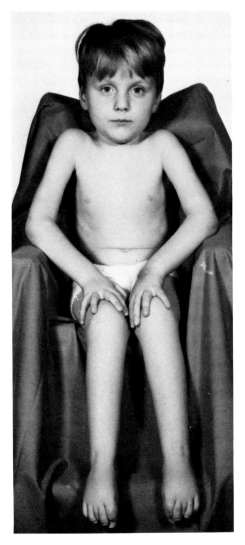

**Fig. 3-6.** Patient with group 2 Werdnig-Hoffmann disease has profound proximal and truncal weakness. There is wasting of shoulder girdle. He is unable to stand without braces. (From Swaiman, K. F.: Anterior Horn Cell and Cranial Motor Neuron Disease. In Swaiman, K. F., and Wright, F. S.: The practice of pediatric neurology, St. Louis, 1975, The C. V. Mosby Co., p. 945.)

difficulty with the gait is progressive and necessitates confinement to a wheelchair in the second decade. Deep tendon reflexes may be present early but disappear. Patellar deep tendon reflexes are often lost first, but the ankle tendon reflexes may remain for a relatively long period. It may not be possible to differentiate these patients from those with juvenile proximal hereditary muscular atrophy (Kugelberg-Welander disease).

In one series of cases, six of eight patients were able to stand without support between the ages of 1 and 2. Only two of the eight walked alone (Byers and Banker, 1961). In another group, 10 of the 15 children walked alone (Gamstorp, 1967). Scoliosis is the most prevalent orthopedic problem in the later stages of groups 2 and 3 (Schwentker and Gibson, 1976).

DIAGNOSTIC CONSIDERATIONS. Reports of patients with a benign form of this disease must be evaluated cautiously. In one series, only 65% of 32 patients had neurogenic features on electromyographic examination (Wijngaarden and Bethlem, 1973). In comparison, in the largest series compiled mostly from the literature, virtually all patients had electromyographic evidence of neurogenic features (Namba, Aberfeld, and Grob, 1970). The latter report summarized 375 such cases reported by others and seven cases observed by the authors. Overall, 36% of the patients had onset of the disease before age 2 years, 48% between the ages of 2 and 18 years, and 16% over age 18. In the authors' series, most patients with infantile onset manifested the first symptom at about 12 months as delay or difficulty in walking. (This demonstrates the skewing of the distribution from that reported for groups 1 and 2.) In 25 patients (25% of those with infantile onset), lack of muscle tone or diminished movement was recognized before 12 months of age.

In this series, neurogenic atrophy was diagnosed electrophysiologically in 97% of 211 patients. Findings were normal or inconclusive in four patients with infantile onset and two patients with juvenile onset. Five of these six patients were young children, and

and second years. These children have normal head control and sit unassisted by 6 to 8 months of age. The thigh and hip muscles are weak. Those children who do manage to walk have lumbar lordosis, waddling gait, genu recurvatum, and protuberant abdomen. The in three of the five cases, cooperation during examination could not be obtained. Muscle biopsy in five of the six patients revealed neuropathic muscle atrophy with no evidence of a primary myopathy. The authors stressed the value of electromyography in chronic proximal spinal muscular atrophy (Namba, Aberfeld, and Grob, 1970).

Other studies of large groups of children with spinal muscular atrophy have supported these findings (Pearn, Gardner-Medwin, and Wilson, 1978; Benady, 1978).

A similar disease in animals has been reported (Sandefeldt et al., 1976).

**LABORATORY FINDINGS.** Electromyographic examination reveals findings characteristic of anterior horn cell disease. The study of motor nerve conduction velocity in infants in groups 1 and 2 (progressive spinal muscular atrophy) may reveal slow ulnar and posterior tibial nerve conduction in patients with severe spinal muscular atrophy. In infants with less severe disease, conduction velocity is normal and sometimes even faster (Moosa and Dubowitz, 1976). Sensory action potential delay has been reported in progressive spinal muscular atrophy (Raimbault and Laget, 1972), but no confirmation has been forthcoming. Fibrillation potentials associated with denervation are the best electromyographic criteria of diagnosis (Buchthal and Olsen, 1970). Sensory conduction velocities were normal in the sural or median nerve in patients in all three groups and in patients with juvenile proximal hereditary muscular atrophy (Schwartz and Moosa, 1977).

Chronic polyneuropathy may masquerade as spinal muscular atrophy; therefore examination of motor and sensory conduction velocity in the peripheral nervous system is essential. This is particularly true in children with prolonged survival who have group 2 and group 3 progressive spinal muscular atrophy (Goebel, Zeman, and De Myer, 1976).

Increased activity of serum creatine phosphokinase (CPK) has occasionally been reported but is not of the magnitude reported in myopathic or myositic diseases. The studies of elevated serum enzyme activity in infantile spinal muscular atrophy often have not involved age-matched control groups and therefore may be misleading.

MORPHOLOGY. Detailed studies of children in group 3 are not available, but there are many studies of children in the younger groups. Pathologic changes do not vary among the three groups except for those changes associated with a chronic course. Because many of the children have prolonged anoxia shortly before death, the relationship between the primary disease process and the nonspecific changes reported in the cerebral hemispheres and the cerebellum is uncertain.

The motor nuclei of the cranial nerves are involved in varying degrees, except for that of cranial nerve III. Cranial nerve V is usually severely affected, with evidence of central chromatolysis and neuronophagia, although clinical manifestations are rare. Cranial nerve VI is similarly involved but to a lesser degree; again, clinical manifestations are uncommon (Byers and Banker, 1961). In clinical groups 1 and 2, the motor nucleus of cranial nerve VII (facial nerve) is usually involved; central chromatolysis, neuronophagia, nerve cell loss, and gliosis are prominent pathologic findings but clinical manifestations are unusual. More cells are lost from the nucleus of cranial nerve VII than from that of cranial nerve V or VI. The nucleus ambiguus, the motor nucleus for cranial nerves IX, X, and XI, is also commonly involved. The motor nucleus of cranial nerve XII is severely affected and its involvement is usually apparent clinically.

On a number of occasions, infants with clinical and autopsy findings of progressive spinal muscular atrophy have had associated abnormalities of the cerebellum, including hypoplasia. In addition, some have had severe mental retardation (Norman and Kay, 1965; Weinberg and Kirkpatrick, 1975; Goutiéres, Aicardi, and Farkas, 1977).

Examination of the spinal cord reveals compromise of the anterior horn cells. There

**Fig. 3-7.** Anterior horn of cervical spinal cord of patient with group 1 Werdnig-Hoffmann disease. There is marked decrease in number of neurons and many of those remaining are shrunken. Increase in number of nuclei is reflection of mild astrocytosis. Nissl stain.

is selective loss of the larger cells, especially of the ventromedial group (Fig. 3-7). Some cells are pyknotic, and neuronophagia is prevalent. Only a slight increase in glial cells and mild gliosis are noted.

Although sensory changes are not a component of the clinical pattern, postmortem studies reveal myelin loss in the posterior columns, particularly of fibers originating in the lumbar area. Changes in the sensory ganglia in the lumbar area indicate sensory neuron degeneration (Marshall and Duchen, 1975; Carpenter et al., 1975).

Examination of the muscles reveals uniform involvement except of the diaphragm, sternothyroid, and sternohyoid muscles.

HISTOPATHOLOGIC MUSCLE STUDIES. Microscopic study of muscle tissue removed at biopsy reveals group lesions of affected fibers interspersed with normal fiber bundles (Fig. 3-8). In comparison with normal tissue, the affected fibers are smaller in diameter and fat tissue is more abundant between the fiber bundles. Disproportionate preservation of large rounded fibers in the denervated fasciculi has been found (Byers and Banker, 1961), but changes in the muscle spindle have not been reported.

Histochemical study of the anterior horn cells for enzyme activities in the Embden-Meyerhof pathway and tricarboxylic acid cycle shows that most cells are not deficient in enzyme activity. Indeed, involved cells, identifiable by chromatolytic changes, show an increase in the activity of several enzymes, including nicotinamide-adenine dinucleotide phosphate diaphorase (Huttenlocher and Cohen, 1966). Electron microscopic studies reveal abnormalities present in axons that impinge on the anterior horn cells (Chou and Fakadej, 1970). Increased numbers of mitochondria have also been found in the anterior horn cells, which explains the enzyme changes. Degeneration of the anterior horn cells may be a phenomenon secondary to disease of the axons of the internuncial neurons or of a more rostral segment of the corticospinal pathway.

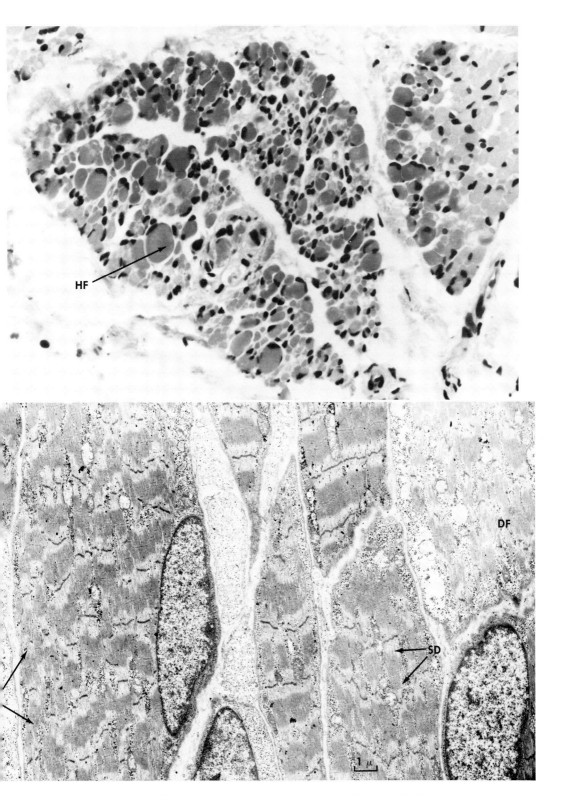

**Fig. 3-8.** Proximal muscle from 3-month-old infant with group 1 Werdnig-Hoffmann disease.
**A,** Cross section demonstrating marked variation of fiber size. There are many rounded, atrophic fibers with a few large hypertrophied fibers *(HF)* and many smaller atrophic fibers (H &
E; ×425.). **B,** Ultrastructural appearance showing small fibers, sarcomere disruption, *SD,*
and degenerating fiber, *DF* (×7,000.). (Courtesy Dr. Stephen A. Smith.) (From Swaiman,
K. F.: Anterior horn cell and cranial motor neuron disease. In Swaiman, K. F., and Wright,
F. S.: The practice of pediatric neurology, St. Louis, 1975, The C. V. Mosby Co., p. 943.)

ELECTRON MICROSCOPIC CHANGES IN NEUROGENIC MUSCULAR ATROPHY. Electron microscopic studies of muscle from patients with progressive infantile spinal muscular atrophy reveal changes similar to those in the adult (Aran-Duchenne) type and in peripheral neuropathy. The outer membranes of the atrophic fibers remain intact and usually retain their normal structural configuration. Although there are fewer mitochondria, they appear to be normal and retain their customary anatomic relationship with one another. Occasionally the mitochondria in atrophic fibers are swollen, the nuclei are irregular in shape, and the outer nuclear membrane is cleaved from the inner nuclear membrane. Single membranes, appearing to be lysosomal in origin, surround collections of granules. Many of the lysosomes are interspersed among the myofibrils, but others are grouped near the nuclei close to the Golgi apparatus. Many thin filaments are usually visible in the subsarcolemmal areas. Free granules, probably ribosomes, occur in association with these filaments.

Many fibers show loss of filaments from their myofibrils, changes typical of denervation atrophy. Other atrophic fibers contain clumps of the thin filaments often seen in young myoblasts. This configuration suggests a process of active regeneration or cessation of maturation (Shafiq, Milhorat, and Gorycki, 1967).

In studying muscle tissue from seven children with spinal muscular atrophy, another investigator noted the presence of three types of muscle cells: normal cells, small cells with a large central nucleus appearing as older myoblasts, and cells resembling myotubules containing a common basement membrane. The last two types were thought to represent an arrest in maturation rather than an atrophic process (Fidziańska, 1974).

**GENETIC FINDINGS.** Sporadic cases of infantile spinal muscular atrophy are frequently seen. The Byers and Banker classification may actually comprise different clinical groups with different genetic patterns, but this possibility has not been substantiated.

In almost all of the large published series, the infantile form of the disease is inherited on an autosomal recessive basis. The clinical characteristics and pattern of progression of the disease usually do not vary among affected family members. When variation does occur, the manifestations do not extend over the large range of clinical possibilities.

Spinal muscular atrophy has been reported in second cousins. It has been proposed that a genetic variant of the disease is present in which an autosomal dominant trait requires an allelomorphic activator gene to become phenotypically apparent (Zellweger, Schneider, and Schuldt, 1969). The hypothesis is that three alleles are present on the locus of the spinal muscular atrophy gene: a, a', and A. Allele a is the normal gene occurring in most individuals. Allele a', called an activator gene, occurs commonly but less often than allele a. The third, allele A, a mutant gene, rarely occurs. Allele A carries spinal muscular atrophy as a dominant trait but requires the presence of the activator gene a' before the disease can be expressed phenotypically.

Electromyographic studies in parents of patients with the disease, primarily in groups 1 and 2, reveal a tendency toward increased amplitude of the action potential in the quadriceps and deltoid muscles (Emery, Anderson, and Noronha, 1973). Larger studies of such parents are needed to assess further these findings, in the hope that the carrier state can be detected.

**TREATMENT.** The most serious orthopedic problem among patients with spinal muscular atrophy is scoliosis. Spinal deformities tend to develop in nonwalkers earlier than in walkers. Most curves are thoracolumbar in location. Surgical correction should be undertaken only after careful consideration (Schwentker and Gibson, 1976). Vigorous preoperative and postoperative physical therapy is necessary to prevent loss of strength or function after spinal fusion.

Many patients benefit from powered chairs, lifts, special mattresses, and accessible environmental controls. Spinal orthoses usually will not prevent or retard scoliosis but may help the patients to sit. Lightweight orthoses for the legs occasionally facilitate walking (Wilkins and Gibson, 1976).

No definitive therapy is available. Supportive care, including pulmonary drainage and antibiotic administration, may be necessary during upper respiratory infections. The patients are usually of normal intelligence, and special provisions for transportation are frequently necessary to assure appropriate educational experience.

### Juvenile proximal hereditary muscular atrophy (Kugelberg-Welander disease, juvenile spinal muscular atrophy)

The initial report of this condition described a dozen patients with a juvenile type of proximal hereditary muscular atrophy

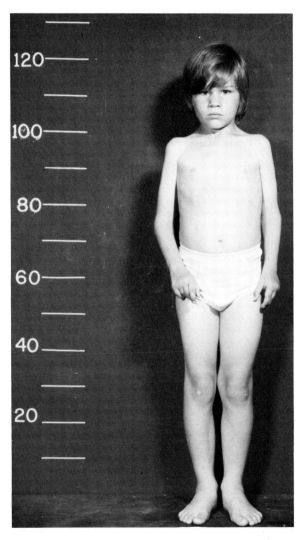

**Fig. 3-9.** Patient with juvenile proximal hereditary muscular atrophy (Kugelberg-Welander disease) manifests mild generalized weakness, but in addition he has marked weakness and atrophy of proximal shoulder girdle.

originally believed to be limb-girdle muscular dystrophy (Kugelberg and Welander, 1956). The condition is now known to be secondary to anterior horn cell involvement and has a pattern of weakness similar to that of infantile spinal muscular atrophy.

CLINICAL FINDINGS. Onset occurs between ages 2 and 17 years with symptoms resembling group 3 infantile spinal muscular atrophy (Amick, Smith, and Johnson, 1966). Patients initially have impaired gait secondary to weakness of the hip and thigh muscles (Fig. 3-9); they can no longer run, jump, or climb stairs normally. Eventually, classic Gowers' sign develops. The legs are usually involved first, the arms much later. Only cranial nerves XI and XII are involved. Fasciculations of the tongue and moderate weakness of the sternocleidomastoid muscles may be apparent. Deep and superficial sensations are normal.

Atrophy begins in the quadriceps muscles and is evident next in the shoulder girdle and upper arms. The forearm muscles atrophy later, with more severe involvement in the flexor muscles than in the extensor muscles. The fingers and hands are not involved. The feet and legs are only slightly affected and rarely undergo severe atrophy, even late in the course of the disease. Because the gastrocnemius muscles are little involved but the quadriceps muscles are severely atrophied, an erroneous diagnosis of pseudohypertrophy of the calf muscles may be made. The deep tendon reflexes at the knee are lost early but those of the ankles persist until later.

Progressive external ophthalmoplegia has been reported in patients with typical proximal hereditary muscle atrophy as well as in a patient with prolonged anterior horn cell disease beginning at birth (Pachter et al., 1976; Aberfeld and Namba, 1969). Cardiac arrhythmias and congestive heart failure have also been reported (Tanaka et al., 1976).

Juvenile spinal muscular atrophy runs a slowly progressive course. Eight to nine years after onset of symptoms, some patients lose the ability to walk, but many can still walk 20 or more years after onset, and one patient could walk 40 years after onset.

LABORATORY FINDINGS. Microscopic study of muscle tissue removed at biopsy reveals the group lesions of anterior horn cell disease. Electromyographic examination shows fibrillation potentials and loss of the normal number of motor-unit potentials in the affected muscles. Giant potentials, larger in amplitude and of longer duration than normal motor-unit potentials, are also present.

The disease often appears to be transmitted as an autosomal recessive trait, but several instances of autosomal dominant transmission have been recorded (Armstrong, Fogelson, and Silberberg, 1966; Tsukagoshi et al., 1966; Cao et al., 1976). X-linked occurrence of proximal spinal atrophy and bulbar muscular atrophy has been reported in adult males (Kennedy, Alter, and Sung, 1968).

The infantile and juvenile forms probably represent different portions of the spectrum of spinal muscular atrophy with onset at birth or years later.

### Other forms of motor neuron-induced muscular atrophy

A condition best termed "facioscapulohumeral neurogenic atrophy" has been reported on several occasions (Fenichel, Emery, and Hunt, 1967; Furukawa and Toyokura, 1976). One parent and children manifested atrophy of the muscles of the shoulders, neck, and face, beginning in the second decade. One child, a girl, had some involvement of the hip girdle. The disorder may be confused readily with facioscapulohumeral dystrophy, but the electromyogram is consistent with anterior horn cell disease.

Spinal muscular atrophy in a scapuloperoneal distribution, called scapuloperoneal atrophy, has been reported (Emery, Fenichel, and Eng, 1968) and occurs in both sporadic and X-linked cases (Mawatari and Katayama, 1973). Difficulties often begin in the first decade, although later onset and slower progression have also been reported (Kaeser, 1965).

Chronic spinal muscular atrophy, often distal in distribution, occurs on a familial basis. The disease process may be inherited as an autosomal dominant trait (Vignaendra and Thiam Ghee, 1976; Nelson and Amick, 1966). The clinical manifestations, including atrophy, may appear at the end of the first or beginning of the second decade.

### Progressive bulbar paralysis of childhood (Fazio-Londe disease)

Decrease in motor cells in cranial nerve nuclei is clearly evident in progressive bulbar paralysis (Gomez, Clermont, and Bernstein, 1962), a condition that may be hereditary (Fazio, 1892; Londe, 1893). Involvement of the anterior horn cells in the cervical and upper thoracic cords accompanies other abnormalities, including loss of neurons in the dentate nucleus. Cranial nerve VII is virtually always affected and the nuclei of cranial nerves III, IV, VI, VII, X, and XII may be involved. Age of onset varies but may be as early as age 3.

Postmortem examination suggests that bulbar paralysis is only part of the spectrum of progressive lower motor neuron disease. Major degenerative changes were found in the brain stem, and histologic evidence of anterior horn cell disease was present, although clinical signs were not evident (Alexander, Emery, and Koerner, 1976).

### Möbius' syndrome

Möbius' syndrome is a nonprogressive condition that consists of facial palsy, usually bilateral, and bilateral involvement of cranial nerve VI. The upper face is usually involved more than the lower face. Partial external ophthalmoplegia is common; usually medial rectus action with resultant convergence is noted (Fig. 3-10).

Patients usually have conjugate eye movements in the vertical plane and occasionally ptosis. Besides dysfunction of cranial nerves

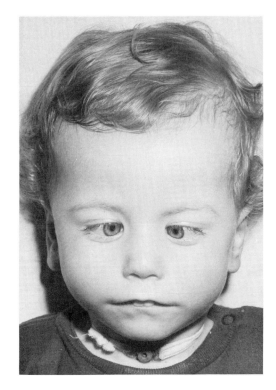

**Fig. 3-10.** Patient with Möbius' syndrome. He has bilateral cranial nerve VI as well as bilateral cranial nerve VII paresis. He also has associated swallowing difficulties and recurrent pneumonitis, which prompted insertion of tracheostomy tube 2 months before this photograph was taken.

VI and VII, abnormalities of cranial nerves V, X, XI, and XII are common. The pectoral muscles may be absent. The condition has been reported in twins.

Symptoms usually result from lack of development or deterioration of the motor cells of the involved cranial nerves. However, the process may not always be nuclear in origin but may be supranuclear or the result of myopathic abnormalities (Pitner, Edwards, and McCormick, 1965; Van Allen and Blodi, 1960). Many of the reported cases probably represent myotonic dystrophy and congenital nonprogressive myopathies. A number of investigators have noted a parallel with the diverse anatomic classifications appropriate for arthrogryposis.

### Amyotrophic lateral sclerosis

Amytrophic lateral sclerosis is a progressive degenerative disease that affects the corticospinal tracts, the motor nuclei of the lower medulla, and the anterior horn cells of the spinal cord. It may begin in the first 2 decades of life and progress slowly thereafter (Markand and Daly, 1971; Nelson and Prensky, 1972). The juvenile form may represent a point on the continuum of anterior horn cell disease between progressive bulbar paralysis of childhood and adult amyotrophic lateral sclerosis.

Atrophy and fasciculations of the tongue and distal muscles of the hands are usually present, and spasticity of the legs is common. Progression of the bulbar symptoms causes death, usually within a few years after their onset. Both sporadic and hereditary cases have been described in children. Many of the cases seen in the first decade have the same course as group 3 infantile spinal muscular atrophy (De Barsy and Mouchette, 1967; Gamstorp, 1967).

Inclusion cells that appear to be derived from Nissl substance have been noted in sporadic juvenile cases (Nelson and Prensky, 1972). A hereditary form has been reported, with onset usually in adulthood (Thomson and Alvarez, 1969). Studies of a Japanese family with this form revealed many hyaline inclusion bodies in the cytoplasm of the remaining motor nerve cells. These bodies consisted of a halo and a core composed of protein and lipids. Electron microscopic studies reveal that the halos are composed of radial filaments and the cores of filaments and granular bodies, similar to Lewy bodies. In this family the hereditary pattern was autosomal dominant (Takahashi, Nakamura, and Okada, 1972).

### Benign congenital hypotonia

Infants with the conditions subsumed under the title benign congenital hypotonia are weak and hypotonic in the neonatal period but improve as they mature (Gordon, 1966; Greenfield, Cornman, and Shy, 1958; Wal-

ton, 1957). The symptomatology and etiology vary.

The initial report described 17 children with hypotonia at birth or shortly thereafter. By age 10, eight had recovered completely and nine had improved markedly (Walton, 1957). No evidence of progressive muscular dystrophy, progressive spinal muscular atrophy, mental retardation, or upper motor unit disease was present.

Of the eight who recovered, all had deep tendon reflexes when initially examined, although the reflexes were difficult to elicit in three. Only two of these children had electromyographic examination. In both cases, excess polyphasic potentials were present. Muscle tissue from biopsies in two members of this group was normal on microscopic examination.

Of the nine children who recovered incompletely, three had no deep tendon reflexes, and electromyographic examination showed excess short-duration potentials. Four of the nine underwent muscle biopsy.

The electromyographic findings in benign congenital hypotonia suggest myopathic disease, and at least some of these children may have nonprogressive congenital myopathies. Nerve conduction studies provide more precise diagnosis. At biopsy, muscle tissue does not show any morphologic alteration, but recent histochemical studies have shown prominent grouping of type I fibers in some cases.

A diagnosis of benign congenital hypotonia should be withheld until clinical and laboratory observations have excluded specific neuromuscular entities or central nervous system involvement, including intellectual retardation (Dubowitz, 1968).

The term "universal hypoplasia of muscle" has been used to describe infants who are weak and hypotonic at birth and improve slightly over the years. Deep tendon reflexes are usually present. Although muscle mass is thought to be decreased, little objective documentation exists (Ford, 1966; Rabe, 1964). No abnormalities on laboratory examination have been reported. Occasional family incidence is apparently the only difference between this group of patients and the incompletely recovered group described as having benign congenital hypotonia by Walton.

### Arthrogryposis multiplex congenita

Arthrogryposis multiplex congenita is a syndrome, present at birth, that comprises multiple contractures of the joints of the arms and legs. Four general pathologic types have been delineated: (1) anterior horn cell arthrogryposis, (2) peripheral neurogenic arthrogryposis, (3) myopathic arthrogryposis, and (4) arthrogryposis of the intrinsic joints and capsules. In a large series of cases, studies utilizing serum enzyme activity, electromyography, determination of nerve conduction velocity, and muscle biopsy show the anterior horn cell type to be the most common. The other three types are discussed here as a matter of convenience.

ANTERIOR HORN CELL ARTHROGRYPOSIS. Anterior horn cell arthrogryposis results from profound decrease in the number of anterior horn cells in the cervical and lumbar enlargements. Usually the infant's arms rotate inward and extend at the elbows. The forearms are often pronated, with ulnar deviation at the wrists. The hands and fingers are flexed, the latter tightly. The thighs are usually flexed at the hips and externally rotated. The knees may be flexed or extended, but the feet almost always have an equinovarus deformity. The limbs appear thin and the joints enlarged by comparison (Fig. 3-11). The patella may be unusually small or absent. Heart malformations, inguinal hernias, cleft palate, scoliosis, and rigidity of the temporomandibular joint may also be present (Adams, Denny-Brown, and Pearson, 1962). Examination of the joints shows a small degree of passive movement and occasionally some active movement. The patients are profoundly weak and are hypotonic within a decreased range of motion. Deep tendon reflexes are absent, and electromyographic studies reveal the abnormalities of anterior horn cell impairment.

The few pathologic studies of the involved muscles show them to be decreased in size (Drachman and Banker, 1961) or absent (Adams, Denny-Brown, and Pearson, 1962). Some hip contractures appear to result from unopposed contraction of the iliopsoas muscles. Although there are few changes in endomysial connective tissue, perimysial connective tissue may be greatly increased. The muscle spindles are normal.

One case has been reported with total involvement of the limbs and absence of the anterior horn cells in the lumbosacral enlargement. A few anterior roots were seen in the lumbosacral area. The number of anterior horn cells was greatly decreased in the thoracolumbar and cervical areas. The remainder of the cord was normal.

Arthrogryposis has been found in more than one generation in a family. It has been reported in one member in each of two sets of identical twins (Drachman and Banker, 1961).

Treatment of patients with arthrogryposis, most of whom appear to have had the neurogenic variety, frequently produces sufficient alignment and stability of the lower extremities through surgical procedures so that independent ambulation is possible (Fisher et al., 1970). Some improvement of upper extremity function is generally possible by the employment of nonoperative methods.

NEUROGENIC ARTHROGRYPOSIS. Neurogenic arthrogryposis is ordinarily considered to be secondary to anterior horn cell disease, but on rare occasion the anterior spinal roots are the site of the primary lesion. Two infants have been described with multiple articular rigidity consistent with arthrogryposis multiplex congenita: flexed elbows, extended wrists, acute flexion of the knee and hip joints, and bilateral pes equinovarus. Both had siblings with similar contractures, establishing a familial pattern.

Subsequent studies revealed nodular fibrosis of the anterior spinal roots of the en-

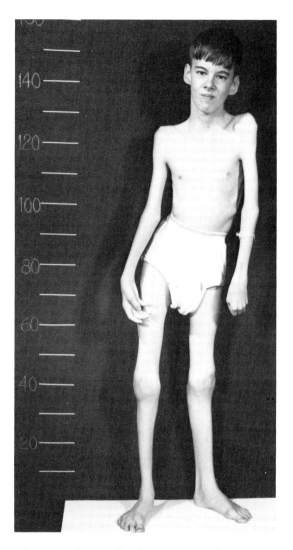

**Fig. 3-11.** Patient with anterior horn cell arthrogryposis with accompanying muscle wasting, which is particularly prominent in distal arms and legs. He has undergone a number of orthopedic procedures.

tire spinal cord and absence of myelin and axis cylinders. A few anterior horn cells showed central chromatolysis, thought to be secondary to the anterior root lesions. The pattern in skeletal muscle was that of neurogenic muscular atrophy. Most muscles of the extremities were replaced extensively by fat, and at times it was difficult to identify muscle tissue as such (Bargeton et al., 1961; Pena et al., 1968). A few neurons in the anterior horn cell region showed dark staining of the nucleus and cytoplasm and mild shrinkage,

but these findings were thought to be of little pathologic importance.

MYOPATHIC ARTHROGRYPOSIS. Myopathic arthrogryposis is often associated with hypotonia and with absent or barely detectable deep tendon reflexes (Banker, Victor, and Adams, 1957). Contractures similar to those of the neurogenic form are present. Differentiation from the neurogenic form is often possible on the basis of flexion rather than extension of the elbow and knee joints.

It is likely that many neonates with myopathic arthrogryposis have myotonic dystrophy (Sarnat, O'Connor, and Byrne, 1976). The legs are predominantly affected in these patients. Often these patients have loose, wrinkled skin and lack subcutaneous tissue. Weakness of the neck muscles may affect the ability to flex the head. Children with the myopathic form of arthrogryposis may have increased serum CPK activity, and electromyographic findings are consistent with myopathic involvement.

Few studies of muscle tissue have been reported in this form of arthrogryposis. Muscle fibers may vary greatly in size and the endomysial connective tissue may be increased.

Myopathic arthrogryposis also occurs in lambs, who have blindness and varying degrees of agenesis of the cerebral hemispheres (Whittem, 1957).

ARTHROGRYPOSIS OF THE INTRINSIC JOINTS AND CAPSULES. Little has been written about arthrogryposis of the intrinsic joints and capsules. After careful evaluation, most of these cases probably fall into the neurogenic and myopathic categories.

Experimental procedures using intravenous injection of Coxsackievirus A-2 into chick embryos result in viral infection of the muscle cells and subsequent disappearance of muscle tissue. Sequelae include ankylosis of joints; this finding suggests that arthrogryposis can result from a primary myopathy with paralysis (Drachman et al., 1976).

A syndrome of arthrogryposis known as Kuskokwim disease has been reported in the Alaskan Eskimo and is named for the river delta where the original cases were found (Petajan et al., 1969). The patients have multiple contractures of the joints, most often affecting the knees and ankles. The primary difficulty appears to be in the connective tissue. Evidence of myopathy, neuropathy, or motor cell disease is not present. The disease is manifested in the first decade of life and appears to be transmitted as an autosomal recessive trait.

Contractures at the elbows and knees may be present in the first few months of life. Internal tibial torsion and severe planovalgus

are common. The deep tendon reflexes are present in the biceps muscles and ankles but may be absent in the triceps muscles and knees. Flexion hip contractures are also present. At least one patient had a small cataract at age 3; cataracts are rare in adults.

X-ray studies have shown cysts in the proximal long bones of several patients. Several, too, have had pigmented nevi and decreased corneal reflexes, but the association of these findings with arthrogryposis remains to be firmly established. Arthrogryposis may be associated with webbed-neck, Klippel-Feil deformity and anomalies of the genitourinary system (Beckerman and Buchino, 1978).

### Infantile neuroaxonal dystrophy

Infantile neuroaxonal dystrophy, first described by Seitelberger (1952), is a degenerative disease of childhood with onset in late infancy (Huttenlocher and Gilles, 1967). The child usually develops normally during the first year. Thereafter there is onset of slowly progressive weakness, muscle atrophy, and hypotonia. There are also signs and symptoms of corticospinal tract involvement, urinary retention, and visual and sensory defects, including nystagmus, optic atrophy, and blindness. Seizures occasionally occur. The disease is inherited as an autosomal recessive trait and a familial pattern is often noted (Duncan et al., 1970)

The course of the disease is protracted over a period of years. Contractures of arms and legs and progressive bulbar difficulties are common. Most children die before age 12. Rare juvenile cases occur (Vuia, 1976).

The electroencephalogram shows diffuse, fast background activity with superimposed multifocal spikes and wave complexes without a characteristic pattern. No abnormalities of the spinal fluid or serum electrolytes have been reported. Electromyographic study reveals evidence of anterior horn cell disease. The abnormalities noted in the peripheral nerves consist of occasional globular, ovoid, or fusiform swelling along the course of the axons, which usually increase to more than twice their normal diameter. These structures are amorphous, opaque, refractile, darkly eosinophilic, and often fragmented.

Electron microscopic studies reveal asymmetric destruction of the myelin sheath, regional separation of the remaining laminae, and existence of dystrophic axons and motor end-plates, including axonal spheroids. Such spheroids have also been described in Hallervorden-Spatz syndrome, mucoviscidosis, congenital biliary atresia, presenile dementia (Alzheimer's disease), congenital ataxia in lambs, avitaminosis E, and intoxications (Martin and Martin, 1972).

One report of electron microscopic studies suggests that the spheroids are formed by a unique mechanism involving accumulation of a macromolecular substance that is synthesized in the neuron and transported to the nerve endings. At first the substance appears amorphous, then aggregates into characteristic angulated membranous profiles. The investigators have suggested that these findings indicate a derangement of the pathway of synthesis or packaging of neurotransmitters or their receptors (Mei Liu, Larson, and Mizuno, 1974).

Pathologic studies reveal eosinophilic spheroids in the central and autonomic nervous systems (Berard-Badier et al., 1974) and iron-containing pigment in the basal ganglia. There is also cerebellar degeneration with associated neuronal, myelin, and glial changes (Haberland, Brunngraber, and Witting, 1972).

Biochemical studies show abnormalities in the white matter, primarily marked reduction in cerebrosides. Analysis of the gray matter reveals normal ganglioside composition but reduction in the glycoprotein-carbohydrate content and glycosaminoglycan level (Haberland, Brunngraber, and Witting, 1972).

### Cerebellothalamospinal degeneration

A 23-month-old child who died with signs of hyperreflexia and spasticity has been described. His sister died of a similar disorder. Postmortem examination revealed chromato-lytic changes of the anterior horn cells and brain stem nuclei, as well as changes of the cells of the thalamus and cerebellum (Norman and Kay, 1965).

## INFECTIOUS DISEASES
### Poliomyelitis

Poliomyelitis is a viral disease that has its greatest clinical effect on the central nervous system. Nonparalytic poliomyelitis is the most common form and to a large degree is clinically indistinguishable from other meningoencephalitides.

CLINICAL FEATURES.   Poliomyelitis is caused by three immunologically different types of virus that do not produce cross-immunity; infection with a specific type results in permanent immunity to that type. Immunization with killed virus and attenuated live-virus vaccines has effectively ended the large-scale epidemics of the disease that formerly occurred in the summer and early fall. The nonepidemic form most commonly affects children, while the epidemic form more often involves an older population.

The viruses are transmitted from human to human, primarily by secretions of the upper respiratory tract and by fecal contamination. Infection with Coxsackieviruses has resulted in clinical manifestations similar to those of paralytic poliomyelitis (Grist, 1962; Jarcho, Fred, and Castle, 1963).

Malaise, usually accompanied by muscular pains or stiffness, heralds the onset. Headaches are often noted, and symptoms of upper respiratory infection are very common in children. As the disease progresses, the patient may have some degree of nuchal rigidity and low-grade fever. Muscular tightness then becomes evident, predominantly in the hamstring, thigh, and neck. Boys are more often involved than girls.

Poliomyelitis, characterized by a triad of fever, nuchal rigidity, and spasm of the back muscles, may occur in infants less than 1 year old (Abramson and Greenburg, 1955). Under 1 year of age, spinal involvement is more common than bulbar involvement. Bulbar symptoms are more common in boys than in girls.

The course of the disease may be slowly progressive or fulminating, but the more rapid the progression, the more severe the eventual involvement. The anterior horn cells are the prime target of the virus and motor weakness is usually present. The weakness is usually asymmetric and scattered. After age 1 year the incidence of quadriplegia and trunk muscle weakness is higher.

Life is seriously threatened when bulbar involvement results in embarrassment of the respiratory, autonomic, and circulatory centers of the brain stem and in profound weakness of the muscles of respiration and swallowing. Fulminating bulbar poliomyelitis with rapid involvement of the cardiorespiratory centers of the brain stem has a poor prognosis (Auld, Kevy, and Eley, 1960; Baker, Matzke, and Brown, 1950).

Poliomyelitis has occurred in utero on several occasions and may lead to death in the neonatal period (Pugh and Dudgeon, 1954).

Of the patients reported in one series, about one-fourth had nonparalytic poliomyelitis, one-half had spinal poliomyelitis, one-eighth had bulbar poliomyelitis, and one-tenth had bulbospinal involvement (Auld, Kevy, and Eley, 1960; Lepow and Spence, 1965).

### LABORATORY FINDINGS

SPINAL FLUID. Spinal fluid examination usually shows pleocytosis with mononuclear cells and normal or slightly elevated protein concentration. Very early in the disease, polymorphonuclear cells may be prevalent. The spinal fluid glucose content is usually normal.

THERAPY. In the presence of bulbar symptoms, mechanical support of respiration and drug support of circulation may be necessary. Early use of tracheostomy is often essential. Marked flaccidity and weakness of the muscles may be replaced by tightness and spasm. Application of passive stretch exercises and heat, together with education of the patient

in using the affected muscles, is very important and may be necessary for months and even years.

### Transverse myelitis associated with viral conditions

Although the signs and symptoms of these conditions are caused by different microorganisms, the clinical picture is similar and allows for a combined general discussion.

The site of involvement is usually the thoracic cord. The illness begins abruptly and progresses rapidly over 24 to 48 hours. Malaise, lethargy, fever, and myalgia may immediately precede or accompany the early symptoms of cord involvement. Back pain at the level of the involved thoracic segments and paresthesias of the legs and trunk are often present. Disruption of the anterior horn cells in the cervical or lumbar enlargements leads to lower motor neuron involvement of the arms or legs (Fig. 3-12). The gross weakness may be temporary or permanent. The most common sequence of symptoms is flaccidity of the legs followed by loss of control in the rectal and bladder sphincters. Sensory loss extending to the level of cord impairment is detectable. There may be hyperalgesia in the transitional zone between involved and uninvolved areas. Interruption of the autonomic pathway results in loss of sweating below the spinal segment of disruption.

Although the symptoms may recede as early as the first week after their onset, usually they persist for several weeks or even months. The flaccidity in the areas below the spinal segment involvement may gradually change to spasticity after several weeks, and the areflexia may be replaced by hyperreflexia accompanied by demonstrable ankle clonus and the presence of Babinski's sign.

Spinal fluid protein concentration may be normal, or if the rootlets or peripheral nerves are involved, slightly elevated. Pleocytosis dominated by lymphocytes is common. The spinal fluid glucose concentration is usually unchanged. Electromyographic findings suggestive of anterior horn cell disease may be present.

A number of viral diseases and infections have been incriminated in transverse myelitis with anterior horn cell involvement. They include rubeola, mumps, varicella, rubella, smallpox, infectious mononucleosis, rabies vaccination, and smallpox vaccination (Blatt and Lepper, 1953; Miller, Stanton, and Gibbons, 1956; Mukherjee, 1965; Paine and Byers, 1953; Silverman, 1949; Tyler, 1957; McCarthy and Amer, 1978).

Neuromyelitis optica (Devic's disease) is a condition characterized by symptoms of myelitis and blindness. Demyelination of the optic nerves results in visual impairment secondary to retrobulbar optic neuritis or optic neuritis. The optic chiasm is usually the area involved (Markham and Otenasek, 1954).

The relationship between viral and other infections and transverse myelitis is not un-derstood. Several lines of evidence suggest that a hyperimmune mechanism may be involved. Other hypotheses have been propounded to explain the presence of postexanthematous and postimmunization encephalitis. Direct viral infection with late onset of cord disruption is the probable underlying mechanism. In rubeola encephalitis, inclusion bodies have been found in central nervous system tissue (Adams, Baird, and Filloy, 1966).

The prognosis for recovery in transverse myelitis is relatively poor. Most patients have significant neurologic residua.

Pathologic studies at autopsy in patients who died early in the course of the illness have revealed perivascular cuffing by lymphocytes around the small veins. Perivenous demyelination, myelomalacia, and cyst formation are present (Greenfield and Norman, 1963; Miller, Stanton, and Gibbons, 1956). Neuromyelitis optica results in severe

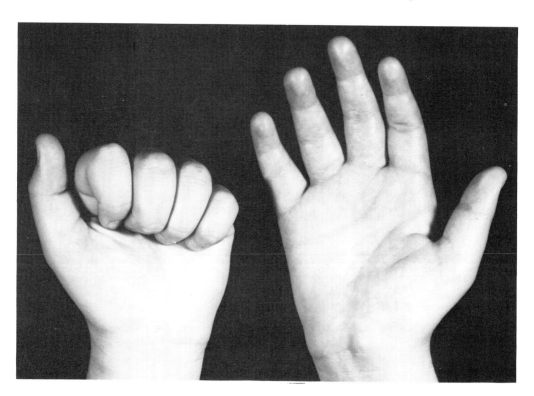

**Fig. 3-12.** Hands of child who had suffered from viral encephalomyelitis. There are atrophy of hypothenar muscles and atrophic changes of skin of fingers.

myelomalacia that follows infarction of the cord.

Transient anterior horn cell dysfunction secondary to phenytoin administration has been reported (Direkze and Fernando, 1977) and may be confused with anterior horn cell disease induced by infection.

## Traumatic causes of anterior horn cell dysfunction

### Spinal cord injury and anterior horn cell impairment

Birth injuries, falls, car accidents, or blows to the spine may cause partial or complete transection of the spinal cord. Various pat-

terns of neurologic deficit ensue. Accompanying fractures or dislocations of the vertebrae are common. The clinical picture is dominated by the effects of interruption of the corticospinal tract, posterior column, and lateral spinothalamic tract. Manifestations include paresis of the limbs, depending on the level of injury, and loss of deep and superficial sensations below the level of injury. Bladder function is almost always compromised.

When the spinal cord is injured in the cervical or lumbosacral enlargements, findings characteristic of anterior horn cell disruption occur in the arms or legs. Trauma is not

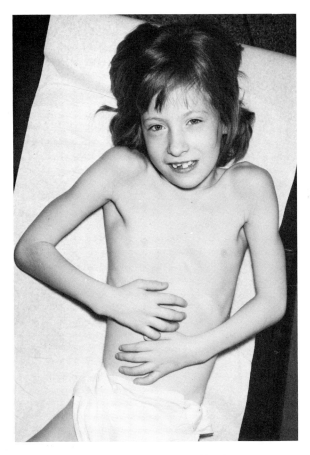

**Fig. 3-13.** Cervical cord trauma was incurred at time of birth. Fingers were often held in uncommon postures resulting from pattern of disruption of anterior horn population of cervical cord. Distal phalanx of right little finger was amputated during infancy because of severe self-mutilation, which was facilitated by sensory deficit. Unopposed action of diaphragm results in pectus excavatum deformity.

likely to cause isolated anterior cell injury unless the anterior spinal artery is the only structure involved.

Trauma associated with difficult delivery, especially breech presentation, usually occurs in the middle and lower cervical segments of the cord (Abroms et al., 1973). Rarely is there radiologic evidence of fracture or dislocation of the spine. These infants are flaccid immediately after birth, but spasticity of the legs may develop later. The patterns of residual motor strength in the arms vary. The injury may be mistaken for bilateral Erb's palsy, but the involvement of the small muscles of the hands and paresis of the legs should suggest the diagnosis of injury to the spinal cord rather than the brachial plexus (Fig. 3-13).

Diaphragmatic respiration unopposed by thoracic muscle results in pectus excavatum. The abdominal muscles are often weak and the abdomen protrudes. Urinary retention and subsequent infection present additional hazards. Horner's syndrome is often present. Impairment or absence of sweating below the levels innervated by the upper thoracic nerves may cause poor control of temperature and lead to hyperthermia, which is troublesome and at times dangerous. Air-conditioning may be mandatory for these infants in the summer.

The relatively high risk of middle or lower cervical cord injuries in breech presentation with persistent hyperextension of the head has been well documented in a review of the literature (Abroms et al., 1973). Of 88 cases reviewed, 21% involved complete transection of the cervical cord. None of the infants delivered by cesarean section sustained spinal cord injury.

No specific treatment is available. Physical and occupational therapy may be of value.

### Metabolic conditions

In Tay-Sachs disease, the anterior horn cells are involved by the storage of ganglioside $GM_2$, and their impairment often leads to hypotonia and weakness. The disease picture is dominated by myoclonic seizures and blindness associated with a cherry red spot in the macula (Swaiman, 1975).

Beta-hydroxyisovaleric aciduria and beta-methylcrotonylglycinuria have been found in the urine of patients with a clinical condition reminiscent of spinal muscular atrophy. Hyperglycinemia was associated with pathologic findings in the anterior horn cells and pyramidal tract in the first decade and perhaps as early as the first 2 years of life. The patients appeared to have a defect in glycine-serine interconversion (Bank and Morrow, 1972).

### Vascular conditions
#### Anterior spinal artery occlusion

The anterior spinal artery arises from the junction of the vertebral arteries and transverses the anterior median sulcus the full length of the spinal cord. Radicular arteries are divided into anterior and posterior radicular arteries. The anterior spinal artery receives blood from the anterior radicular arteries that enter with the nerve roots between the third cervical and third lumbar segments (Fig. 3-14). The anterior spinal artery in turn is further divided into many sulcal branches that pierce the central gray matter, supply the anterior horn cells, and then divide into numerous small penetrating vessels that supply the white matter of the lateral and anterior columns. The penetrating branches of the anterior spinal artery are end arteries; if they are compromised, the anterior half of the spinal cord becomes ischemic or infarcted.

The two posterior spinal arteries have a different anatomic relationship and provide more extensive collateral circulation; therefore compromise of the posterior spinal arteries does not usually cause severe clinical impairment.

The manifestations of occlusion of anterior spinal artery blood flow have been described (Steegman, 1952). Compromise of the anterior spinal artery is most common in arteriosclerotic vascular disease in adults, but cer-

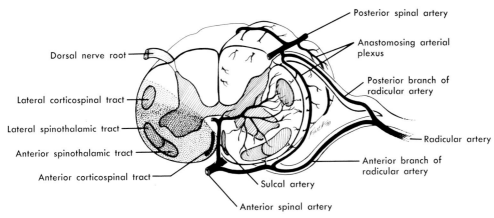

**Fig. 3-14.** Anterior spinal artery supplies most of anterior portions of spinal cord as well as most of lateral column area of cord (stippled area). Anterior horn cells and lateral spinothalamic tracts are heavily dependent on anterior spinal artery blood supply.

tain conditions in childhood lead to this involvement. Trauma and sometimes infectious conditions often cause anterior spinal artery insufficiency in children (Goebel and Muller, 1977). Embolism and thrombosis from cardiac disease and hypercoagulable states are other etiologic factors (Oller-Navarro, Rivera-Reyes, and Rodriguez-Rivera, 1979).

In studies in rhesus monkeys, obstruction of the blood flow below the first lumbar vertebra results in a lesion that evolves from the central gray matter outward. The infarcts are most severe in the third and sixth lumbar segments. The area above the ligation is relatively uninvolved. The central gray matter is uniformly infarcted. The lesions vary in severity. In the more extensive lesions, the adjacent circumferential white matter is involved; in the most extensive lesions, only a thin rim of the peripheral white matter is preserved. This preservation of the peripheral white matter and sometimes the lateral edge of the anterior horn may be related to the perfusion by pial plexus vessels and vasa corona, both fed by the posterior spinal arteries. This circulation can supply up to half of the outer rim of white matter (Fried and Aparicio, 1973).

The clinical manifestations resulting from anterior spinal artery compromise are related to the level at which the artery is occluded (Steegman, 1952). Occlusion of the anterior spinal artery near its formation from the two vertebral arteries results in brain stem involvement. These findings may be unilateral but are usually bilateral. Often spastic quadriplegia and loss of pain and temperature sensations occur, along with some loss of light touch sensation below the affected level. Involvement of the cervical spinal cord results in flaccid paralysis of the arms because of the disruption of the anterior horn cells in the cervical enlargement. Occlusion of the anterior spinal artery in the area of the lumbar enlargement leads to weakness, atrophy, and loss of deep tendon reflexes in the legs. Loss of pain and temperature sensations is common in the legs.

In certain lesions below the medulla, pain and temperature sensations can be dissociated from light touch sensation. Because the tracts subserving pain and temperature sensations cross in the anterior white commissure of the spinal cord, they are compromised by anterior spinal artery occlusion, whereas the tracts primarily subserving light touch sensation ascend in the cord without crossing and are preserved.

Bladder dysfunction is a frequent occurrence in obstruction of the anterior spinal artery and may prove to be one of the most difficult problems in patient care. Occasionally automatic and sometimes voluntary bladder function returns after a number of weeks.

Differential diagnosis of anterior spinal artery obstruction in children includes consideration of tumors and congenital vascular malformations and anomalies. Vascular syndromes of the spinal cord are sometimes seen in children in association with coarctation of the aorta (Owens and Swan, 1963; Darwish, Archer, and Modin, 1979). During operation, normal blood flow must be established from the proximal to the distal portions of the aorta. To facilitate this correction, a narrowed section of the aorta must be removed and an adequate anastomosis developed. In the thoracic area, one and sometimes two radicular arteries arise from the aorta; these support blood flow of the anterior spinal artery through radicular branches. If, during operation, the radicular artery is permanently severed or clamped for a prolonged period, the clinical picture of anterior spinal artery occlusion may occur (Weenink and Smilde, 1964).

Although sensory deficits may initially be severe after ischemia induced in this manner, they tend to recede in the first weeks after operation, but the motor deficits remain. The deficits appear to result primarily from anterior horn cell impairment, and this phenomenon has been regarded as demonstrating the principle that the anterior horn cells are in the region of highest oxidative metabolic dependency in the spinal cord (Dodson and Landau, 1973).

At times the anterior spinal artery syndrome occurs in patients with coarctation of the aorta who have not had surgery (Weenick and Smilde, 1964).

### Spinal cord vascular anomalies

Arteriovenous malformations of the spinal cord are relatively infrequent in the first 2 decades of life (Tobin and Layton, 1976); therefore infarction as a result of thrombosis and hemorrhage associated with vascular anomalies of the spinal cord are relatively

rare. When infarction occurs, pain is present in the back or abdomen with gradual or sudden loss of all sensation and strength in the legs. After 12 to 24 hours, the legs become flaccid and control of the urinary bladder is lost (Buchanan and Walker, 1941). Several weeks later, the flaccidity of the limbs changes to spasticity. Priapism has sometimes been reported. Often at operation, a large mass of pulsating vessels is present in the spinal canal.

The anterior horn cells are involved, but involvement of the corticospinal and spinothalamic tracts makes the clinical picture predominantly one of pain and temperature sensation loss and upper motor neuron impairment, with acute flaccidity frequently changing to spasticity after several weeks.

Lumbar puncture shows the cerebrospinal fluid pressure to be normal, and the fluid is xanthochromic or normal in color. Spinal fluid flow is often blocked. If an obstruction is present, the protein concentration is often grossly increased.

Myelography is not consistently reliable enough to predict the extent of the lesion or the degree of anterior or intramedullary component. Therefore angiography should be performed in every patient with an arteriovenous malformation (Tobin and Layton, 1976). On the basis of angiographic pattern, three types of lesions have been described: single coiled vessel, glomus, and juvenile.

Success of surgical procedures is dependent on residual damage, number of feeding vessels, and extent and pattern of the vascular mass.

### REFERENCES

Aberfeld, D. C., and Namba, T.: Progressive ophthalmoplegia in Kugelberg-Welander disease, Arch. Neurol. **20:**253, 1969.

Abramson, H., and Greenburg, M.: Acute poliomyelitis in infants under one year of age: epidemiological and clinical features, Pediatrics **16:**478, 1955.

Abroms, I., et al.: Cervical cord injury secondary to hyperextension of the head in breech presentations, Obstet. Gynecol. **41:**369, 1973.

Adams, J. M., Baird, C., and Filloy, L.: Inclusion bodies in measles encephalitis, J.A.M.A. **195:**290, 1966.

Adams, R. D., Denny-Brown, D., and Pearson, C. M.:

Disease of muscle, ed. 2, New York, 1962, Paul B. Hoeber, Inc., p. 310.

Alexander, M. P., Emery, E. S., III, and Koerner, F. C.: Progressive bulbar paresis in childhood, Arch. Neurol. **33**:66, 1976.

Alpers, B., and Comroe, B.: Syringomyelia with choked disk, J. Nerv. Ment. Dis. **73**:577, 1931.

Amick, L. D., Smith, H. L., and Johnson, W. W.: An unusual spectrum of progressive spinal muscular atrophy, Acta Neurol. Scand. **42**:275, 1966.

Armstrong, R. M., Fogelson, M. H., and Silberberg, D. H.: Familial proximal spinal muscular atrophy, Arch. Neurol. **14**:208, 1966.

Auld, P. A., Kevy, S. V., and Eley, R. C.: Poliomyelitis in children, N. Engl. J. Med. **263**:1093, 1960.

Baker, A. B., Matzke, H. A., and Brown, J. R.: Poliomyelitis. III. Bulbar poliomyelitis: study of medullary function, Arch. Neurol. Psychiatry **63**:257, 1950.

Bank, W. J., and Morrow, G., III: A familial spinal cord disorder with hyperglycinemia, Arch. Neurol. **27**:136, 1972.

Banker, B. Q., Victor, M., and Adams, R. D.: Arthrogryposis multiplex due to congenital muscular dystrophy, Brain **80**:319, 1957.

Bargeton, E., et al.: Etude anatomique d'un cas d'arthrogrypose multiple congénitale et familiale, Rev. Neurol. **104**:479, 1961.

Beckerman, R. C., and Buchino, J. J.: Arthrogryposis multiplex congenita as part of an inherited symptom complex—2 case reports and a review of literature, Pediatrics **61**:417, 1978.

Benady, S. G.: Spinal muscular atrophy in childhood: review of 50 cases, Dev. Med. Child Neurol. **20**:746, 1978.

Berard-Badier, M., et al.: Infantile neuroaxonal dystrophy or Seitelberger's disease: IV. Autonomic nervous system involvement: electron microscopic study in two siblings, Acta Neuropathol. **28**:261, 1974.

Berke, J. P., and Magee, K. R.: Craniofacial dysostosis with syringomyelia and associated anomalies, Arch. Neurol. **33**:63, 1976.

Bertrand, G.: Dynamic factors in the evolution of syringomyelia and syringobulbia. In Proceedings of the Congress of Neurological Surgeons, Baltimore, 1973, The Williams & Wilkins Co., p. 322.

Blatt, N. H., and Lepper, M. H.: Reactions following antirabies prophylaxis: report on sixteen patients, Am. J. Dis. Child. **86**:395, 1953.

Buchanan, D. N., and Walker, A. E.: Vascular anomalies of the spinal cord in children, Am. J. Dis. Child. **61**:928, 1941.

Buchthal, F., and Olsen, P. Z.: Electromyography and muscle biopsy in infantile spinal muscular atrophy, Brain **93**:15, 1970.

Byers, R. K., and Banker, B. Q.: Infantile muscular atrophy, Arch. Neurol. **5**:140, 1961.

Cao, A., et al.: A family of juvenile proximal spinal muscular atrophy with dominant inheritance, J. Med. Genet. **13**:131, 1976.

Carpenter, S., et al.: Pathologic involvement of sensory neurons in Werdnig-Hoffmann disease, Neurology **25**:364, 1975.

Chou, S. M., and Fakadej, A. V.: Ultrastructure of chromatolytic motoneurons in a case of Werdnig-Hoffman disease, Neurology **20**:381, 1970.

Cowie, T. N.: Diastematomyelia with vertebral column defects, observations on its radiological diagnosis. Br. J. Radiol. **24**:156, 1951.

Darwish, H., Archer, C., and Modin, J.: The anterior spinal artery collateral in coarctation of the aorta. A clinical angiographic correlation, Arch. Neurol. **36**: 240, 1979.

De Barsy, A. M., and Mouchette, S.: Sur la sclerose laterale amyotrophique infantile sporadique, Encephale **61**:45, 1967.

Di Chiro, G., et al.: Computerized axial tomography in syringomyelia, N. Engl. J. Med. **292**:13, 1975.

Direkze, M., and Fernando, P. S. L.: Transient anterior horn cell dysfunction in diphenylhydantoin therapy, Eur. Neurol. **15**:131, 1977.

Dodson, W., and Landau, W.: Motor neuron loss due to aortic clamping in repair of coarctation, Neurology **23**:539, 1973.

Drachman, D. B., and Banker, B. Q.: Arthrogryposis multiplex congenita, Arch. Neurol. **5**:77, 1961.

Drachman, D. B., et al.: Experimental arthrogyrposis caused by viral myopathy, Arch. Neurol. **33**:362, 1976.

Dubowitz, V.: The floppy infant. A practical approach to classification. Dev. Med. Child. Neurol. **10**:706, 1968.

Duncan, C., et al.: Peripheral nerve biopsy as an aid to diagnosis in infantile neuroaxonal dystrophy, Neurology **20**:1024, 1970.

Emery, A., Anderson, A., and Noronha, M.: Electromyographic studies in parents with children with spinal muscular atrophy, J. Med. Genet. **10**:8, 1973.

Emery, E. S., Fenichel, G. M., and Eng, G.: A spinal muscular atrophy with scapuloperoneal distribution, Arch. Neurol. **18**:129, 1968.

Fazio, M.: Ereditarietá della paralisi bulbare progressiva, Riforma Med. **8**:327, 1892.

Fenichel, G. M., Emery, E. S., and Hunt, P.: Neurogenic atrophy simulating facioscapulohumeral dystrophy, Arch. Neurol. **17**:257, 1967.

Fidziánska, A.: Ultrastructural changes in muscle in spinal muscular atrophy—Werdnig-Hoffmann's disease, Acta Neuropathol. **27**:247, 1974.

Fischer, E. G., Welch, K., and Shillito, J., Jr.: Syringomyelia following lumboureteral shunting for communicating hydrocephalus, J. Neurosurg. **41**:96, 1977.

Fisher, R. L., et al.: Arthrogryposis multiplex congenita: a clinical investigation, J. Pediatr. **76**:255, 1970.

Ford, F. R.: Diseases of the nervous system. In Infancy, childhood and adolescence, ed. 5, Springfield, Ill., 1966, Charles C Thomas, Publisher, p. 1221.

Fried, L., and Aparicio, O.: Experimental ischemia of the spinal cord: histologic studies after anterior spinal artery inclusion, Neurology **23**:289, 1973.

Furukawa, T., and Toyokura, Y.: Chronic spinal muscular atrophy of facioscapulohumeral type, J. Med. Genet. **13**:285, 1976.

Gamstorp, I.: Progressive spinal muscular atrophy with onset in infancy or early childhood, Acta Paediatr. Scand. **56**:408, 1967.

Gardner, W. J.: Hydrodynamic mechanism of syringomyelia: its relationship to myelocele, J. Neurol. Neurosurg. Psychiatry **28**:247, 1965.

Gardner, W. J.: Myelomeningocele. The results of rupture of the embryonic neural tube, Cleve. Clin. Q. **27**:88, 1960.

Goebel, H. H., and Muller, J.: The unusual features of traumatic neurogenic muscular atrophy in the infant: an anatomic study, Neuropaediatrie **8**:274, 1977.

Goebel, H. H., Zeman, W., and De Myer, W.: Peripheral motor and sensory neuropathy of early childhood, simulating Werdnig-Hoffmann disease, Neuropaediatrie **7**:182, 1976.

Gomez, M., Clermont, V., and Bernstein, J.: Progressive bulbar paralysis in childhood (Fazio-Londe's disease), Arch. Neurol. **6**:317, 1962.

Gordon, N.: Benign congenital hypotonia: a syndrome or a disease? Dev. Med. Child. Neurol. **8**:330, 1966.

Goutières, F., Aicardi, J., and Farkas, E.: Anterior horn cell disease associated with ponto-cerebellar hypoplasia in infants, J. Neurol. Neurosurg. Psychiatry **40**:370, 1977.

Greenfield, J. G., and Norman, R. M.: Demyelinating diseases. In Blackwood, W., et al, editors: Greenfield's neuropathology, Baltimore, 1963, The Williams & Wilkins Co., p. 477.

Greenfield, J. G., Cornman, T., and Shy, G. M.: The prognostic value of the muscle biopsy in the "floppy infant," Brain **81**:461, 1958.

Grist, N. R.: Type A7 Coxsackie (type 4 poliomyelitis) virus infection in Scotland, J. Hyg. **60**:323, 1962.

Guinter, R. H., Hernried, L. S., and Kaplan, A. M.: Infantile neurogenic muscular atrophy with prolonged survival, J. Pediatr. **90**:95, 1977.

Haberland, C., Brunngraber, E. C., and Witting, L. A.: Infantile neuroaxonal dystrophy, Arch. Neurol. **26**:391, 1972.

Hilal, S. K., Marton, D., and Pollack, E.: Diastematomyelia in children: radiographic study of 34 cases, Radiology **112**:609, 1974.

Huttenlocher, P. R., and Cohen, R. B.: Oxidative enzymes in spinal motor neurons in Werdnig-Hoffmann disease, Neurology **16**:398, 1966.

Huttenlocher, P. R., and Gilles, F. H.: Infantile neuroaxonal dystrophy, Neurology **17**:1174, 1967.

Jackson, M.: Familial lumbosacral syringomyelia and the significance of developmental errors of spinal cord and column, Med. J. Austr. **1**:433, 1949.

James, C. C., and Lassman, L. P.: Diastematomyelia, Arch. Dis. Child. **39**:125, 1964.

Jarcho, L. W., Fred, H. L., and Castle, C. H.: Encephalitis and poliomyelitis in the adult due to coxsackievirus group B, type 5, N. Engl. J. Med. **268**:235, 1963.

Kaeser, H. E.: Scapuloperoneal muscular atrophy, Brain **88**:407, 1965.

Kennedy, W., Alter, M., and Sung, J.: Progressive proximal spinal and bulbar muscular atrophy of late onset, Neurology **18**:671, 1968.

Kugelberg, E., and Welander, L.: Heredo-familial juvenile muscular atrophy simulating muscular dystrophy, Arch. Neurol. Psychiatry **75**:500, 1956.

Lassman, L. P., Michael, J. C., and Foster, J. B.: Hydromyelia, J. Neurol. Sci. **7**:149, 1968.

Lepow, M. L., and Spence, D. A.: Effect of trivalent oral poliovirus vaccine in an institutionalized population with varying natural and acquired immunity to poliomyelitis, Pediatrics **35**:236, 1965.

Leyden, E.: Ueber hyderomyelus und syringomyelie, Virchows. Arch [Pathol. Anat.] **68**:1, 1876.

Londe, P.: Paralysie bulbaire progressive infantile et familiale, Rev. Med. **13**:1020, 1893.

Markand, O. N., and Daly, D. D.: Juvenile type of slowly progressive bulbar palsy: report of a case, Neurology **21**:753, 1971.

Markham, J. W., and Otenasek, F. J.: Neuromyelitis optica simulating cord tumor: report of a case with review of nine additional cases, Arch. Neurol. Psychiatry **72**:758, 1954.

Marshall, A., and Duchen, L. W.: Sensory system involvement in infantile spinal muscular atrophy, J. Neurol. Sci. **26**:349, 1975.

Martin, J. J., and Martin, L.: Infantile neuroaxonal dystrophy, Eur. Neurol. **8**:239, 1972.

Mawatari, S., and Katayama, K.: Scapuloperoneal muscular atrophy with cardiopathy, Arch. Neurol. **28**:55, 1973.

McCarthy, J. T., and Amer, J.: Postvaricella acute transverse myelitis: case presentation and review of literature, Pediatrics **62**:202, 1978.

Meacham, W.: Surgical treatment of diastematomyelia, J. Neurosurg. **27**:78, 1967.

Mei Liu, H., Larson, M., and Mizuno, Y.: An analysis of the ultrastructural findings in infantile neuroaxonal dystrophy (Seitelberger's disease), Acta Neuropathol. **27**:201, 1974.

Mellins, R., et al.: Respiratory distress as the initial manifestation of Werdnig-Hoffmann disease, Pediatrics **53**:33, 1974.

Miller, H. G., Stanton, S. B., and Gibbons, S. L.: Parainfectious encephalomyelitis and related syndromes, Q. J. Med. **25**:428, 1956.

Moes, C. A., and Hendrick, E. B.: Diastematomyelia, J. Pediatr. **63**:238, 1963.

Moosa, A., and Dubowitz, V.: Motor nerve conduction velocity in spinal muscular atrophy of childhood, Arch. Dis. Child. **51**:974, 1976.

Mukherjee, S. K.: Involvement of anterior horn of spinal cord in infectious mononucleosis, Br. Med. J. **1**:1112, 1965.

Namba, T., Aberfeld, D., and Grob, D.: Chronic proximal spinal muscular atrophy, J. Neurol. Sci. **11**:401, 1970.

Nelson, J. S., and Prensky, A. L.: Sporadic juvenile amyotrophic lateral sclerosis, Arch. Neurol. **27**:300, 1972.

Nelson, J. W., and Amick, L. D.: Heredofamilial progressive spinal muscular atrophy: a clinical and electromyographic study of a kinship, Neurology **16**:306, 1966.

Netsky, M.: Syringomyelia: a clinical pathologic study, Arch. Neurol. Psychiatry **70**:741, 1953.

Norman, R. M., and Kay, J. M.: Cerebellothalamospinal degeneration in infancy: an unusual variant of Werdnig-Hoffmann disease, Arch. Dis. Child. **40**:302, 1965.

Oller-Navarro, J. L., Rivera-Reyes, L., Rodriguez-Rivera, A. A.: Juvenile diabetic myelopathy. A 14-year-old girl with juvenile diabetes mellitus complicated by acute transverse myelopathy, Clin. Pediatr. **18**(1):60, 1979.

Oppenheim, H.: Ueber allgemeine und localisierte Atonie der Muskulatur (Myatonie) im frühen Kindesalter, Maandshr. Psych. Neurol. **8**:232, 1900.

Owens, J. C., and Swan, H.: Complications in the repair of coarctation of the aorta, J. Cardiovasc. Surg. **4**:816, 1963.

Pachter, B. R., et al.: Congenital total external ophthalmoplegia associated with infantile spinal muscular atrophy. Fine structure of extraocular muscle, Invest. Ophthalmol. **15**:320, 1976.

Paine, R. S., and Byers, R. K.: Transverse myelopathy in childhood, Am. J. Dis. Child. **85**:151, 1953.

Pearn, J.: Fetal movements and Werdnig-Hoffmann disease, J. Neurol. Sci. **18**:373, 1973.

Pearn, J. H., Gardner-Medwin, D., and Wilson, J.: A clinical study of chronic childhood spinal muscular atrophy: a review of 141 cases, J. Neurol. Sci. **38**:23, 1978.

Pena, C. E., et al.: Arthrogryposis multiplex congenita, Neurology **18**:926, 1968.

Petajan, J., et al.: Arthrogryposis syndrom (Kuskokwin disease) in the Eskimo, J.A.M.A. **209**:1481, 1969.

Pitner, S., Edwards, J., and McCormick, W.: Observations on the pathology of the Moebius syndrome, J. Neurol. Neurosurg. Psychiatry **28**:362, 1965.

Pugh, R. C., and Dudgeon, J. A.: Fatal neonatal poliomyelitis, Arch. Dis. Child. **29**:381, 1954.

Rabe, E. F.: The hypotonic infant, J. Pediatr. **64**:422, 1964.

Raimbault, J., and Laget, P.: L'apport de l'electrol-yographie au diagnostic de l'amyotrophie spinale infantile de Werdnig-Hoffmann, Pathol. Biol. **20**:287, 1972.

Romanes, G. J.: The motor cell columns of the lumbosacral spinal cord of the cat. J. Comp. Neurol. **94**:313, 1951.

Sandefeldt, E., et al.: Animal model of human disease—infantile spinal muscular atrophy, Werdnig-Hoffmann disease, Am. J. Pathol. **82**:649, 1976.

Sarnat, H. B., O'Connor, T., and Byrne, P. A.: Clinical effects of myotonic dystrophy on pregnancy and the neonate, Arch. Neurol. **33**:459, 1976.

Schwartz, M. S., and Moosa, A.: Sensory nerve conduction in the spinal muscular atrophies, Dev. Med. Child. Neurol. **19**:50, 1977.

Schwentker, E. P., and Gibson, D. A.: The orthopaedic aspects of spinal muscular atrophy, J. Bone Joint Surg. **58**:32, 1976.

Seitelberger, F.: Eine unbekannte Form von infantiler lipoidspeicher Krankhirt des Gehirns, Proc. First Int. Congr. Neuropath. **3**:323, 1952.

Shafiq, S. A., Milhorat, A. T., and Gorycki, M. A.: Fine structure of human muscle in neurogenic atrophy, Neurology **17**:934, 1967.

Silverman, A. C.: Mumps complicated by the preceding myelitis, N. Engl. J. Med. **241**:262, 1949.

Spiro, A. J.: Minipolymyoclonus: a neglected sign in childhood spinal muscular dystrophy, Neurology **20**:1124, 1970.

Steegman, A. T.: Syndrome of the anterior spinal artery, Neurology **2**:15, 1952.

Swaiman, K. F.: Diseases of amino acid metabolism and associated conditions. In Swaiman, K. F., and Wright, F. S.: *The practice of pediatric neurology,* St. Louis, 1975, The C. V. Mosby Co., p. 359.

Takahashi, K., Nakamura, H., and Okada, E.: Hereditary amyotrophic lateral sclerosis, Arch. Neurol. **27**:292, 1972.

Tanaka, H., et al.: Cardiac involvement in the Kugelberg-Welander syndrome, Am. J. Cardiol. **38**:528, 1976.

Thomson, A. F., and Alvarez, F. A.: Hereditary amyotrophic lateral sclerosis, J. Neurol. Sci. **8**:101, 1969.

Tobin, W. D., and Layton, D. D.: The diagnosis and natural history of spinal cord arteriovenous malformations, Mayo Clin. Proc. **51**:637, 1976.

Tsukagoshi, H., et al.: Kugelberg-Welander syndrome with dominant inheritance, Arch. Neurol. **14**:378, 1966.

Tyler, H. R.: Neurological complications of rubeola (measles), Medicine **36**:147, 1957.

Van Allen, M., and Blodi, F.: Neurologic aspects of the Moebius syndrome, Neurology **10**:249, 1960.

Vassilopoulos, D., and Emery, A. E.: Quantitative histochemistry of the spinal motor neurone nucleus during human fetal development, J. Neurol. Sci. **32**:275, 1977.

Vignaendra, V., and Thiam Ghee, L.: A family with neurogenic atrophy of the distal muscles of the upper limbs, Med. J. Aust. **2:**639, 1976.

Vuia, O.: Neuroaxonal dystrophy, a juvenile-adult form, Clin. Neurol. Neurosurg. **79:**307, 1976.

Walton, J. N.: The limp child, J. Neurol. Neurosurg. Psychiatry **20:**144, 1957.

Weenink, H. R., and Smilde, J.: Spinal cord lesions due to coarctio aortae, Psychiatr. Neurol. Neurochir. **67:**259, 1964.

Weinberg, A. G., and Kirkpatrick, J. B.: Cerebellar hypoplasia in Werdnig-Hoffmann disease, Dev. Med. Child. Neurol. **17:**511, 1975.

Whittem, J. H.: Congenital abnormalities in calves; arthrogryposis and hydranencephaly, J. Path. Bact. **73:**375, 1957.

Wijngaarden, G., and Bethlem, J.: Benign infantile spinal muscular atrophy, Brain **96:**163, 1973.

Wilken, K. E., and Gibson, D. A.: The patterns of spinal deformity in Duchenne muscular dystrophy, J. Bone Joint Surg. **58**(1):24, 1976.

Williams, B., and Timperley, W. R.: Three cases of communicating syringomyelia secondary to midbrain gliomas, J. Neurol. Neurosurg. Psychiatry **40:**80, 1977.

Williams, B.: Difficult labour as a cause of communicating syringomyelia, Lancet **2:**51, 1977.

Zellweger, H., Schneider, H., and Schuldt, D. R.: A new genetic variant of spinal muscular atrophy, Neurology **19:**865, 1969.

# CHAPTER 4

# Disorders of peripheral nerves and spinal nerve roots

## Peripheral nerve apparatus

A peripheral nerve is formed from axons originating from cell bodies within the central nervous system or from sensory or automatic ganglia outside the central nervous system (Fig. 4-1). Thus three types of fibers function within each peripheral nerve:

1. Sensory fibers from dorsal root ganglia
2. Motor fibers from the anterior horn cells
3. Autonomic fibers from cell bodies within the central nervous system and from the autonomic ganglia

The motor and autonomic fibers form the anterior or ventral root; the sensory fibers form the posterior or dorsal root. The anterior and posterior roots join to form the peripheral nerve containing these axons of differing function. The anterior and posterior roots merge just distal to the dorsal root ganglion and exit from the foramen.

The primordia of the spinal nerves appear early in embryologic development as the neural groove closes to form the neural tube. When the neural tube is formed, certain cells near the superior margins remain independent and form the neural crest. These neural crest cells are the anlagen of sensory ganglia of the spinal nerves, the cranial nerves of sensory function, and indirectly the sympathetic ganglia.

From the mantle layer of the developing spinal cord, some of these cells differentiate into neuroblasts, which functionally become nerve cells. Fibers from neuroblasts within the ventrolateral portion of the mantle layer form the anterior roots of the spinal nerves, while fibers from neuroblasts in the dorsal root ganglia form the posterior roots of the spinal nerves. The fibers from the dorsal root ganglia are initially bipolar but become unipolar with connections to various peripheral receptors.

Neuroblasts that have migrated from the neural crest and the neural tube form the sympathetic ganglia.

The peripheral nerve acquires a cellular sheath as it develops. Cells of ectodermal origin, or Schwann cells, migrate with the developing nerve and form the cellular covering known as the neurilemmal sheath. The migrating Schwann cells gradually spread over the growing nerve, forming the myelin sheath by wrapping their cytoplasm in circular, concentric layers around the axon. Generally, development of this sheath begins near the neuron and progresses peripherally.

The myelin covering the axon is divided into segments by the nodes of Ranvier. Each segment contains one Schwann cell nucleus. Myelin consists of alternating layers of Schwann cell membrane. In unmyelinated fibers, the axons indent the Schwann cell membrane but concentric layering does not develop. The axons are grouped in

79

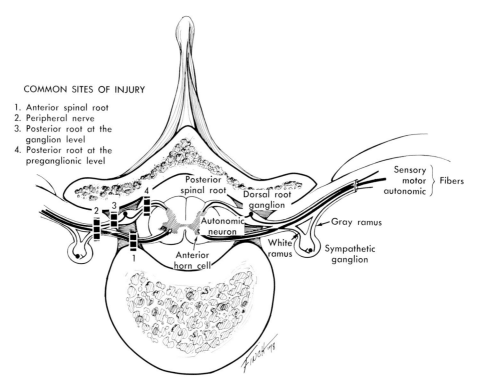

COMMON SITES OF INJURY

1. Anterior spinal root
2. Peripheral nerve
3. Posterior root at the ganglion level
4. Posterior root at the preganglionic level

**Fig. 4-1.** Schematic representation of peripheral nerve apparatus illustrating functional groups of fibers and common sites of injury in anterior spinal root *(1)*, peripheral nerve *(2)*, posterior root at the ganglion level *(3)*, and preganglionic level *(4)*.

bundles within the peripheral nerve, and each axon is supported by delicate connective tissue called endoneurium. Each bundle of axons is surrounded by firmer connective tissue called the perineurium. Surrounding many bundles of axons is the epineurium, a connective tissue layer continuous with adjacent connective tissue. The peripheral nerve trunks receive nutrient arteries at intervals along their length to form an anastomotic chain on the surface of or within the nerve bundles.

The cell body is the anatomic site for maintaining the viability of the axons and consequently of the peripheral nerve. Many pathologic processes can affect the peripheral nerve in different areas—the axon, its myelin sheath, or the interstitial connective tissue. Any one of these sites may bear the brunt of the pathologic process, or they may all be affected to some degree. If the cell body is destroyed, the entire axon degenerates. If the axon is interrupted distal to its cell body, only the distal portion of the nerve degenerates in a process known as wallerian or axonal degeneration. Primary involvement of the Schwann cell interferes with the integrity of the myelin, and segmental demyelinization ensues. Classic segmental demyelinization occurs in diphtheritic and lead neuropathies.

**Clinical characteristics of peripheral nerve involvement**

Peripheral neuropathies may be classified according to the clinical course of the disease (acute, subacute, or chronic), the type and distribution of functional impairment (motor, sensory, autonomic, or mixed), the pathologic involvement (such as primary involvement of axon, Schwann cell, or interstitial tissue), or a combination of these features. Finally, classification may be based on the presumed etiology. The term "neuropathy" signifies a disorder of nerve function without regard for the etiologic or pathologic features. The term "neuritis" should be used only if the pathophysiologic disorder is known to be inflammatory in origin. If more than one nerve is involved, the term "polyneuropathy" is used. Although no single system of classification is satisfactory for clinical purposes, one based on etiology appears to be workable.

Disorders of the peripheral nerves are classified as traumatic, toxic, infectious, metabolic-degenerative, vascular, congenital, and neoplastic. A few disorders of idiopathic origin present a typical clinical syndrome and are easily recognizable. However, the origin of a peripheral neuropathy often remains obscure despite a thorough diagnostic search. Table 4-1 represents an etiologic classification of some of the known disorders of the peripheral nerve.

Initially the diagnostic approach seeks to confirm the presence of a peripheral neurop-

**Table 4-1.** Etiologic classification of disorders of peripheral nerves and spinal roots

Congenital
  Congenital hypomyelination neuropathy
  Congenital indifference to pain
  Congenital sensory neuropathy (HSN* II)
  Congenital sensory neuropathy with anhidrosis (HSN IV)
  Familial dysautonomia (Riley-Day syndrome; HSN III)
  Hereditary sensory radicular neuropathy (HSN I)
  Nonprogressive sensory neuropathy
  Progressive sensory neuropathy
Idiopathic
  Bell's palsy
  Guillain-Barré syndrome
  Recurrent neuropathy
Infectious
  Herpes
Metabolic-degenerative
  Abetalipoproteinemia (Bassen-Kornzweig syndrome)
  Ataxia-telangiectasia
  Chédiak-Higashi syndrome
  Diabetes mellitus
  Friedreich's ataxia
  Giant axonal neuropathy
  Globoid cell leukodystrophy (Krabbe's disease)
  Hypertrophic interstitial neuritis (Dejerine-Sottas disease, HMSN† III)
  Alpha-lipoproteinemia (Tangier disease)
  Metachromatic leukodystrophy
  Peroneal muscular atrophy (Charcot-Marie-Tooth disease, HMSN I)
  Porphyria
  Refsum's disease (heredopathia atactica polyneuritiformis, HMSN IV)
  Uremia
  Vitamin deficiencies

Neoplastic
  Hodgkin's disease
  Leukemia
  Neurofibromatosis
  Spinal cord tumor
Toxic
  Antibiotic-induced neuropathy
  Antimetabolite-induced neuropathy
  Botulism
  Diphtheria
  Heavy-metal intoxication
  Neuropathy related to glue sniffing
  Postimmunization neuropathy
  Postinjection sciatic nerve palsy
Traumatic
  Birth injury involving brachial plexus, radial, or obturator nerves
  Childhood brachial plexus injury
Vascular
  Dermatomyositis
  Lupus erythematosus
  Polyarteritis nodosa
  Rheumatoid arthritis
  Scleroderma

*HSN, hereditary sensory neuropathy.
†HMSN, hereditary motor sensory neuropathy.

athy. The cause may be apparent from the history, associated physical signs, or specific laboratory investigation.

The characteristic symptoms of peripheral nerve involvement are weakness and sensory impairment. Usually the weakness is more pronounced distally. The diagnosis of neuropathy is suggested by the presence of impairment of either superficial sensation (touch, pain, and temperature) or deep sensation (vibration or position sense) or both. However, sensory signs may be minimal or lacking in certain diseases, such as peroneal atrophy. Since pathologic processes often have a predilection for certain portions of the peripheral nerve (roots or ganglia) or of the mixed peripheral nerve that contains motor, sensory, or autonomic fibers, careful examination of the functions served by these portions may aid in determining the site of the lesion.

Fig. 4-1 depicts impairment at different anatomic portions of the peripheral nerve. If a lesion occurs in the anterior root (site *1* in the figure), the predominant finding is weakness without sensory loss. Symptoms of this lesion may be difficult to distinguish from those of anterior horn cell disease. Tendon reflexes are diminished or absent, but the decrease of reflex activity may not parallel the degree of weakness. Muscle atrophy may be severe; fasciculations are rare. A careful search should be made for signs of autonomic instability, such as changes in skin color or temperature or a noticeable lack of sweating. Distal weakness, fasciculations (rarely), and manifestations of autonomic dysfunction are signs of an anterior root lesion that are rarely present in anterior horn cell disease. Electromyography may show a decrease in motor nerve conduction velocity in the affected nerves.

A lesion at site *2* results in a combination of motor, sensory, and autonomic signs. The degree of involvement may vary, with motor weakness predominating, but some sensory impairment (touch, pain, vibration, or position sense) is often demonstrable. The tendon reflexes are depressed or absent.

A lesion at site *3* causes a sensory neuropathy. Interruption of the afferent limb of the reflex arc impairs tendon reflexes. Any sensation may be involved. Characteristically the sensory loss has a glove-stocking distribution, that is, extending from the distal portion of the extremity toward the elbow or knee. Motor nerve conduction velocity is normal while sensory nerve conduction or latency may be impaired.

A lesion at site *4* is clinically identical to a lesion at site *3*, but these lesions may be differentiated by the histamine test. The flare portion of the triple response to intradermal injection of histamine (1:100 concentration) depends on an intact connection between the dorsal root ganglion and the peripheral nerve. Therefore, if the lesion involves or is distal to the ganglion (site *3*), no flare response occurs. Conversely, if the lesion is proximal to the ganglion (site *4*), a flare response occurs.

A lesion at site *4* may result from primary involvement of the spinal cord, with interruption of the reflex arc and extension of the pathologic process into the dorsal root fibers. Consequently, peripheral nerve involvement may be minimal in comparison with other neurologic signs resulting from spinal cord disease.

Peripheral nerve involvement is differentiated from anterior horn cell and primary muscle disease by the presence of sensory or autonomic symptoms and signs, characteristic distal weakness, and infrequent fasciculations.

The clinical diagnosis of a peripheral nerve disorder is readily made by the presence of sensory or autonomic signs. A careful search is often necessary to detect minimal sensory impairment. In the infant or young child, electrodiagnostic evaluation of sensory latency may provide additional clues to the site of origin of the disease. When weakness is the only manifestation of peripheral nerve disorder, electromyography can clearly demonstrate, by delayed motor conduction velocity, the location of the disorder in the peripheral nerve.

When clinical findings indicate involvement of the peripheral nerve, the course of the disease may suggest the differential diagnosis. An acute onset is common in toxic, infectious, or vascular processes. Metabolic and degenerative diseases usually have an insidious onset and chronic course.

## Idiopathic neuropathies
### Guillain-Barré syndrome

The Guillain-Barré syndrome was first described in the nineteenth century, but the etiology is yet to be defined. The confusion is evident by the profusion of descriptive terms, such as acute febrile neuritis, acute ascending spinal paralysis, acute polyneuritis, infectious neuronitis, and acute inflammatory polyradiculoneuropathy. However, development of diagnostic criteria based on the main clinical features allows for formulation of a reasonable differential diagnosis, identification of a common etiology, development of reliable prognostic data, and assessment of various treatment programs.

The following diagnostic criteria (McFarland and Heller, 1966; Osler and Sidell, 1960) present the salient features of the Guillain-Barré syndrome.
1. The paralysis may follow a nonspecific infection, but an illness known to be associated with polyradiculoneuropathy, such as herpes zoster or diphtheria, should not be present.
2. Findings should include diffuse lower motor unit paralysis, rapid or gradual in onset and with symmetric involvement.
3. Sensory involvement may be present but is generally less severe than the motor weakness.
4. Cerebrospinal fluid (CSF) examination should contain fewer than 10 white cells/cu mm.
5. CSF protein concentration should equal or exceed 60 mg/dl.

**CLINICAL FEATURES.** Reported in children from 16 months to 15 years of age, Guillain-Barré syndrome has a typical pattern of clinical manifestations (Low, Schneider, and Carter, 1958; Peterman, et al., 1959). In up to 75% of cases a nonspecific antecedent infection is present, commonly a respiratory or gastrointestinal infection (Kennedy et al., 1978). Guillain-Barré syndrome may be associated with childhood diseases such as rubella, rubeola, mumps, and infectious mononucleosis. Pain or paresthesia heralds onset of the paralysis in about 50% of patients. The pain often occurs in the legs or feet but may also be present in the hands. In most patients, paralysis begins in the lower extremities and ascends. The course of the paralysis is characterized by gradual onset with progression of symptoms over days to several weeks.

Cranial nerve involvement occurs in about half of the cases. Bilateral paralysis of cranial nerve VII (facial nerve) is most frequent, although other cranial nerves may be involved. Bilateral papilledema has been reported in a few cases but differs from that in optic neuritis, which is accompanied by loss of visual acuity. Dysphagia has been reported in a small number of patients, implicating cranial nerves IX and X. Paralysis of the extraocular muscles, especially the lateral rectus, has been reported but is unusual (Fisher syndrome) (Ricker and Hertel, 1976).

The tendon reflexes are depressed or absent, but the cutaneous reflexes (abdominal, cremasteric) are generally present. Weakness is more pronounced in the distal muscles, often most prominently in the extensor muscles. The weakness is symmetric in distribution, but homologous muscles are not necessarily involved to the same degree. When there is complete flaccid paralysis, no differentiation can be made.

Sensory examination is difficult in young children. Even when the examination is adequate, generally only minimal involvement is evident. Position sense is often impaired first, followed by impairment of vibration, touch, pain, and temperature sensations. The early paresthesias tend to be intermittent. Muscle tenderness and nuchal rigidity may be present. Urinary incontinence or retention of urine occurs in about 20% of cases.

Urinary symptoms often occur during the stage of active progression of the paralysis and are transient. Persistent urinary dysfunction suggests spinal cord involvement.

Differential diagnosis should include processes known to be neurotoxic, such as diphtheria and poliomyelitis; lead, arsenic, and thallium poisoning; acute porphyria; childhood diseases; tick paralysis; and sarcoidosis. Several features differentiate poliomyelitis from Guillain-Barré syndrome. In poliomyelitis, there is often a specific infectious prodromal stage accompanied by fever and prominent signs of meningeal irritation. The paralysis peaks within a few days and tends to be asymmetric and limited. Tendon reflexes are decreased and asymmetric, depending on the weakness. Sensation is normal. The CSF cell count and protein concentration are usually elevated.

The clinical course of Guillain-Barré syndrome is somewhat variable. The weakness often develops over several days or even weeks, or it may progress rapidly to produce flaccid quadriplegia. The patient may recover as early as 2 weeks after onset; most patients show significant recovery by 4 to 8 weeks. The mortality rate is 3% to 4%.

The most serious development in a patient with Guillain-Barré syndrome is impairment of respiratory function as a result of weakness of the intercostal muscles. Severe respiratory distress occurs when both intercostal and diaphragmatic muscles are involved. If the deltoid and biceps muscles are weak, the disease process is close to the origin of the phrenic nerve and respiratory distress should be anticipated. Increase in the rate of respiration and use of accessory muscles of respiration signal its presence.

Patients with impaired respiratory capacity should be monitored by measuring tidal volume. Cyanosis and restlessness indicate impending respiratory failure. If the respiratory capacity decreases or the patient has difficulty handling secretions, a tracheotomy is necessary and a respirator should be used to assist or maintain respiration. Further treatment during the acute stage involves maintaining hydration and good nutrition to assure adequate renal function. To avoid stasis pneumonia, the immobilized patient should be turned to promote bronchial drainage. Urinary catheterization may be necessary for a short period as the weakness progresses and causes some urinary retention. Active physical therapy is contraindicated during the progressive stage of the illness. However, appropriately placed footboards and trochanteric pads minimize development of contractures and skin ulcers and facilitate recovery and rehabilitation.

Autonomic dysfunction is common in Guillain-Barré syndrome (Lichtenfeld, 1971). Hypertension, lability of blood pressure, postural hypotension, electrocardiographic changes, and facial flushing may occur. Hypertension apparently results from an alteration in the sympathetic nervous system and the production of high levels of catecholamines (Mitchell and Meilman, 1967). The hypertension may be transient and is often associated with tachycardia. Respiratory compromise should be excluded as a cause. If hypertension persists, treatment with reserpine (0.2 to 0.5 mg/day) or hydralazine hydrochloride (0.75 mg/kg/day) is indicated.

The serum calcium concentration should be carefully monitored from the beginning of the illness. If it increases as a result of prolonged immobilization, measures to reduce calcium intake and promote incorporation of calcium into bone should be undertaken.

The prognosis for recovery is generally quite good. About 65% of patients recover completely. The rest show some persistent weakness and atrophy of the muscles of the legs and feet (Eberle et al., 1975; Gordon et al., 1977).

**LABORATORY FINDINGS.** The peripheral white blood count, differential count, and erythrocyte sedimentation rate are normal unless lung or bladder infection is present. CSF pressure is normal, but the protein concentration is always elevated at some time during the illness. Protein concentration usually is greatest during the second week; however, it may rise for several weeks and then gradually return to normal over a period of months. There is no positive correlation between the severity of the disease and the rate of rise or the absolute value of the protein concentration.

The CSF cell count is below 10 mononuclear cells/cu mm. If the CSF cell count is elevated, the possibility of primary bacterial or viral infection should be considered. The serum calcium concentration may be elevated if the patient has been immobilized for a long period. Hyponatremia with inappropriate secretion of antidiuretic hormone has been reported (Posner et al., 1967).

In most cases, electromyography reveals the characteristic pattern of peripheral nerve involvement. The motor nerve conduction velocity decreases a few weeks after onset and is often more impaired distally (Fig. 4-2). In one study of 26 patients (Peterman et al., 1959), the nerve conduction time was reduced in all patients 8 weeks after onset. Delayed motor nerve conduction suggests diffuse involvement of the peripheral nerve by a demyelinating process. Fibrillation potentials may be seen after the second or third week of illness and represent axonal degeneration. A few patients have normal motor

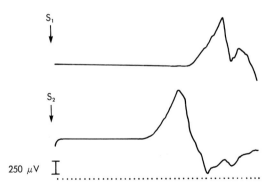

**Fig. 4-2.** Motor nerve conduction velocity in patient with Guillain-Barré syndrome showing prolonged latencies, prolonged evoked potential duration, and decreased evoked potential amplitude. ($S_1$) stimulation at elbow; ($S_2$) stimulation at wrist. Interval between dots is 1 msec.

nerve conduction velocity during the first weeks of the illness (Eisen and Humphreys, 1974).

**PATHOPHYSIOLOGY.** Pathologic findings at autopsy (Haymaker and Kernohan, 1949) vary with the stage of the disease. The main site of involvement is the proximal portion of the peripheral nerve distal to the dorsal ganglion. The predominant feature is acute, severe edema of the spinal roots. Following the acute stage, the axons and myelin sheaths degenerate and are infiltrated by inflammatory lymphocytes (Fig. 4-3). Although demyelinization appears to be the predominant pathologic feature, axonal or wallerian degeneration occurs in many nerve fibers. Lesions in the dorsal root ganglia vary, but chromatolysis of nerve cells is usually present to some degree. In the central nervous system, the main pathologic finding is central chromatolysis of the anterior horn cells, thought to be secondary to lesions in the nerve fibers.

Guillain-Barré syndrome has been considered an immunologic disorder (Behan et al., 1972). Humoral antibodies, IgM immunoglobulins, have been found along myelin sheaths in affected patients. In addition, delayed hypersensitivity mechanisms may play a role. Abnormal lymphoid cells with active DNA synthesis have been noted in peripheral blood. They resemble the mononuclear cells found in response to a variety of antigenic stimuli and presumably are capable of antibody production (Hart, Hanks, and Mackay, 1972). Ultrastructural features suggest that the circulating mononuclear cells are indistinguishable from some of the cells infiltrating the nerve roots (Whitaker et al., 1970).

**TREATMENT.** Guillain-Barré syndrome has been treated with corticotropin and corticosteroids (Heller and DeJong, 1963), but the efficacy of these drugs has been questioned. Some patients have reportedly become worse with such treatment. In a double-blind study of 16 patients, the time from onset of illness to recovery was less in patients treated with steroids (Swick and McQuillen, 1976).

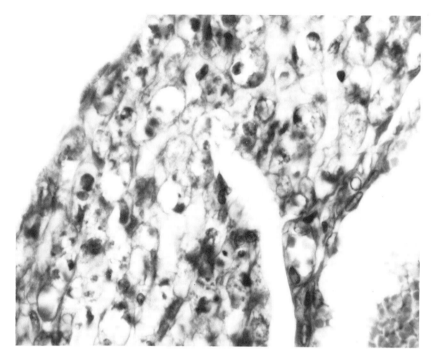

**Fig. 4-3.** Anterior nerve roots of cervical spinal cord from a patient with Guillain-Barré syndrome. Rarefaction and vacuolization of the anterior roots are caused by swelling and loss of myelin sheaths and axons. Luxol-fast blue-PAS stain.

In general the shortest recovery time is associated with the slowest conduction velocity (McQuillen, 1971). There are inadequate control studies in the use of immunosuppressive agents (Rosen and Vastola, 1976).

### Facial paralysis (lower motor neuron facial paralysis, Bell's palsy)

Sir Charles Bell in 1821 described the anatomy of the facial nerve and differentiated its function from that of the trigeminal nerve. He also recognized several cases of facial paralysis associated with trauma or infection. Bell's palsy is a lower motor unit facial paralysis of undetermined cause. Complete or partial weakness of the entire side of the face results from involvement of the facial nerve (cranial nerve VII).

Knowledge of the functional anatomy of the facial nerve is essential to the accurate diagnosis of this type of paralysis. The facial nerve is a mixed nerve containing motor and sensory fibers that serve the muscles of expression, taste, lacrimation, salivation, and an auditory reflex (Fig. 4-4). A lesion at any point from the facial nerve nucleus in the pons to the termination of the nerve in the facial muscles causes facial paralysis. Idiopathic facial paralysis presumably results from edema and inflammation of the facial nerve as its passes through the facial canal within the temporal bone.

**CLINICAL FEATURES.** Often the first manifestation of facial paralysis is pain localized to the ear on the affected side. The paralysis may have a sudden onset and progress rapidly over a few hours. Generally, the child has had only a mild upper respiratory infection before onset of the paralysis and has otherwise been well. The parents may first notice that the child's face is pulled to one side while the opposite affected side is flat and immobile. The child has difficulty closing the eye, drinking, and eating. When paralysis is

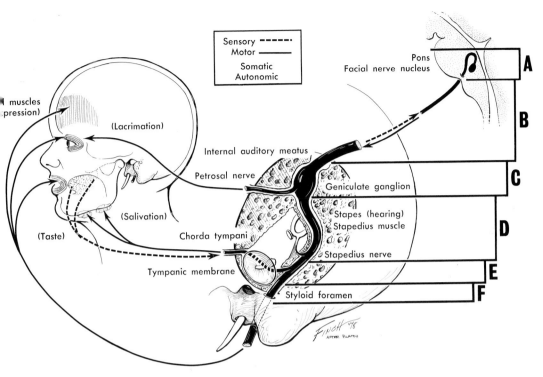

**Fig. 4-4.** Functional anatomy of facial nerve (cranial nerve VII), a mixed nerve with both motor and sensory components. *A* through *F*, possible sites of facial nerve injury. (See Table 4-3.)

complete, the affected side of the face sags and there may be excessive tearing. In a crying infant, the intact or normal side pulls downward.

Differentiation between peripheral facial paralysis and central facial paralysis is often simple. Peripheral nerve paralysis involves the muscles of the entire side of the face, including the forehead and the muscles about the eye; central facial paralysis affects only the lower portion of the face. The reason for this anatomic difference is that the portion of the facial nucleus supplying the frontalis, orbicularis oculi, and corrugator muscles is innervated from both hemispheres; therefore in the presence of a lesion of one cerebral hemisphere, the nucleus supplying the muscles of the upper portion of the face is innervated from the unaffected hemisphere.

The diagnosis of idiopathic facial paralysis is one of exclusion. Table 4-2 lists some of the common causes of lower motor unit facial

**Table 4-2.** Etiologic classification of facial paralysis (peripheral or motor unit)

Congenital
　Absence of cranial
　　nerve VII nuclei
Idiopathic
　Bell's palsy
　Melkersson's syndrome
Infectious
　Encephalitis
　Guillain-Barré syndrome
　Herpes zoster (Ramsay Hunt syndrome)
　Mastoiditis
　Meningitis
　Osteomyelitis
　Otitis media
　Parotitis
　Poliomyelitis
Metabolic
　Hypothyroidism
　Idiopathic infantile
　　hypercalcemia
　Osteopetrosis
Traumatic
　Birth
　　Forceps pressure
　　Fracture
　　Pressure from maternal sacrum
　　Postnatal fracture
Neoplastic
　Brain stem tumor
　Local tumors
　Neurofibromatosis
Vascular
　Brain stem malformation
　Hypertension (renal disease frequent)

**Table 4-3.** Clinical localization of facial nerve lesions*

| Anatomic site | Facial muscle movement | Taste | Lacrimation | Salivation | Hyperacusis |
|---|---|---|---|---|---|
| Nucleus (A) | Impaired | Normal | Normal | Normal | Present |
| Pons to internal auditory meatus (B) | Impaired | Normal | Impaired | Impaired | Present |
| Geniculate ganglion (C) | Impaired | Impaired | Impaired | Impaired | Present |
| Ganglion to stapedius nerve (D) | Impaired | Impaired | Normal | Impaired | Present |
| Stapedius nerve to chorda tympani (E) | Impaired | Impaired | Normal | Impaired | Absent |
| Below chorda tympani (F) | Impaired | Normal | Normal | Normal | Absent |

*Letters refer to designations in Fig. 4-4.

paralysis. The history is significant in ruling out many of these conditions (Manning and Adour, 1972).

Congenital facial paralysis is a bilateral condition evident at or shortly after birth and usually associated with similar involvement of cranial nerve VI or its nucleus (Möbius' syndrome). History of a traumatic delivery indicates possible fracture of the skull. Most commonly, facial paralysis in the newborn infant results from pressure on the facial nerve by the prominence of the maternal sacrum (Hepner, 1951). A cardiofacial syndrome consists of a unilateral partial lower facial weakness and congenital heart disease (Cayler, Blumenfeld, and Anderson, 1971). The facial weakness involves only the lip depressors, most commonly the angulus oris muscle. This entity probably represents hypoplasia of the muscle (Nelson and Eng, 1972).

The lack of fever and of signs of an infectious process generally rules out infection. In Guillain-Barré syndrome, facial paralysis is most often bilateral. Skull x-ray films should substantiate the diagnosis of osteopetrosis. Other causes can be determined on the basis of examination.

When possible, the discrete functions of the facial nerve should be tested to determine the site of the lesion. Table 4-3 summarizes the clinical findings in relation to the anatomic sites of pathologic abnormality. In typical Bell's palsy the facial muscles of one side of the face are completely or partially paralyzed so that the patient cannot wrinkle the forehead, close the eye, or retract the corner of the mouth in attempting to smile (Fig. 4-5). In order to test taste, the examiner asks the child to protrude the tongue, holds the tongue with a piece of gauze, and then alternately applies to the anterior edge of the tongue solutions of salt, sugar, vinegar, and quinine to test the taste sensations of salty, sweet, sour, and bitter, respectively. The patient's tongue should not be allowed to retract into the mouth during the examination because the test solutions will be dispersed, yielding faulty results.

A disturbance in lacrimation may be detected by visual inspection. If the pathways of lacrimation are intact, excessive tearing often occurs in the ipsilateral eye as a result of corneal irritation secondary to absence of the blink reflex. Diminished lacrimation is difficult to detect by inspection. The nasolacrimal reflex may be tested by stimulating the nasal mucosa with a piece of cotton, which normally causes intense lacrimation on the stimulated side. Diminished response is a reliable indicator of lacrimal hypofunction. The Schirmer's test measures tear formation. Whatman filter paper (No. 41) strips are hooked over the lower lid margins bilaterally and the amount of paper moistened in 5 minutes is compared.

Sophisticated audiologic study is necessary to assess stapedius nerve function accurately.

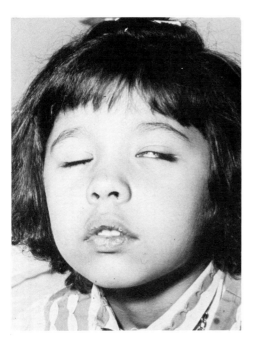

**Fig. 4-5.** Patient with paralysis of left facial nerve (cranial nerve VII) resulting in paralysis of left side of face and inability to close eye tightly or retract corner of mouth forcibly.

Involvement of the stapedius nerve may be suspected if the patient complains of increased auditory acuity or sensitivity to low tones in the ear on the paralyzed side.

**LABORATORY FINDINGS.** Laboratory findings include a normal peripheral white cell count, differential count, and erythrocyte sedimentation rate, and normal CSF pressure and protein concentration. Skull films, including views of the internal auditory meatus, should be obtained to rule out skull fracture, osteomyelitis, mastoiditis, increased intracranial pressure, calcification, and osteopetrosis.

Electrodiagnostic techniques have been used to predict the prognosis and course of facial paralysis. These studies have included measurement of conduction velocity in the facial nerve (Langworth and Taverner, 1963), detection of the level or threshold of response to stimulation (Campbell et al., 1962), and electrical stimulation of the tongue (Peiris and Miles, 1965). Signs of nerve degeneration are detectable as early as 72 hours after onset of paralysis by measuring the nerve threshold to electrical stimulation. Before 72 hours, electrodiagnostic techniques do not detect reliable signs of degeneration. Prognosis for recovery has been assessed by the electrically elicited blink reflex (orbicularis oculi reflex). Return of the reflex before loss of distal facial nerve excitability is associated with a good clinical recovery (Kimura, Giron, and Young, 1976).

In a study to determine concomitant peripheral nerve involvement (Chaco, 1973), 16% of affected patients had subclinical neuropathy evidenced by reduced motor conduction velocity in both the facial nerves and the median and ulnar nerves.

**TREATMENT.** Treatment of idiopathic facial paralysis has included a variety of drugs, such as vasodilators, ascorbic acid, prednisone, prednisolone, and adrenocorticotropic hormone (ACTH). In addition, surgical decompression has been recommended in some cases.

Some control studies of different therapies have been performed, others have been equivocal, and yet others have been interrupted because the results of therapy necessitated abandonment of the original experimental design. ACTH was favored originally by Taverner and co-workers (1966); however, in 1971 their data suggested that prednisolone was more effective (Taverner, Cohen, and Hutchinson, 1971). Prednisone appears to relieve pain and improve facial function (Adour et al., 1972; Adour and Wingerd, 1974). Aberrant blink reflexes can be demonstrated in many patients following facial nerve degeneration (Kimura, Rodnitzky, and Okawara, 1975). The effects of therapy must be compared with the natural history of idiopathic facial paralysis. The natural course of the disease suggests that about 60% of patients recover completely. In the rest, signs of facial nerve degeneration develop together with postparalytic features such as partial paralysis of individual muscles, loss of a variety of associated movements, and facial contractures.

At present, the most prudent treatment in children appears to be a 10-day course of prednisone therapy after other pathologic conditions have been excluded (Wolf et al., 1978). The patient is treated with prednisone, 60 mg per square meter of body surface per day for 3 days, and the dosage is tapered in 7 days. If the paralysis is only partial, no treatment is needed.

In the older child, it is possible to obtain accurate electrodiagnostic information. If the child is seen 5 days or more after onset of the paralysis and the electrical excitability is normal, no treatment is needed, because in all likelihood the child has a physiologic conduction block of the facial nerve and will recover completely without treatment. Unfortunately, in the first 24 to 72 hours after onset, such a prediction is not possible.

If the patient cannot close the eye, a bland ophthalmic ointment should be instilled several times a day and the eye covered with a patch to protect the cornea against drying. In addition, electrical stimulation of the paralyzed muscles several times a day may prevent atrophy of the denervated muscles until either the physiologic block disappears or the nerve regenerates. No adequately controlled study has been made to verify the benefits of electrical stimulation; its use is strictly empirical.

The value of surgical decompression of the nerve in the facial canal is uncertain. In one study (Mechelse et al., 1971), no difference from medically treated patients could be demonstrated in surgically treated patients in the second or third week after onset of paralysis. Certainly, patients with no evidence of denervation or with only partial denervation, as measured electrodiagnostically, do not need surgery. Until means exist to identify at the onset of paralysis those patients in whom the prognosis is poor, the question of surgical decompression versus medical treatment will not be resolved.

### Recurrent facial paralysis

Recurrent facial paralysis, especially on the same side, should suggest the possibility of underlying tumor or malformation. In addition, Melkersson's syndrome (Saberman and Teta, 1966; Stevens, 1965) should be considered. This syndrome, often familial, consists of a triad of recurrent facial paralysis, recurrent facial swelling, and deep fissuring of the tongue (lingua plicata).

## Neuropathies caused by trauma
### Brachial plexus injury

One of the most common types of brachial plexus injury occurs in the newborn infant. Duchenne in 1872 (reported in 1883) ascribed the injury to trauma at delivery. It remained for Erb (1874) to localize the trauma to the fifth and sixth cervical nerves or the site of their union.

Lesions of the brachial plexus are best understood in relation to its anatomy (Fig. 4-6). The brachial plexus originates from the anterior primary rami of spinal segments C5, C6, C7, C8, and T1. From these rami are formed the three trunks of the brachial plexus. The upper trunk contains fibers from spinal segments C5 and C6. The middle trunk is an extension of the undivided C7 ramus. The lower trunk is formed principally from fibers of segments C8 and T1. Each trunk divides into an anterior and a posterior division, and from these divisions the cords of the brachial plexus are formed. The lateral cord is formed from the anterior division of the upper and middle trunks, the medial cord from the anterior division of the lower trunk, and the posterior cord from the posterior division of all three trunks.

Knowledge of the origin of the peripheral nerves facilitates delineation of the site of a lesion within the plexus. Table 4-4 summarizes the origin of the major peripheral nerves from the different portions of the plexus—the spinal rami, trunks, and cords. From the undivided spinal rami arise the dorsal scapular and long thoracic nerves. The dorsal scapular nerve (C5) innervates the levator scapulae and rhomboid muscles. The long thoracic nerves (C5 to C7) innervate the serratus anterior muscles. If these muscles remain functional after an injury to the

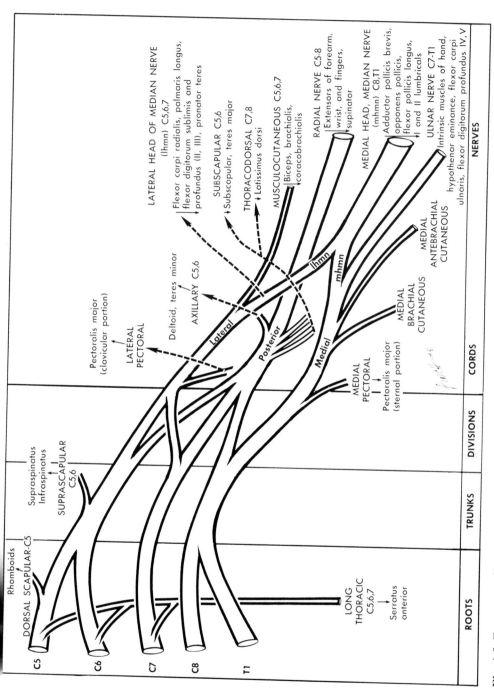

**Fig. 4-6.** Formation of brachial plexus from anterior primary rami of spinal segments C5, C6, C7, C8, and T1. These rami form the three trunks of brachial plexus: upper, middle, and lower. Each trunk then divides into an anterior and a posterior division. The divisions combine to form the lateral, medial, and posterior cords.

**Table 4-4.** Origin of major peripheral nerves from brachial plexus

| Origin | Nerve | Muscle |
|---|---|---|
| Spinal<br>Root | Dorsal scapular (C5)<br>Long thoracic (C5, 6, 7) | Rhomboid<br>Serratus anterior |
| Trunk<br>Upper | Suprascapular (C5, 6) | Supraspinatus, infraspinatus |
| Cords<br>Lateral | Musculocutaneous (C5, 6, 7)<br>Lateral head of median<br>    nerve (C5, 6, 7)<br>Lateral pectoral (C5, 6, 7) | Biceps, brachialis, coracobrachialis<br>Flexor carpi radialis, palmaris longus, flexor digitorum<br>    sublimus and profundus (II, III), pronator teres<br>Pectoralis major (clavicular portion) |
| Medial | Ulnar (C7-T1)<br><br>Medial head of median<br>    nerve (C8-T1)<br>Medial pectoral (C8-T1) | Intrinsic muscles of hand, hypothenar eminence, flexor<br>    carpi ulnaris, flexor digitorum profundus (IV, V)<br>Abductor pollicis brevis, opponens pollicis, flexor polli-<br>    cis longus, first and second lumbricals<br>Pectoralis major (sternal portion) and minor |
| Posterior | Axillary (C5, 6)<br>Radial (C5-C8)<br>Subscapular (C5, 6)<br>Thoracodorsal (C7, 8) | Deltoid, teres minor<br>Extensors of forearm, wrist and fingers, supinator<br>Subscapular, teres major<br>Latissimus dorsi |

upper brachial plexus, the lesion is distal to the origin of the spinal rami.

The suprascapular nerve, the only nerve of significance arising from the trunk (upper) level of the brachial plexus, innervates the supraspinatus and infraspinatus muscles (C5 and C6).

Most peripheral nerves originate from the various cords of the plexus. The nerves and muscles and principal muscle groups are listed in Table 4-4. The lateral cord is the source of the musculocutaneous nerve, the lateral head of the median nerve, and the lateral pectoral nerve. The medial cord forms the ulnar nerve, medial pectoral nerve, and the medial head of the median nerve. The posterior cord gives rise to the subscapular, thoracodorsal, axillary, and radial nerves. Haymaker and Woodhall (1962) have detailed the anatomy of the brachial plexus.

**BIRTH INJURY.** In the newborn infant, brachial plexus injury results from traction on an extremity during breech delivery or traction on the head and neck in vertex delivery (Adler and Patterson, 1967). The history of an infant with brachial plexus injury often reveals a complicated delivery associated with a long, hard labor. There may be other evidence of trauma, such as fracture of the clavicle or humerus or dislocation of the humerus. The affected infant usually has a high birth weight (over 9 pounds) and often the mother was heavily sedated during labor.

Brachial plexus injury is generally apparent at delivery; the manifestation depends on the level of injury to the plexus. In the most common form, injury occurs to the fifth and sixth cervical rami or upper trunk of the plexus, and the paralysis involves the upper arm, most often the right arm. This injury has been referred to as Erb's palsy or Duchenne-Erb palsy (Fig. 4-7). The infant characteristically lies with the humerus adducted and internally rotated; the elbow is extended with the forearm pronated and wrist flexed occasionally. Paralysis involves the deltoid, supraspinatus, infraspinatus, biceps, brachialis, brachioradialis, and supinator muscles and the extensors (C6 portion) of the wrists and fingers. The ipsilateral portion of the diaphragm may also be paralyzed if C4 is also involved. Biceps and radioperiosteal reflexes are absent; the grasp reflex is present. When the Moro's reflex is elicited, the movement

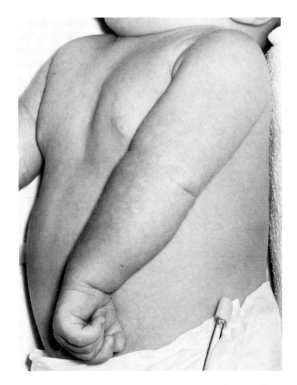

**Fig. 4-7.** Infant with Erb's palsy. Note characteristic position of arm: elbow extended and adducted, humerus internally rotated, forearm pronated, and wrist flexed. (From Wright, F. S.: Neuropathies in childhood. In Swaiman, K. F. and Wright, F. S.: The practice of pediatric neurology, St. Louis, 1975, The C. V. Mosby Co., p. 968.)

of the arms is asymmetric. Scapular winging from serratus anterior impairment is common. Sensation is normal except for a small area over the deltoid muscle and radial aspect of the forearm (distribution of the musculocutaneous nerve).

Injury of the lower trunk of the plexus, C8 and T1, causes weakness of the forearm and hand (Klumpke's paralysis), compromising the extensors of the forearm, flexors of the wrists and fingers, and intrinsic muscles of the hand. Horner's syndrome is often present on the affected side because of involvement of the sympathetic fibers that traverse the T1 primary nerve ramus on the ipsilateral side. In Klumpke's paralysis (Fig. 4-8), the child typically has the elbow flexed, forearm supinated, wrist extended, and a clawlike deformity of the hand, with hyperextension of the metacarpophalangeal joints. The triceps

reflex is depressed; the grasp reflex is absent. The response to pinprick and touch in the palm may be decreased.

A severe injury involving the entire plexus causes complete paralysis of the arm. It hangs limply from the shoulder and is areflexic, with sensory loss extending to the middle of the upper arm. In severe brachial plexus injury, associated spinal cord damage may be present with subsequent disturbance of the corticospinal tract, anterior horn cells, and sensation. The roots of the brachial plexus may be avulsed from the spinal cord, or the roots or trunk of the plexus may be severely stretched. In either case, hemorrhage may be present. In avulsion, there may be some bleeding into the subarachnoid space. Thus blood in the spinal fluid of a patient with brachial plexus injury suggests a grave prognosis. The presence of Horner's syn-

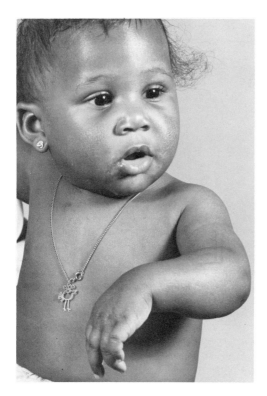

**Fig. 4-8.** Infant with lower brachial plexus injury (Klumpke's paralysis) with involvement of extensors of forearm and wrist. Note characteristic position of arm: elbow flexed, wrist flexed, and clawlike deformity of the hand.

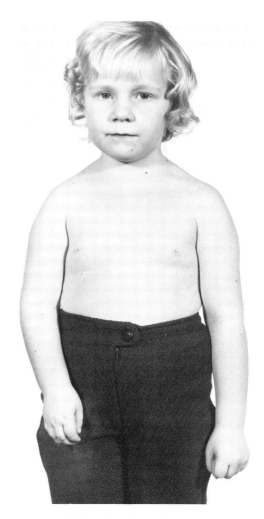

**Fig. 4-9.** Child with right Erb's palsy. Note late sequellae: deltoid muscle atrophy and shortening of arm.

drome usually indicates intraspinal avulsion of the T1 root. In severe injury the torn nerve roots may be identified on the myelogram because dye extends into a diverticulum of the spinal dura at the site of avulsion.

In an upper brachial plexus injury, the primary lesion occurs where the fifth and sixth cervical nerves join the upper trunk of the plexus. If, at examination, there is any active movement of the affected muscles, the prognosis is generally good. These children tend to improve rapidly by the end of the first week of life and often recover completely. In a follow-up study of infants with brachial plexus injury, 30% recovered by 6 months with minimal residual weakness, 55% showed fair recovery by 12 months, and 15% had severe residual weakness (Eng, 1971). Persistent abnormalities included atrophy,

weakness, atrophy of scapula and shortening of humerus, contractures, peculiar posturing of the arm in adduction, and tightness in internal rotation (Fig. 4-9).

Brachial plexus injury must be differentiated from a central nervous system lesion. A cerebral lesion usually involves the leg as well as the arm; the reflexes are present, even hyperactive, and there may be changes in the infant's awareness or alertness. A spinal cord lesion is characterized by limited bilateral weakness, sensory loss over the trunk, corticospinal tract involvement, and sometimes urinary bladder abnormalities. Skeletal fractures can be detected by appropriate x-ray studies.

TREATMENT. Treatment of upper brachial plexus paralysis requires minimal active physical therapy in the first few days of life. Seven to ten days after the injury, all joints must be put through full range of motion several times a day to maintain mobility and prevent contractures. The arm should not be rigidly immobilized. However, it is important to support the wrist with a splint to prevent flexion contractures and maintain the fingers in proper position. Electrotherapy with galvanic current stimulation to induce strong muscle contraction has been recommended to prevent muscle fibrosis. However, controlled studies are not available.

In lower brachial plexus injury, the forearm and hand should be splinted to maintain appropriate posture. However, full range of motion exercises should be performed at all joints several times a day to prevent contractures.

Surgical exploration is generally of little value because of the avulsive nature of the injury. If the lesion is located in the distal plexus, surgical intervention may be indicated for removal of a hematoma or for neurolysis of adhesions.

Intensive physical therapy is indicated when spontaneous improvement ceases. Residual deformity, such as internal rotation of the shoulder or clawhand, may necessitate surgical correction (Ransford and Hughes, 1977).

**INJURY IN OLDER CHILDREN.** In older children the brachial plexus is subject to injury from falls, dislocation of the humerus into the axilla, fracture, and pressure palsy, which may result from wearing a cast (Fig. 4-10). The diagnosis is evident from the history of the injury, and the site of involvement is determined by careful examination of the muscles innervated by the brachial plexus.

Paralytic brachial neuritis (Parsonage-Turner syndrome), an unusual form of brachial plexus dysfunction of unknown etiology, has been described in children by Magee

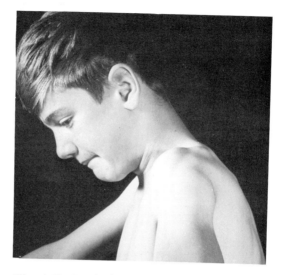

**Fig. 4-10.** Brachial plexus injury in older child manifested by atrophy of deltoid and supraspinatus muscles. Lesion was diffuse throughout the plexus but involved primarily upper trunk and posterior cord.

and DeJong (1960). This disease may appear in the first decade of life but primarily affects adults. Clinical features are often sufficiently typical to permit diagnosis. There is no evidence of fever or sign of infection. Trauma in these patients is usually minimal and is not thought to be etiologically related. The characteristic feature is sudden onset of sharp burning pain in the shoulder and neck, radiating down the arm or extending to the scapular area. Pain gradually increases in severity and then subsides within hours or days. Often after the pain has disappeared, the patient experiences weakness in the muscles of the shoulder girdle on one or both sides. Examination commonly reveals weakness of the deltoid, supraspinatus, infraspinatus, biceps, and serratus anterior muscles. However, any single muscle or combination of muscles innervated by the brachial plexus may be involved. Sensory loss is minimal and often occurs in the distribution of the axillary or radial nerves. X-ray studies of the spine are normal. CSF protein concentration is usually normal, although an elevated concentration has been reported in a few cases. The prognosis is generally good but recovery is slow.

Injury to the lower brachial plexus may also result from congenital abnormalities of structures within the thoracic outlet, such as a cervical rib, abnormalities of the thoracic vertebrae, or shortening of the scalene muscle. Such pressure palsy generally affects the lower portion of the plexus as it passes over the first rib. The child may complain of paresthesias or pain in the fingers in areas innervated by the ulnar nerve. Examination reveals weakness and sensory change in the fourth and fifth fingers. The arterial pulse may be diminished on the affected side; the examiner may accentuate this sign by raising the patient's arm to an abducted position. Treatment consists of surgical removal of the cervical rib or compressing scalene muscle.

### Neonatal injury to other nerves

In the newborn, trauma to other peripheral nerves is rare. Direct trauma to the radial nerves has produced paralysis (Feldman, 1957). The presence of necrosis in the subcutaneous fat over the course of the radial nerve suggests the diagnosis. No common etiologic factor has been determined. Examination shows wristdrop as the main result of injury to the radial nerve. Treatment consists of frequent application of passive range of motion exercise and use of a splint. Recovery occurs within 4 to 12 weeks.

Except for injection injuries, traumatic peripheral nerve paralysis in the legs during the newborn period is rare. However, injury to the obturator nerve has been reported (Craig and Clark, 1962). The typical posture is external rotation of the lower leg and abduction at the hip, with the knee flexed. Active internal rotation and adduction of the thigh are impaired, and active extension of the knee is moderately limited. There is no sensory loss. The disorder presumably results from the position of the infant in utero. Sustained traction and subsequent neural ischemia result in physiologic block. The paralysis disappears in 10 to 14 days.

## Neuropathies caused by toxic materials

Toxic neuropathy can result from a variety of materials accidentally obtained or intentionally administered as medical treatment. The history often suggests the diagnosis. Acute onset of symptoms and signs of sensory disturbance and weakness should suggest a peripheral neuropathy of toxic origin. Accidentally ingested medications, a history of pica, the use of antibiotics for an intercurrent infection, or recent immunization may point to the cause. In taking the history, the examiner should seek evidence of exposure to unusual substances, such as glue sniffing (Korobkin et al., 1975). Vincristine is a potent neurotoxin (Rosenthal and Kaufman, 1974).

Antibiotics and antimetabolites have been implicated in the etiology of peripheral neuropathy. It is often difficult to differentiate between the effect of the primary disease for which the drug is used and the toxic effect of the drug itself. A presumptive diagnosis is made on the basis of a temporal relationship between onset of peripheral neuropathy and administration of the drug followed by recovery after its discontinuance.

A severe sensory and mild motor neuropathy associated with acute ketotic diabetes mellitus has developed following rodenticide ingestion (Prosser and Karam, 1978).

### Postinjection nerve paralysis

Sciatic nerve involvement follows injection of neurotoxic materials into the buttocks of neonates, especially premature infants (Gilles and French, 1961; Hudson, McCandless, and O'Malley, 1950; Mills, 1949). Drugs clinically implicated include penicillin, streptomycin, tetanus antitoxin, B vitamins, vitamin K, bismuth, mercury, quinine, tetracycline, sulfisoxazole, and diethanolamine. Experimental intraneural injections of penicillin, peanut oil, and streptomycin have sometimes caused axonal degeneration and fibroblastic proliferation. The diagnosis should be strongly suspected if the history documents one or more gluteal injections of a

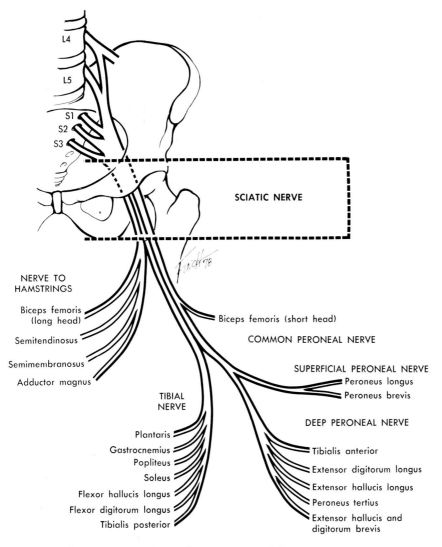

**Fig. 4-11.** Formation of sacral plexus showing origin of the sciatic nerve, its branches, and muscles innervated by the sciatic nerve.

potentially neurotoxic substance before the appearance of the sciatic paralysis.

Paralysis is apparent one to several days after the injection. Generally the infant has been treated for an intercurrent infection, such as otitis media or pneumonia. It is important to exclude infections known to be neurotoxic, such as poliomyelitis, diphtheria, and herpes zoster. In the newborn infant, paralysis may result from intra-arterial injection of a drug into the umbilical artery (San Agustin, Nitowsky, and Borden, 1962), an abnormal birth presentation, or a congenital bony anomaly (Lester and McAlister, 1970).

The causes postulated for sciatic nerve injury include drug hypersensitivity, direct penetration of the needle into the nerve, ischemia of the nerve, and direct injection of neurotoxic substance into the nerve. The last is the most probable, since it explains the fibroblastic proliferation and axonal degeneration with intraneural scarring.

Knowledge of the muscles innervated by the sciatic nerve (Fig. 4-11) is essential for clinical examination. The sciatic nerve is derived from the sacral plexus formed by the primary rami of L4, L5, S1, S2, and S3. Although the sciatic nerve forms a single trunk, it has three component parts. The most lateral portion is the common peroneal nerve. Medial to this is the tibial nerve. The nerve to the hamstring muscles occupies the most medial side of the sciatic trunk. The sciatic nerve exits from the pelvis through the greater sciatic foramen. In the buttock the sciatic nerve is protected by the gluteus maximus muscle. However, at the lower aspect of the buttock, it becomes more superficial and occupies a position between the adductor magnus and the hamstring muscles. Above the popliteal fossa the sciatic nerve divides into the tibial and common peroneal nerves.

The common peroneal nerve proceeds laterally to the posterior aspect of the head of the fibula, where it subsequently wraps around the neck of the fibula and divides into a superficial and deep peroneal nerve. The superficial peroneal nerve innervates the peroneus longus and brevis muscles. It supplies sensation to the anterior and lateral side of the leg and the dorsum of the foot. The deep peroneal nerve innervates the tibialis anterior, extensor digitorum longus, extensor hallucis longus, and extensor digitorum brevis muscles. It also supplies the peroneus tertius and first dorsal interosseous muscles. The deep peroneal nerve has a limited sensory field, confined to an area on the dorsum of the foot between the great and second toes. The nerve to the hamstring muscles supplies the adductor magnus, semimembranosus, semitendinosus, and long head of the biceps femoris muscles.

The tibial nerve innervates the gastrocnemius, plantaris, soleus, popliteus, and tibialis posterior muscles. The tibial nerve at the level of the soleus muscle continues as the posterior tibial nerve and innervates the flexor digitorum longus and flexor hallucis longus muscles. The tibial nerve supplies sensation to the sole of the foot and back of the heel, extending up the back of the leg.

CLINICAL FEATURES. Pain and dysesthesia of the foot may be present. These symptoms may be so severe that the child will not walk or allow the foot to be touched. The most common sign is footdrop. Plantar flexion and inversion of the foot are characteristic. The patient is unable to dorsiflex the foot, either against resistance or when attempting to walk on the heels.

Inability to walk on the toes is a sign of weakness of the gastrocnemius muscle. However, the only manifestation of tibial nerve involvement may be absence or diminution of the ankle tendon reflex. Weakness of the hamstring muscle is evident when the patient attempts to flex the affected leg against resistance. Hamstring muscle weakness indicates involvement of the sciatic nerve before its division into the tibial and peroneal nerves. Muscle atrophy of the leg may be severe. In sciatic nerve paralysis of long duration, growth failure of the leg and foot is striking (Fig. 4-12). Loss of pain or touch sensation may be detected over the lateral aspect of the leg, extending over the dorsum of the foot when the peroneal nerve is involved and over the sole of the foot and up the back of the leg when the tibial nerve is involved.

In infants, definitive findings on muscle or sensory testing are difficult to obtain. If the sciatic paralysis is severe, the diagnosis is apparent from the footdrop and diminished leg movement. If paralysis is mild, electromyography is helpful in diagnosis. Denervation of muscles in the distribution of the sciatic nerve is evidence of axonal degeneration. Electromyography localizes the pathologic findings to the involved portion of the sciatic nerve. Lack of clinical signs or electromyographic evidence implicating the hamstring or gastrocnemius muscles does not rule out sciatic nerve involvement, for only the peroneal portion of the sciatic nerve may be affected during its course through the buttock.

Differential diagnosis should include neurotropic infectious disease, intoxication, and spinal cord tumor. A spinal cord tumor is un-

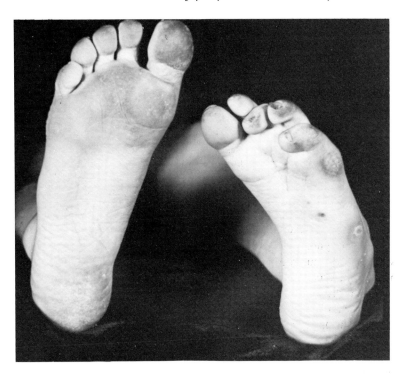

**Fig. 4-12.** Growth retardation and plantar flexion and inversion deformities of the left foot resulting from sciatic nerve injection paralysis.

likely if the lower motor unit findings are unilateral and there is no evidence of progression of symptoms or involvement of other cord structures, such as the pyramidal tract.

The prognosis for recovery is usually poor. In general, only one third of the patients with this lesion recover completely. Footdrop often persists without improvement. Deep gluteal granuloma is also a poor prognostic sign and is the only indication of surgical exploration. If no improvement occurs over 6 to 12 months, operation may be considered, although results are disappointing. The aim of surgery is to remove the granuloma and adhesions about the nerve. Physical therapy should be directed toward restoring function and preventing contractures. Surgical reconstruction by tendon transplant may be appropriate.

TREATMENT. Prevention of sciatic nerve paralysis is crucial. Injections into the gluteal muscles should not be made. In recent years, the use of the lateral thigh as an injection site has reduced the incidence of postinjection sciatic nerve paralysis.

### Postimmunization neuropathy

Neurologic complications after prophylactic immunization have been reported following the use of virtually all biologic substances (Miller and Stanton, 1954). The complications may affect any part of the nervous system from the cerebral cortex to the peripheral nerve, and although they are rare, they must be taken into account in the differential diagnosis. Peripheral neuropathy has been associated with prophylactic injections for tetanus (toxoid, antitoxin), pertussis, diphtheria, rubella, typhoid, and Schick test and with use of the triple vaccine for diphtheria, pertussis, and tetanus. Substances containing horse serum often affect the brachial plexus.

CLINICAL FEATURES. Postrubella immunization polyneuropathy presents with two types of pain syndromes (Kilroy et al., 1970; Schaffner et al., 1974). The first syndrome is characterized by paresthesias and pain, usually awakening the child at night or in the early morning hours and involving the arm, wrist, or hand. The second syndrome affects the legs. The child usually complains upon awakening in the morning of pain in the popliteal fossa and is reluctant to bend the legs. The child walks with a crouching gait on tiptoes (catcher's crouch posture). Postrubella immunization polyneuropathy syndromes occur with a mean latency of 40 days (range 7 to 99 days). The arm syndrome symptoms last up to a week and do not return. Weakness and carpal tunnel syndrome have been reported in some of the children. The leg syndrome lasts longer and may recur. In approximately 6% of children, severe recurrences of the leg syndrome may be seen as late as 33 months after immunization. Studies demonstrate decreased nerve conduction velocities at the time of the acute illness. Polyneuropathy has been noted to occur after both natural rubella infection and rubella immunization. However, the leg syndrome has not been reported after natural rubella infection. One major difference between the neuropathy of natural rubella and that following immunization is the latent period. In the natural infection, the latent period is short, with the neuropathy beginning while the exanthem is present; in the post immunization neuropathy, the latent period is variable but relatively long.

**PATHOPHYSIOLOGY.** Pathologic findings include edema of the peripheral nerves and ganglion cells followed by degeneration.

### Neuropathy associated with antibiotics and antimetabolites

Many drugs have been implicated in the etiology of peripheral neuropathy. It is frequently difficult to differentiate between the effect of a primary disease for which the drug is being used and the toxic effect of the drug. The temporal relationship of the occurrence of the peripheral neuropathy with the administration of the drug and subsequent recovery after discontinuing the drug are useful guidelines.

Peripheral neuropathy has been described primarily in adult and adolescent patients being treated with isoniazid for tuberculosis (Pegum, 1952; Jones and Jones, 1953). Clinically these patients have paresthesias in the feet and hands. They develop weakness, muscle tenderness, and often have a footdrop. Tendon reflexes are reduced in the affected limbs. The neuropathy appears to be related to the dosage, and it occurs most commonly with the use of high doses. The basic mechanism in the production of this form of peripheral neuropathy is an interference with pyridoxine (Biehl and Vilter, 1954). This form of peripheral neuropathy occurs more commonly in individuals who metabolize isoniazid slowly. Pathologically both myelinated and unmyelinated fibers show axonal degeneration (Ochoa, 1970).

In the face of renal dysfunction, the administration of certain drugs may cause a peripheral neuropathy. Treatment with nitrofurantoin has resulted in mild peripheral neuropathy characterized by pain and paresthesia, especially in the lower extremities (Collings, 1960). Patients suffering from this condition exhibited mild weakness, decreased tendon reflexes, and impaired vibration sense. Pathologically there has been degeneration of myelin sheaths.

Administration of chloramphenicol in high dosages for a prolonged period of time has resulted in blurring of vision and paresthesias. Examination has revealed optic neuritis and absent tendon reflexes (Joy, Scalettar, and Sodee, 1960).

Treatment with kanamycin may produce deafness, blurring of vision, and weakness. The weakness has resulted from a curarelike neuromuscular blockade. However, one report has been made of local injection into the extradural space in the region of the cauda equina, with resulting peripheral neuropathy characterized by severe sensory and motor loss (Freemon, Parker, and Greer, 1967). This complication has not been described following systemic therapy, but kana-mycin is potentially neurotoxic for the pe-ripheral nerves.

Vincristine used in the treatment of leu-kemia and neuroblastoma can produce a pe-ripheral neuropathy (Morress, D'Agostino, and Jarcho, 1967; Windmiller et al., 1966; and Casey et al., 1973). At times it is difficult to distinguish between the effect of the drug and the effect of the disease for which the drug is used. However, vincristine neurop-athy is clearly related to the dose of the drug. Paresthesias are the most common initial symptoms, usually starting in the hands fol-lowed later by symptoms in the feet. On ex-amination, the most common sign is loss of Achilles tendon reflex and depression of oth-er tendon reflexes. Superficial sensory loss is mild. Vibratory sensation is reduced and po-sition sense is generally normal. Weakness of the hands and leg cramps are the first signs of motor involvement. Most commonly ex-tensor muscles of the fingers and wrists are severely involved. Bilateral footdrop is com-mon and some patients are unable to walk or stand without support. Neuropathy im-proves when the drug is stopped or the dose is reduced. Weakness subsides rapidly and the tendon reflexes improve but may re-main depressed or absent. Electromyog-raphy demonstrates some reduction in maxi-mum motor conduction velocity and dener-vation characterized by fibrillation poten-tials. Compound action potential amplitude and sensory nerve action amplitude are re-duced. Axonal degeneration is the dominant pathology (McLeod and Penny, 1969).

### Neuropathy associated with heavy-metal intoxication

Although intoxication with heavy metals is less common in children than in adults, the patient's history should be carefully explored for exposure to insecticides, sprays, and dusts, and for the occurrence of pica.

Lead intoxication in children generally produces an encephalopathy. However, pe-ripheral neuropathy may precede the de-velopment of encephalitic symptoms, and if the incipient neuropathy is recognized, early treatment may prevent the development of central nervous system complications (Seto and Freeman, 1964). A history of pica, espe-cially involving the eating of paint chips or plaster, should immediately alert the physi-cian to the possibility of lead intoxication (Lin-Fu, 1973). Lead neuropathy most com-monly produces a motor neuropathy with only mild sensory impairment. In contrast to adults, children with lead intoxication more commonly present with footdrop rather than wristdrop. The patients are generally pale and irritable and have a symmetric distal weakness of both extremities. Bilateral foot-drop and wristdrop are common. Examina-tion may reveal a mild diffuse weakness as well as the symmetric distal weakness. The tendon reflexes are usually absent. Motor nerve conduction velocities are reduced.

The diagnosis is suggested by the history of pica. The presence of anemia and basophilic stippling of red blood cells and/or radiopaque material in the gut constitute strong pre-sumptive evidence. X-ray studies of long bones may disclose dense metaphyseal bands (Fig. 4-13). The diagnosis is confirmed by elevated lead concentration in the blood (greater than 60 $\mu$gm Pb/100 gm whole blood). In addition, coproporphyrin and $\Delta$-aminolevulinic acid are increased in urine. Urinary catecholamine metabolites may be altered (Silbergeld and Chisolm, 1976). Treatment consists of removal of the source of lead and the combined use of the chelat-ing agents edathamil calcium disodium (EDTA); 2, 3-dimercaptopropanol (BAL); and D-penicillamine (Chisholm 1968, 1970).

Arsenic intoxication may occur through in-advertent exposure to insecticides (Heyman et al., 1956). If intoxication is acute, nausea, vomiting, and diarrhea will predominate, while neurologic symptomatology will be minimal. Following exposure to arsenic, brawny desquamation over the trunk and ex-tremities with hyperkeratotic scaling on the palms and soles are often seen. Skin changes usually occur 1 to 6 weeks after the acute ex-posure. In cases of chronic arsenic intoxica-

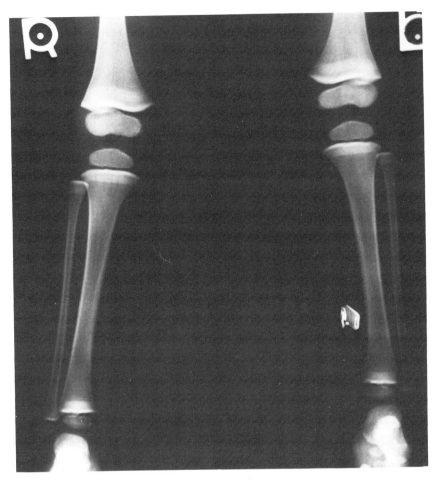

**Fig. 4-13.** Lead poisoning. Note increased thickness and density in metaphyseal zones of long bones.

tion, the neurologic symptoms predominate. Changes in the skin and nail beds occur quite late. One to three weeks following exposure, the patient may complain of paresthesias, and after several days, weakness develops in the feet and legs. Examination reveals symmetric distal weakness, often severe. Sensory examination shows a decrease of all sensations in a glove-stocking distribution. The tendon reflexes are depressed. After several weeks the patient may develop leg edema and the brawny desquamation and hyperkeratotic scaling of the skin. In addition, 6 weeks following exposure, transverse white striae are seen in the fingernails (Mees'

lines). Arsenic poisoning rarely produces cranial nerve involvement (Friedman and Olsen, 1941), and the CSF protein concentration is normal. These latter two features differentiate arsenic toxicity from the classic Guillain-Barré syndrome. The peripheral neuropathy apparently results from an interference with the metabolism of pyruvate. Pathologically there is degeneration of myelin and axons and increased fibrosis and cellularity (Chhuttani, Chawla, and Sharma, 1967). Treatment consists of administration of BAL in repeated courses or of penicillamine.

Thallium salts are used commonly in pesticides and depilatories. Thallium intoxication occurs in children following accidental ingestion of rodent poison or depilatory substances. Although a peripheral neuropathy may result from thallium intoxication, more commonly profound central nervous system symptomatology develops (Sunderman, 1967). In addition, acute gastrointestinal symptoms of vomiting, diarrhea, and abdominal pain occur within hours after the ingestion of the poison. Alopecia occurs 10 to 15 days after ingestion and constitutes a cardinal diagnostic sign of thallium intoxication.

## Neuropathies caused by toxins
### Diphtheria

Diphtheria is an acute infectious disease caused by *Corynebacterium diphtheriae*. Neurologic symptoms result from a toxin elaborated by the organism (McDonald and Kocen, 1975).

**CLINICAL FEATURES.** A classic form of polyneuropathy occurs with diphtheria (Brown, 1952), easily recognized by a typical progression of symptoms and signs. The history of a sore throat and serosanguineous nasal discharge prior to the onset of the weakness are characteristic. The initial symptoms are the development of nasal speech and swallowing difficulty, with some regurgitation of food because of paralysis of the muscles of the palate. After 3 to 4 weeks the patient may complain of blurring of vision as a result of the paralysis of the ciliary muscle with loss of accommodation. After 4 to 6 weeks the patient experiences diplopia as the paralysis involves the eye muscles. The patient then develops weakness of the extremities and trunk and may complain of numbness and tingling in the extremities.

Examination reveals exudate and membrane formation in the pharynx. Paralysis of the palate and extraocular muscles and dilated pupils with loss of accommodation are found. In addition, the patient may demonstrate the typical findings of the Guillain-Barré syndrome, with profound flaccid weakness of the extremities and diminished to absent tendon reflexes. The sensory modalities of touch, pain, vibration, and position sense are impaired. The patient may also have signs of congestive heart failure.

**LABORATORY FINDINGS.** A throat culture (special media—Loeffler's) should be taken to demonstrate the organism. Electrocardiographic changes, which occur in 50% of the patients, vary from slow conduction to an A-V conduction block. Examination of the CSF may show the characteristic increase in protein concentration with a normal cell count.

**PATHOPHYSIOLOGY.** The pathology consists of a segmental demyelinization in the anterior and posterior spinal roots with degeneration of posterior root ganglion cells (Fisher and Adams, 1956). The demyelinization is restricted to short segments, and the axon cylinders are generally spared. Wallerian degeneration is not prominent, and there is no evidence of inflammatory cells.

**TREATMENT.** Treatment consists of the administration of penicillin and diphtheria antitoxin and the general measures discussed under treatment of the Guillain-Barré syndrome, including maintenance of respiration, hydration, and nutrition. A tracheostomy may be needed if the child has difficulty in swallowing. The prognosis for recovery is good, although full recovery may be delayed for several months.

### Botulism

Botulism results from acute food poisoning caused by the ingestion of food containing toxin of *Clostridium botulinum* (Tyler, 1963; Cherington, 1974; Dowell, 1978). *Bacillus botulinus* is a gram-positive, spore-bearing, anaerobic bacillus. Heterologous toxins are produced by different strains. Seven types have been described, with types A, B, and F most often associated with human disease. The diagnosis is established by demonstration of the botulinum toxin in serum or stools of affected patients and in suspected foods. A potential source of *C. botulinum* ingestion by infants is honey.

**CLINICAL FEATURES.** The incubation period is short, usually a matter of a few hours, and the disease begins with nausea, vomiting, and diarrhea. The first neurologic symptoms are blurring of vision or double vision. Other cranial nerves are involved in rapid progression, producing dizziness and difficulty in hearing, swallowing, and speaking. The patients often complain of a dry mouth and sore throat. If these swallowing difficulties are severe, the patient develops airway obstruction and dyspnea and cyanosis. In addition, generalized muscular weakness develops, commonly appearing on the second day of illness.

On examination the patients are usually mentally alert but occasionally may be somnolent. Examination of the cranial nerves reveals fixed dilated pupils, paralysis of extraocular muscles, and ptosis. In addition, bilateral facial weakness and weakness of pharyngeal muscles occur. There is usually generalized symmetric weakness, which is initially proximal. The tendon reflexes may be normal initially but become depressed as weakness develops. No sensory involvement is present. The course of botulism is rapidly downhill. Death often ensues within 1 or 2 weeks.

Botulism has been described in infancy (Pickett et al., 1976; Berg, 1977; and Clay et al., 1977). Botulism should be suspected in any infant with acute, acquired hypotonia and weakness. Infantile botulism develops between 3 and 18 weeks of age; patients demonstrate lethargy, irritability, poor feeding, constipation, and generalized weakness. Examination reveals generalized hypotonia and weakness. The infants often are unable to suck or swallow. They have sluggish pupillary responses or dilated, fixed pupils. Bilateral ptosis or complete external ophthalmoplegia may be present. Facial diplegia, poor suck, and an absent gag reflex demonstrate involvement of cranial nerves VII, IX, and X. In addition to the abnormal pupillary responses, delayed gastric emptying and paralytic ileus represent further autonomic nervous system involvement.

The differential diagnosis of botulism should include Guillain-Barré syndrome, myasthenia gravis, tick paralysis, diphtheria, poliomyelitis, heavy metal intoxication, Leigh's syndrome, polymyositis, polyneuropathy, organophosphate poisoning, neomycin sulfate toxicity, belladonna poisoning, excessive magnesium, and deficient calcium.

**LABORATORY FINDINGS.** Results of routine laboratory studies, including CSF examination, are normal. An electrocardiogram may show T wave abnormalities. Electromyographic studies are important in diagnosis. Motor nerve conduction velocity is normal; however, the amplitude of the evoked compound muscle action potential is reduced. Needle electrode examination shows small-amplitude, short-duration, numerous potentials for the amount of contraction. Occasional fibrillation and positive sharp waves are seen (Clay et al., 1977). Repetitive nerve stimulation yields two types of responses dependent upon the severity of clinical manifestations. In severely affected individuals, a low-amplitude motor action potential is seen with a decremental response at low rates of stimulation and an insignificant incremental response at high rates of stimulation. In mildly affected patients, the evoked compound muscle action potential amplitude is normal with no decremental response at low rates of stimulation and a significant incremental response at higher rates of stimulation (Oh, 1977).

**TREATMENT.** Treatment should be aimed at providing respiratory support as needed. The infants may require ventilation for periods of weeks to months. The outcome of infantile botulism has been uniformly good. Most infants survive with normal development. Death has been reported in adults but rarely in infants. An antitoxin has not been effective in botulism related to types A and B but may be effective in type E botulism. Guanidine hydrochloride has been used in adult patients, but unfortunately it appears to be effective only in extraocular and limb paralysis with little effect on the paralysis of the respiratory muscles (Cherington, 1974).

Guanidine appears to enhance the release of acetylcholine from nerve terminals.

## Neuropathies due to infections
### Herpes

Herpes zoster is a viral infection that produces weakness in association with a vesicular eruption affecting the peripheral nerves in the distribution of the eruption (Kendall, 1957; Dayan, Ogul, and Graveson, 1972; Thomas and Howard, 1972; Gardner-Thorpe, Foster, and Barwick, 1976). Herpes zoster results from activation of a latent varicella virus (Weller and Witton, 1958). This infection may follow or be associated with spinal cord trauma, spinal cord tumor, lymphatic leukemia, and Hodgkin's disease. Herpes simplex infection may also involve the peripheral nervous system (Layzer and Conant, 1974).

The incubation period ranges from 7 to 21 days. The patient experiences fever and malaise with pain or increased skin sensitivity over the distribution of the affected nerve. After several days, a rash appears that develops into groups of vesicles. The vesicular eruption often appears at the midline and spreads distally in a sensory dermatome pattern distribution. Lesions are found commonly on the trunk. The arms and legs may be involved, but the lesions rarely go below the knee or elbow.

The nervous system may be involved at several anatomic levels. Paralysis may be localized to a single nerve because of herpetic involvement of the anterior root. The spinal cord may be involved, resulting in a transverse myelitis with spasticity and sensory impairment. Encephalitis can be associated with herpes zoster. Lastly, there may be a Guillain-Barré syndrome, with flaccid paralysis developing shortly after the appearance of the rash (Knox, Levy, and Simpson, 1961).

Pathologically there is inflammation and necrosis of the posterior root ganglia, resulting in wallerian degeneration of the peripheral nerves. In a series of sural nerve biopsies at varying intervals after the onset of herpes zoster, the earliest pathologic changes were focal wallerian degeneration, resulting from inflammation of the ganglia and nerve fibers (Zacks, Langfitt, and Elliott, 1964). In addition, there is loss of axon cylinders and degeneration of myelin. The late stage of the zoster infection is characterized by proliferation of collagen and the formation of fibrous tissue with few remaining myelinated fibers.

## Neuropathies associated with metabolic diseases
### Diabetes

Diabetic neuropathy refers to several different disorders of the peripheral nervous system (Thomas, 1973). The most common form is a slowly progressive, symmetric, distal sensory polyneuropathy involving the lower extremities. Less common are the mononeuropathy and multiple mononeuropathies, including the cranial nerve lesions, isolated peripheral nerve lesions, and mononeuropathy multiplex, in which the onset is more rapid, motor involvement is more severe than sensory involvement, and recovery is the rule. Autonomic neuropathy is a symmetric polyneuropathy.

Pathologically, distal symmetric polyneuropathy is characterized by loss of myelinated and unmyelinated fibers, segmental demyelinization, proliferation of Schwann cells, and increase in connective tissue (Thomas and Lascelles, 1966; Thomas and Eliasson, 1975).

Peripheral neuropathy with predominant sensory symptoms and signs is commonly seen in the adult diabetic. Several studies of diabetic children have attempted to determine the nature and incidence of a peripheral neuropathy. Lawrence and Locke (1963) in a study of 15 diabetic children, found evidence on physical examination for a peripheral neuropathy in 13 patients. The nerve dysfunction was characterized by a peripheral polyneuropathy with a bilaterally symmetric involvement of the distal portion of the lower extremities manifested by decreased or absent ankle tendon reflexes, mild to moderate weakness of the small muscles of the feet, and a stocking-type sensory loss in the lower extremities. In 2 children, there was a bilateral motor mononeuropathy affecting only the common peroneal nerve.

Complete nerve conduction studies and neurologic examinations were performed in a large series of 107 unselected diabetic children (Gamstorp et al., 1966). Eleven patients were considered to have evidence of peripheral nerve disease, 23 had equivocal findings, and 73 had no demonstrable abnormalities. The diabetic children with peripheral neuropathy characteristically had late onset, long duration, and generally poor control of their diabetes. The incidence of peripheral neuropathy was thus approximately 10%. A study of 85 diabetic children revealed abnormal peroneal nerve conduction velocity in 9% of the patients. In these cases, there was no clinical evidence of neuropathy, retinopathy, nephropathy, or other diabetic complications generally associated with vascular change (Eeg-Olofsson and Petersen, 1966).

These studies of diabetic children regarding the presence of a peripheral neuropathy have delineated two groups: one group with overt clinical signs and symptoms of a peripheral neuropathy, and a second subclinical group in which peripheral neuropathy is diagnosed only by electrodiagnostic studies of nerve conduction velocity. The latter group may become symptomatic with increased duration of the diabetes.

A decrease in nerve myoinositol concentration has been implicated in the pathogenesis of diabetic polyneuropathy (Winegrad and Greene, 1976).

### Acute intermittent porphyria

Acute intermittent porphyria is a rare inborn error of metabolism inherited as an autosomal dominant and characterized by an increased level of Δ-aminolevulinic acid synthetase with increased excretion of Δ-aminolevulinic acid and porphobilinogen (Tschudy, 1965). The disease is unusual before puberty, although several childhood cases have been reported (Barltrop, 1964; Bleifer and Alphas, 1959). The youngest patient reported was an 8-month-old infant (Lysaught and McCleery, 1955).

The classic clinical manifestations include acute, severe colicky abdominal pain, neurologic manifestations, and psychiatric disturbances. The neurologic manifestations result from both central and peripheral nervous system impairment. In the peripheral neuropathy, motor weakness predominates, although all sensory modalities may be involved. The motor weakness is generally asymmetric and scattered. However, the disease may produce a generalized flaccid paralysis, with facial diplegia resembling Guillain-Barré syndrome. The upper limbs are often affected initially and proximal muscles may be more involved than distal ones. Paresthesias may precede or coincide with the weakness. The tendon reflexes are diminished or absent. Cranial nerve dysfunction is common, involving cranial nerves III, VII, X, and rarely V, XI, and XII. Urinary retention or incontinence may develop. Mental changes are common and include confusion, delirium, and hallucinations (Ackner et al., 1962; Wochnik-Dyjas, Niewiadomska, and Kostrzewska, 1978).

Pathologically the peripheral nerves show axonal degeneration and patchy demyelinization (Cavanagh and Mellick, 1965). Pathologic changes have been noted in the anterior horn cell of the spinal cord with loss of nerve cells and chromatolysis.

No treatment is known. Acute intermittent porphyria may be triggered by administration of barbiturates and other anticonvulsants such as phenytoin, methsuximide, and ethotoin. Drugs must be withheld as much as possible from patients with acute intermittent porphyria.

The diagnosis is made clinically by the presence of acute abdominal pain and bizarre neurologic and psychiatric manifestations and by determination of excessive urinary excretion of porphobilinogen (Watson and Schwartz, 1941), uroporphyrin, and Δ-aminolevulinic acid. Electromyography shows signs of denervation with normal motor nerve conduction velocity.

The differential diagnosis includes the Guillain-Barré syndrome and lead poisoning.

### Uremia

Polyneuropathy has been described in patients with chronic renal failure. Clinically uremic polyneuropathy is rare in childhood; it occurs more frequently in the adult patient. Uremic neuropathy in adults is related to the duration and severity of renal failure. Children differ from adults in that there is no correlation between the severity of renal failure and the nerve conduction velocity (Arbus et al., 1975). The peripheral neuropathy is characterized by dysesthesias, especially painful burning sensations in the feet, followed by symmetric sensory loss and a slowly progressive weakness. Involvement is more distal than proximal. The pathologic lesion is an axonal degeneration and secondary demyelinization (Dyck et al., 1971). In children with chronic renal failure, although clinical symptomatology has not been apparent, decreased nerve conduction velocity and neural hypoexcitability have been documented (Wright and McQuillen, 1973) by electrodiagnostic studies (Asbury, Victor, and Adams, 1963). Parathyroid hormone has been implicated as a uremic toxin (Avram, Feinfeld, and Huatuco, 1978).

### Vitamin deficiency

Vitamin $B_1$, or thiamine, is a water-soluble vitamin that functions as a coenzyme in carbohydrate metabolism. Deficiency of this vitamin in either the mother or infant produces congenital or infantile beriberi disease (Van Gelder and Darby, 1944). This disease is rare in the United States. Congenital beriberi occurs in infants born of mothers who are severely deficient in thiamine. Infantile beriberi occurs generally within the first 3 months of life and is characterized by anorexia, vomiting, and lethargy (Varavithya, Dhanamitta, and Valyasevi, 1975).

On examination, the infant is pale and listless and often has edema of the extremities. Cranial nerve examination may show ptosis and optic atrophy. The laryngeal nerves may be paralyzed, resulting in a characteristic hoarse cry. The heart may be enlarged with evidence of cardiac failure. The infant shows generalized hypotonia and weakness. The tendon reflexes are depressed or absent. Sensation is normal.

The diagnosis may be suspected on the basis of a history of poor dietary intake in either the mother or infant. Because thiamine functions as a coenzyme in carbohydrate metabolism, a deficiency of this vitamin results in elevation of the serum pyruvic acid concentration. The elevated serum pyruvic acid concentration is presumptive evidence for thiamine deficiency. In addition, thiamine deficiency may be diagnosed by finding decreased activity of red blood cell transketolase (Dreyfus, 1962). Fibroblast transketolase abnormality has been described in Wernicke-Korsakoff syndrome with neuropathy (Blass and Gibson, 1977). Pathologically the peripheral nerves show degeneration of myelin and the axon cylinder.

Pernicious anemia is a macrocytic anemia produced by the deficiency of vitamin $B_{12}$, resulting from failure of gastric mucosa secretion of intrinsic factor (Lampkin and Schubert, 1968; McNicholl and Egan, 1968). There are congenital and juvenile forms of pernicious anemia as well as the more common adult forms. In the adult form of the disease, the characteristic features are absence of intrinsic factor, achlorhydria, gastric mucosal atrophy, and presence of antibodies to gastric mucosa and to intrinsic factor. Congenital pernicious anemia differs from the adult form by the early age of onset, usually around 1 year of age; the absence of intrinsic factor but normal gastric mucosa and acidity; and absence of antibodies to intrinsic factor or to gastric mucosa. The juvenile form may be associated with either the features of the congenital type or typical adult features. The adult form of pernicious anemia may be associated with endocrine abnormalities, especially involving the thyroid, parathyroid, and adrenal glands.

Pernicious anemia may produce profound neurologic dysfunction, including abnormalities of the spinal cord, brain, or peripheral nerve. The brunt of the disease appears to affect the spinal cord, especially the dorsal and lateral columns, producing a subacute combined degeneration. The neurologic abnormalities in childhood may be mild, with only the absence of tendon reflexes and diminished vibration and position sense. In the congenital form of pernicious anemia, the characteristic clinical findings are intermittent vomiting and lethargy. There may be a regression in motor development, with loss of previously acquired motor skills. The infants often show a striking failure of growth. A more severe neurologic involvement may occur in an unrecognized case of pernicious anemia treated only with folic acid. Pearson and associates (1964) have described an infant who developed severe progressive lethargy and irritability that resulted in coma, with absence of all reflexes and Cheyne-Stokes respiration. These neurologic abnormalities responded dramatically to the intramuscular injection of vitamin $B_{12}$.

Pathologically there is degeneration and demyelinization of the spinal cord, especially the dorsal and lateral columns. The peripheral nerves may undergo degeneration of the myelin sheaths.

The diagnosis is suspected from bone marrow biopsy with demonstration of a megaloblastic anemia. The demonstration of vitamin $B_{12}$ deficiency, secondary to absence of intrinsic factor, may be determined by the Schilling test, which measures the absorption or excretion of vitamin $B_{12}$, both with and without added intrinsic factor. In childhood, the neurologic symptoms show striking improvement on treatment with vitamin $B_{12}$. However, many of the patients described have been mentally retarded, and this aspect has not changed appreciably with treatment.

Aronsson and associates (1968) described a patient who developed a rapidly progressive polyneuritis with complete paralysis of all extremities, which responded to large doses of B vitamins. This patient had severe tyrosinosis and had been treated with a diet low in tyrosine and phenylalanine for a prolonged period. The neurologic symptoms appeared to be related to B vitamin deficiency, although the exact B vitamin compound was not delineated.

### Abetalipoproteinemia (Bassen-Kornzweig syndrome)

Abetalipoproteinemia is a disorder characterized by progressive ataxia, retinitis pigmentosa, acanthocytosis (erythrocytes with thorny projections), and low to absent serum beta-lipoproteins (Bassen and Kornzweig, 1950; Gotto et al., 1971; Schwartz et al., 1963). A basic defect is failure to synthesize an apolipoprotein required for the synthesis of very-low-density lipoprotein, low-density lipoprotein, and chylomicrons.

CLINICAL FEATURES. Clinically the early history is dominated by symptoms of intestinal malabsorption, namely, loose, bulky, foul-smelling stools, as well as by slow growth. Neurologic symptoms appear as early as 2 years of age but are more commonly seen after 5 years of age. The cardinal neurologic symptom is progressive ataxia. The patients also develop progressive weakness in the lower extremities.

Neurologic examination may reveal generalized weakness, ptosis, and weakness of extraocular muscles, facial muscles, and tongue, with some twitching movements of the tongue. Retinal changes include pigmentary deposition with macular degeneration. The nystagmus present is probably related to the retinal changes and scotomata. Tendon reflexes are absent. Generalized muscular weakness and muscle wasting may be severe. Sensory examination reveals a profound loss of vibration and position sense. Superficial sensation is also compromised, but to a lesser degree, and touch, pain, and temperature sensations are diminished in a glove-stocking distribution. Finger-to-nose movements, heel-to-shin movements, and rapid alternating movements are all impaired. Truncal ataxia is common. It is difficult to separate cerebellar from posterior column ataxia, because the posterior columns contribute a major portion of the input into the cerebellum; however, the presence of truncal ataxia and titubation are generally considered signs of cerebellar involvement. Babinski's signs may be present. As a result of these neurologic deficits, a wide-based waddling ataxic gait with moderate lordosis ensues. Kyphoscoliosis occurs in about half of the cases, and a pes cavus deformity may be present. Cardiomegaly, arrhythmia, systolic murmur, and congestive heart failure have been described in a few patients.

In the differential diagnosis, Friedreich's ataxia most clearly resembles abetalipoproteinemia. Several other diseases should also be considered, namely, acute intermittent porphyria, Refsum's disease, Fabry's disease, Tangier disease, and hypertrophic interstitial neuritis.

Critchley and associates (1968) have reviewed other syndromes with acanthocytosis and neurologic impairment but without abetalipoproteinemia. The neurologic dysfunction in the adult patient consists of cerebellar ataxia or chorea, while a syndrome closely resembling Friedreich's ataxia is described in a child. Another variation of neurologic disease with acanthocytosis but without change in beta-lipoprotein concentration has been described by Levine and associates (1968). This disease is characterized by neuronal involvement of the central nervous system, including the anterior horn cell and also affecting the dorsal root ganglion cell. The patients are asymptomatic during childhood but have mild weakness with atrophy of the shoulder girdle muscles. The tendon reflexes are decreased or absent.

**LABORATORY FINDINGS.** Laboratory examination reveals several characteristic abnormalities (Kayden, 1972). The red blood cells show spur formation known as acanthocytosis. There is evidence for malabsorption of fats and fat-soluble vitamins. The most characteristic finding is low to absent serum beta-lipoproteins, with markedly reduced serum cholesterol and phospholipids. The concentrations of serum triglycerides are also low. Electromyography reveals fibrillation

and positive wave potentials, and the interference pattern is reduced. Muscle biopsy tissue is normal. The electromyographic and muscle biopsy results do not correlate well with the severe muscle wasting in these patients.

**PATHOPHYSIOLOGY.** The major pathologic changes occur in the spinal cord and cerebellum. Pathologic study (Sobrevilla, Goodman, and Kane, 1964) has shown demyelinization in posterior columns, spinocerebellar pathways, and cerebellum. Loss of anterior horn cells and focal areas of demyelinization in peripheral nerves have also been described.

**GENETICS.** Abetalipoproteinemia is inherited in an autosomal recessive pattern.

**TREATMENT.** Dietary fat restriction and dietary supplementation with fat-soluble vitamins are the only available means of therapy (Muller, Lloyd, and Bird, 1977).

### Familial alpha-lipoprotein deficiency (Tangier disease)

Recurrent neuropathy (Engel et al., 1967; Bale et al., 1971) has been reported in children with alpha-lipoprotein deficiency. The recurrent neuropathy takes the form of fluctuating asymmetric sensory involvement predominantly in the lower extremities, with progressive development of weakness in both distal and proximal muscles. The patient complains of numbness and tingling distally in the extremities; this numbness is followed by weakness. The sensory or motor symptoms generally lessen in time; the weakness also improves, but the patients are left with some mild residual weakness. Children with this disease have unusually large orange-colored tonsils. Intermittent diarrhea may occur.

On examination the striking findings are the presence of hepatosplenomegaly, large tonsils, and lymphadenopathy secondary to accumulation of cholesteryl esters. On neurologic examination there is asymmetric weakness in both the proximal and distal muscle groups associated with minimal muscular atrophy. Pain and temperature may be diminished in the fingers and toes. The tendon reflexes are absent or severely depressed (Kocen, et al., 1967). Electromyography and muscle biopsy are both consistent with the pattern of denervation of muscles. However, the motor nerve conduction velocity is normal or mildly slow. The CSF protein concentration is slightly elevated. Nerve biopsy demonstrates decreased numbers of axons without evidence for axonal degeneration or segmental demyelinization (Kocen et al., 1973).

The characteristic laboratory findings in Tangier disease include low plasma cholesterol content with normal to elevated triglycerides. If these changes are present in the serum, then the alpha-lipoprotein content should be determined. In Tangier disease, the serum alpha-lipoprotein (high-density lipoprotein, HDL) is markedly decreased or absent. There is evidence for cholesterol ester accumulation in the bone marrow and on rectal biopsy. Radioimmunoassay has demonstrated a markedly decreased apolipoprotein A-1 concentration and distribution (Henderson et al., 1978). Since structural abnormalities of the major HDL apoproteins have not been detected, abnormal regulation of synthesis or catabolism may be the basis of the biochemical defect in Tangier disease. Instability of chylomicrons or very-low-density lipoproteins may enhance their phagocytosis by macrophages of the reticuloendothelial system (Herbert et al., 1978). In the differential diagnosis of recurrent neuropathy, Refsum's disease and intermittent porphyria should be considered.

## Metachromatic leukodystrophy (sulfatide lipidosis)

Metachromatic leukodystrophy is a disease of lipid metabolism, characterized by demyelinization and intracellular storage of sulfatide (Austin, 1958). The basic enzymatic defect is an absence of a heat-labile sulfatase (sulfatase A) that prevents the conversion of sulfatide to cerebroside, resulting in increased sulfatide storage (Austin et al., 1964). The lipid accumulates in the brain, peripheral nerve, liver, and kidney. Because of the presence of the abnormal lipid in both the central and peripheral nervous systems, the clinical picture presents the combination of upper motor unit and lower motor unit disease. Classically in the infantile form of metachromatic leukodystrophy, the infant progresses normally for a period of 1 to 2 years and then undergoes progressive deterioration. The onset is often characterized by a decrease in the awareness of surroundings and by an unsteady gait. The gait disturbance results from cerebellar as well as peripheral nerve involvement. There is progressive deterioration, with worsening of the gait difficulty, loss of language function, progressive intellectual deterioration, and late in the illness, spasticity, tremors, and convulsions. A characteristic pattern on neurologic examination is the presence of signs of upper motor unit disease, namely Babinski's signs with or without spasticity, and hypoactive or absent tendon reflexes. A cherry-red spot is occasionally seen on examination of the fundus.

In the older child, metachromatic leukodystrophy often begins with progressive gait disturbance. Intellectual deterioration, manifested by worsening school performance, soon becomes apparent. Spasticity, increased tendon reflexes, clonus, and Babinski's signs characterize the neurologic examination. A decrease or absence of tendon reflexes, as evidence of peripheral nerve involvement, occurs late in the disease.

Nerve conduction studies (Yudell et al., 1967) in patients with metachromatic leukodystrophy have shown a marked reduction in the motor nerve conduction velocity, consistent with segmental demyelinization, in a high percentage of the patients. At the present time, the best diagnostic test is the demonstration of absence of arylsulfatase A activity in the urine or in white blood cells. Another useful test is the demonstration of metachromatic material in sural nerve biopsy tissue and pathologic features of segmental demyelinization as well as a decrease in the number of myelinated fibers. These patients also have a nonfunctioning gallbladder.

The arylsulfatase A test has been useful in diagnosing metachromatic leukodystrophy in asymptomatic siblings of children known to have the condition (Greene, Hug, and Schubert, 1967) and in detecting the carrier state in parents (Dubois, Harzer, and Baumann, 1977).

Treatment with a diet deficient in vitamin A has been suggested (Melchior and Clausen, 1968) but has not been beneficial. Infusion of arylsulfatase A or stimulation of residual activity have been unsuccessful.

### Refsum's disease (heredopathia atactica polyneuritiformis, HMSN IV)

Refsum's disease (Refsum, 1946; Refsum, Salomonsen, and Skatvedt, 1949) is characterized by anorexia, unsteady gait, progressive ichthyosis, and sensorineural hearing deficit. Three of the four children originally described were born of a consanguineous marriage, indicating a recessive inheritance.

**CLINICAL FEATURES.** Examination of the patient shows typical retinitis pigmentosa, deafness, ataxia, polyneuropathy with distal weakness and loss of tendon reflexes, muscular atrophy, and ichthyosis. Mild impairment of touch is often the only sensory change. Intellectual development may be retarded.

**LABORATORY FINDINGS.** The cerebrospinal fluid manifests an albuminocytologic dissociation with a marked increase in total protein. The electrocardiogram is abnormal, with a prolonged Q-T segment and widened QRS complex. Nerve conduction velocity is reduced.

**PATHOPHYSIOLOGY.** Refsum's disease is a disorder of fatty acid metabolism with storage of 3, 7, 11, 15-tetramethyl hexadecanoic acid (phytanic acid) (Richterich, Van Mechelen, and Rossi, 1965). In addition to the preceding clinical findings, the laboratory analysis identifies the disease with a specific metabolic abnormality. Urinary sediment contains epithelial cells and, occasionally, casts that, when stained with Sudan red, show fat drop-

lets both free and within epithelial cells. Chemical analysis of liver, kidney, fat, and skeletal muscle shows large amounts of phytanic acid in brain and systemic organs. Metabolic studies have shown that the accumulation of phytanic acid results from the failure to oxidize exogenous phytanic acid originating in the diet.

Pathologically, interstitial hypertrophic changes with onion-bulb formation, lipid deposits, and intramitochondrial inclusions in Schwann's cells characterize Refsum's disease (Fardeau and Engel, 1969).

**TREATMENT.** Treatment is directed at reduction in the serum phytanic acid level by dietary restriction of phytanic acid (Lundberg et al., 1972; Sahgal and Olsen, 1975).

### Ataxia-telangiectasia

Ataxia-telangiectasia, an autosomal recessively transmitted disease, is characterized by progressive cerebellar ataxia beginning by 2 to 4 years of age, oculocutaneous telangiectasia, and frequent sinopulmonary infections (Boder and Sedgwick, 1963). A deficiency of immunoglobulin A is thought to be the basis for frequent infections (Hansen et al., 1977). The main neurologic abnormalities are those of cerebellar ataxia with bilateral intention tremor, truncal ataxia, titubation, and choreoathetosis. The tendon reflexes are generally depressed or absent. Vibration and position sense may be impaired in other patients. Sensory nerve action potentials may be diminished or absent (Dunn, 1973).

The major pathologic findings (Solitare and Lopez, 1967; DeLeon, Grover, and Huff, 1976) are cerebellar cortical atrophy, demyelinization of the posterior columns, and demyelinization of the dorsal spinocerebellar tracts of the spinal cord.

Robinson (1962) has described a patient with ataxia-telangiectasia, severe muscular weakness, hypotonic extremities, and minimal muscular atrophy of the arms and shoulder. Study of a muscle biopsy was reported to be consistent with severe neuropathy. Other clinical descriptions and pathologic studies of patients with ataxia-telangiectasia suggest that peripheral nerve involvement occurs in the older patients.

### Globoid cell leukodystrophy (Krabbe's disease)

Globoid cell leukodystrophy is a progressive degenerative disease of infancy. This disease, originally described by Krabbe (1916) is inherited as an autosomal recessive trait. The infant develops generalized spasticity, more pronounced in the lower extremities, between 3 and 6 months of age. Feeding becomes difficult, and the infant undergoes progressive loss of awareness of the surroundings. Tonic spasms may be precipitated by sudden noise or bright lights. Examination in the early stage of the disease reveals brisk tendon reflexes and bilateral Babinski's signs. The infant gradually assumes a posture of decorticate rigidity. There may be optic atrophy. In the late stages of the disease, rigidity is replaced by flaccid paralysis with decreased or absent tendon reflexes reflecting peripheral nerve involvement. Motor nerve conduction velocity is reduced. CSF protein concentration is increased.

Peripheral nerve changes have been described including altered myelinization and segmental demyelination (Lake, 1968; Dunn et al., 1969). On light microscopy there is a reduced number of myelinated nerve fibers. Electron microscopic studies demonstrate Schwann cell cytoplasm inclusions, indicating a primary metabolic disorder of the Schwann cell (Bischoff and Ulrich, 1969). The peripheral nerve involvement appears to be a somewhat minor component clinically but does point to the significance of the enzyme deficiency. Biochemical studies demonstrate a deficiency in the enzyme galactocerebrosidase (galactosyl ceramide beta-galactosidase) (Suzuki and Suzuki, 1970).

### Chédiak-Higashi syndrome

The Chédiak-Higashi syndrome is characterized by defective pigmentation of hair and skin, pancytopenia, increased susceptibility to infection, and lymphoreticular malignancy. Mental retardation, seizures, and muscular weakness are among the predominant neurologic manifestations. Lockman and associates (1967) reported a severe peripheral neuropathy related to the accumulation of Chédiak-Higashi granules in the Schwann's cells of the peripheral nerve fibers. The patient described had the typical features of the Chédiak-Higashi syndrome. Over a period of 2 years, the patient developed moderate to severe weakness of the distal muscles of the hands and feet. The tendon reflexes, which were initially present, were lost. No sensory impairment could be detected. The nerve conduction velocity decreased progressively, the weakness became generalized, and there was mild atrophy of the small muscles of the hand.

Light microscopy revealed scattered atrophic muscle fibers. Ultrastructural examination of peripheral nerve revealed massive cytoplasmic particles in giant abnormal lysosomes. The particles were closely associated with the myelin sheaths and unmyelinated nerve fibers.

### Giant axonal neuropathy

Giant axonal neuropathy is a generalized disorder of cytoplasmic microfilaments. The disease begins at 2 to 3 years of age with a clumsy gait and progressive weakness in the legs, arms, and hands. Sensory symptoms are absent (Berg, Rosenberg, and Asbury, 1972; Carpenter et al., 1974).

Most patients have unusual kinky hair (Bolthauser, Bischoff, and Isler, 1977). The muscles subserved by the cranial nerves are normal. Tendon reflexes are absent. The gait is broad-based and ataxic, often with a bilateral footdrop. Moderate to severe weakness is present in the arms and legs, greater in the distal muscles. Sensation is impaired distally in a glove-stocking distribution. Vibration perception and position sense are moderately impaired.

Electromyography reveals normal or increased-duration, high-amplitude motor unit potentials with no evidence of denervation.

| | Peroneal muscular atrophy (HMSN I)* | Hypertrophic interstitial neuritis (HMSN III) | Refsum's disease (HMSN IV) | Friedreich's ataxia | Abetalipoproteinemia |
|---|---|---|---|---|---|
| Onset | Childhood | Infancy | Childhood | Childhood | Childhood |
| Heredity | Dominant | Recessive | Recessive | Recessive | Recessive |
| Course | Progressive | Progressive | Progressive | Progressive | Progressive |
| Symptoms | Awkward walking and running | Slow motor development, ataxia, muscle cramps, double vision, deafness | Anorexia, rough scaly skin, night blindness, deafness, stumbling, unsteady gait | Frequent falling and stumbling, writing difficulty, indistinct speech | Bulky, foul stools, unsteady gait, scotomata |
| **Signs** | | | | | |
| Cranial nerves | Normal | Miosis, nystagmus, deafness | Retinitis pigmentosa | Normal (optic atrophy late) nystagmus | Retinitis pigmentosa, nystagmus, ptosis, strabismus |
| Tendon reflexes | Decrease with age | Areflexic | Areflexic | Areflexic | Areflexic |
| Weakness and atrophy | Anterior tibial and peroneal muscles (hands late) | Distally all limbs, nerves enlarged | Distally, all limbs | Minimal | Generalized |
| Sensory | Normal (slight decrease in position and vibration sense) | Severe loss of all modalities | Variable | Position and vibration sense impaired | Position and vibration markedly impaired, variable loss of touch, pain, and temperature |
| Babinski's sign | Absent | Absent | Absent | Present | Present |
| Skeletal | Pes cavus, hammer toe | Clubfoot, kyphoscoliosis | Short metatarsal | Scoliosis, pes cavus, hammer toe | Scoliosis |
| Cerebellar signs | Absent | Absent | Present—mild | Present | Present |
| **Laboratory findings** | | | | | |
| Blood | | | Phytanic acid increased | | Acanthocytes, low beta-lipoprotein, triglycerides, and cholesterol |
| CSF | Normal | Protein increased | Protein increased | Normal | Normal |
| EKG | Normal | | Prolonged Q-T, wide PRS | Inverted T wave, arrhythmias | May have arrhythmias |
| Motor nerve conduction velocity | Low | Very low | Low | Normal to low | Normal |

*HMSN—Hereditary motor and sensory neuropathy.

Absent responses from the peroneal and posterior tibial nerve stimulation were noted initially.

Sural nerve biopsy demonstrates giant axons filled with packed neurofilaments, segmental demyelinization, and onion-bulb formation (Koch et al., 1977; Peiffer et al., 1977).

## Neuropathies associated with hereditary disease

### Peroneal muscular atrophy (Charcot-Marie-Tooth disease) (HMSN I)

Peroneal muscular atrophy was clearly delineated as an entity in 1886 by the publications of Charcot and Marie in France and Tooth in England (Brody and Wilkins, 1967). Dyck and Lambert (1968a) and Dyck (1975) have discussed and classified the neural muscular atrophies under the general term of hereditary motor and sensory neuropathies (HMSN) (Madrid, Bradley, and Davis, 1977). Dyck has defined seven categories (HMSN I-VII) based on nature of inheritance, age at onset, symptomatology, population of neurons affected, pathology, and biochemical abnormality (Table 4-5).

CLINICAL FEATURES. Peroneal muscular atrophy often appears in the second decade of life, although some difficulty in walking and running may be evident earlier. Foot deformities date from early childhood. Symptoms result from muscle atrophy and weakness in the lower extremities. However, the atrophic process is not limited to muscles innervated by the peroneal nerves but involves the muscles of the lower portion of the thigh and later the small muscles of the hands.

Positive findings are confined to the extremities. There are no abnormalities of the cranial nerves, such as optic atrophy, retinitis pigmentosa, nystagmus, or deafness. The absence of these cranial nerve abnormalities differentiates peroneal muscular atrophy from Refsum's disease, hypertrophic interstitial neuritis (Dejerine-Sottas disease), Friedreich's ataxia, and abetalipoproteinemia.

The physical appearance of the patient

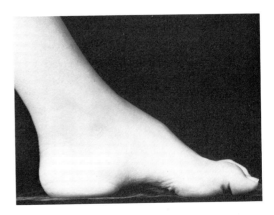

**Fig. 4-14.** Peroneal muscular atrophy. Note mild pes cavus.

suggests the diagnosis. Bilateral symmetric atrophy of the legs in the distribution of the peroneal muscles produces a stork-leg appearance. The patient often has talipes equinovarus or pes cavus, implicating involvement of the intrinsic foot muscles. Because of anterior tibialis and peroneal muscle weakness and abnormalities of the feet (hammer toes, pes cavus) (Fig. 4-14), the patient often walks with a steppage gait. The peroneal, anterior tibial, and sometimes the quadriceps muscles are weak. Tendon reflexes are absent or markedly reduced. Enlargement of the peripheral nerves is palpable in one quarter of affected individuals. As the disease progresses, weakness of the small muscles of the hands becomes evident and clawhand may develop. In rare instances, the disease begins in the hands. The disease progresses slowly and may plateau at any stage but does not appear to shorten life.

The disturbances of sensation are slight, with some decrease in light touch, pain, temperature, vibration, and position sense. Sensory loss usually occurs later than motor dysfunction. Autonomic changes (Jammes, 1972) are characterized by reduced sweating in the legs, low tear production, decreased orthostatic adaptation to tilting, impaired pupillary responses to dim light and drugs, and lowered skin temperature. The postganglionic sympathetic nerve fibers appear to be preferentially affected.

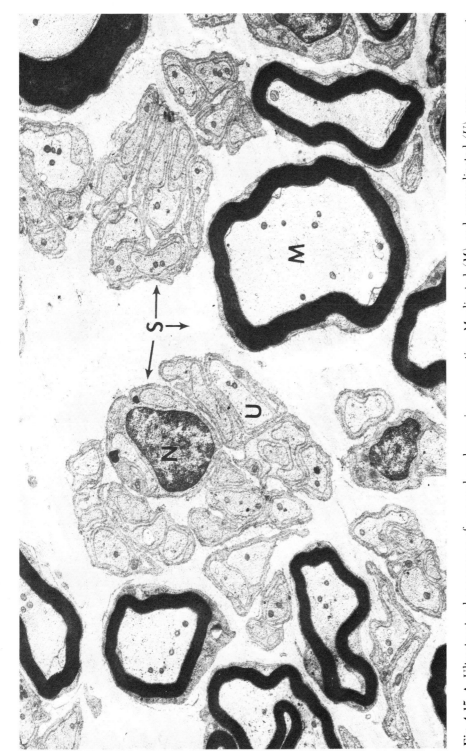

*Continued.*

**Fig. 4-15. A,** Ultrastructural appearance of a normal sural nerve in cross section. Myelinated (*M*) and unmyelinated (*U*) axons are present. Schwann cells (*S*) and their nuclei (*N*) are noted.

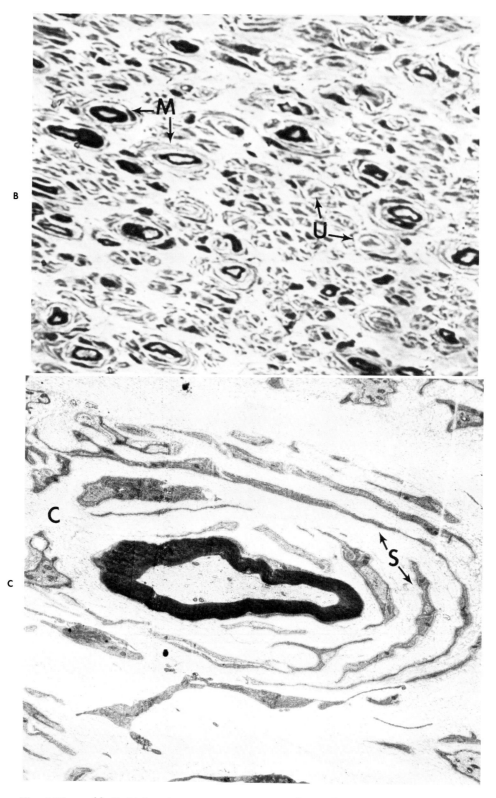

**Fig. 4-15, cont'd. B,** Light microscopic cross section of a sural nerve biopsy from a patient with Charcot-Marie-Tooth disease shows multiple onion bulb formations surrounding myelinated *(M)* and unmyelinated *(U)* axons. **C,** A single myelinated nerve fiber from a patient with Charcot-Marie-Tooth disease is surrounded by multiple layers of Schwann cells *(S)* with excess collagen *(C)* in between. This represents typical ultrastructural appearance of this disease. (**A** and **C,** courtesy Dr. Stephen A. Smith.)

The diagnosis is made from the inheritance pattern, peculiar distribution of muscular atrophy in the lower extremities, and evidence of decreased motor nerve conduction velocity. Table 4-5 outlines the differential diagnostic features of several progressive polyneuropathies. Peroneal muscular atrophy is distinguished by the dominant mode of inheritance, absence of cranial nerve involvement, initial peroneal nerve distribution of weakness, and minimal sensory loss.

**PATHOPHYSIOLOGY.** Pathologic studies in HMSN I have shown an excess of interstitial connective tissue in the peripheral nerve. At biopsy the nerves are abnormally enlarged with decreased numbers of myelinated fibers. Onion-bulb formations are visible in ultramicroscopic preparations (Fig. 4-15). The length and diameter of the internodal segments vary greatly, characteristic of disorders with segmental demyelination. Some axonal degeneration is also present. These changes are not specific, because they also occur in patients with Refsum's disease and hypertrophic interstitial neuritis (Dejerine-Sottas disease).

The anterior roots, and to a lesser degree the posterior ones, show loss of myelinated fibers, degeneration of axons, and fibrosis. In the posterior root ganglia there is loss of large myelinated fibers. In the peripheral nerve trunks there is loss of myelinated fibers and increase of fibrous tissue, usually to a severe degree. Muscles contain groups of atrophic muscle fibers characteristic of denervation. Significant fibrosis of the muscle spindles with loss of intrafusal fibers is common (Hughes and Brownell, 1972).

Degeneration of the dorsal columns, especially the fasciculus gracilis, and loss of anterior horn cells in the lumbar and sacral segments are noted. Recent studies (Dyck, Lais, and Offord, 1974) have demonstrated an increased incidence of demyelinated regions, hypertrophic changes, and loss of large myelinated fibers in the distal portion of the nerve as compared with the proximal portion. These changes appear to result from degeneration of the distal branches of the peripheral sensory neuron ("dying back") and not from selective loss of entire peripheral sensory neurons.

Demonstration of impaired axonal transport of dopamine-β-hydroxylase (Brimijoin, Capek, and Dyck, 1973) has suggested that a primary defect of myelin synthesis or maintenance is not the basis of the pathologic disorder. Alterations in serum phospholipids have been reported (Yao and Dyck, 1978). The current hypothesis is that an unknown metabolic abnormality of the neuron leads to axonal atrophy and secondarily to segmental demyelinization. A concomitant Schwann's cell defect may be present.

**LABORATORY FINDINGS.** Motor nerve conduction velocity measurements clearly demonstrate the site of the pathologic involvement. All individuals with a definite clinical diagnosis of peroneal atrophy have markedly low motor nerve conduction velocities in the ulnar, median, and peroneal nerves (Dyck and Lambert, 1968a). Low conduction velocity can be detected as early as 18 months of age and may be the only evidence of peripheral nerve involvement in a patient with minimal neurologic signs. Sensory nerve action potentials generally cannot be elicited or have a low amplitude and long latency, indicating involvement of the sensory as well as the motor nerves.

**GENETICS.** The disease is most often inherited as a mendelian dominant trait; recessive inheritance has been described. Sporadic cases have also been reported.

**TREATMENT.** Treatment consists of physical therapy to the affected extremities to maintain strength and range of motion and prevent contractures.

### HMSN II

Dyck and Lambert (1968b) have described patients whose clinical manifestations resemble Charcot-Marie-Tooth neuropathy but whose symptoms presumably result from selective degeneration of anterior horn cells and dorsal root ganglion cells (neuronal form). As in Charcot-Marie-Tooth disease, peroneal muscle weakness and atrophy predominate and the inheritance is as an auto-somal dominant trait. The neuronal form (HMSN II) is characterized by later onset of symptoms, no palpable enlargement of peripheral nerves, mild weakness of the small muscles of the hand, and severe weakness and atrophy of the plantar flexor muscles of the ankles. HMSN I is also now considered to result from involvement of the neuron as indicated in the previous section.

The most common presenting symptom is difficulty in walking. About half of the patients have pes cavus; a few have leg pain and cramps. Sensory loss is mild and usually involves the distal aspects of the legs.

The mean conduction velocities of the motor nerves are much higher than those in classic Charcot-Marie-Tooth disease. Those of the ulnar and median nerves are within the normal range but lower than the average velocities in unaffected relatives and controls. Conduction velocity in the peroneal nerve is mildly reduced or borderline. In over half of the patients the digital nerve action potential of the median nerve is unobtainable. Biopsy of the sural nerve may fail to show any histologic evidence of hypertrophic neuropathy or segmental demyelinization.

Patients with Charcot-Marie-Tooth disease may be divided into two distinguishable groups on the basis of nerve conduction velocity, supporting the theory that the disease has a genetic basis (Thomas and Calne, 1974). Most patients have markedly reduced motor nerve conduction velocity, segmental demyelinization, hypertrophic changes on nerve biopsy, and an autosomal dominant pattern of inheritance (HMSN I). The patients with normal or mildly reduced motor nerve conduction velocity who do not have segmental demyelinization on nerve biopsy also have an autosomal dominant pattern of inheritance (HMSN II) (Dyck and Lambert, 1968b).

A sporadic form of progressive spinal muscular atrophy described by Dyck and Lambert (1968b) is characterized by distal symmetric weakness beginning in the leg muscles and later involving the arms. Atrophy

was profound in the muscles of the lower thigh, leg, and foot. Gait disturbance was the earliest, most predominant symptom. Sensory findings were normal; the peripheral nerves were not enlarged. Motor conduction velocities were normal or mildly reduced. This disease is distinguishable from amyotrophic lateral sclerosis by its earlier onset and insidious, prolonged course. In addition, there is no evidence of pseudobulbar, bulbar, or corticospinal tract involvement. Muscle weakness is symmetric, in contrast to the asymmetry usually seen in amyotrophic lateral sclerosis.

### Hypertrophic interstitial neuritis (Dejerine-Sottas disease) (HMSN III)

In 1893 Dejerine and Sottas described a rare form of progressive or recurrent polyneuropathy that they designated progressive hypertrophic interstitial neuritis of childhood.

CLINICAL FEATURES. Most patients manifest symptoms from early infancy, with delayed development of motor landmarks. Walking unaided may not occur until 3 to 4 years of age. The clinical course is usually progressive but may be associated with recurrence and fairly complete remissions. Delay in walking is often the first symptom, followed by progressive weakness in the lower extremities and footdrop. As the disease progresses, symptoms worsen and sensory involvement causes ataxia. Patients often complain of muscle cramps and brief radiating pain. Diplopia, urinary incontinence, and muscle tenderness have been described. Affected individuals often have pes cavus, pes planus, or kyphoscoliosis.

On neurologic examination, many patients have pupillary abnormalities, such as miosis, anisocoria, and irregularity. Nystagmus is common. Hearing loss may be detected. The tendon reflexes are absent; the superficial reflexes may also be absent. Weakness and atrophy are evident, especially in the distal muscles of all extremities. The cardinal clinical feature of hypertrophic interstitial neuritis is the presence of markedly enlarged, firm nerves. Vibration and position sense are markedly impaired, with less severe loss of pain, touch, and temperature sensation. There may be autonomic changes with mottled cyanosis of the extremities and excessive sweating. Static and intention tremors are present bilaterally, and fine motor coordination is impaired.

The differential diagnosis includes many other familial diseases. Peroneal muscular atrophy may be differentiated from hypertrophic interstitial neuritis by the later onset, the absence of severe ataxia and sensory loss, and a dominant inheritance pattern. A distal form of muscular dystrophy is easily recognized by the lack of sensory findings. The absence of palpable enlargement of the nerves and of Babinski's signs readily distinguishes Friedreich's ataxia from hypertrophic interstitial neuritis. Refsum's disease is characterized by retinitis pigmentosa, skin changes, and elevation of the phytanic acid level. Amyloidosis and leprosy do not have the associated skeletal anomalies and may involve other organs, including the skin.

**LABORATORY FINDINGS.** There is a marked decrease in motor nerve conduction velocity, often in the range of 3 to 5 m/sec. These extremely low values are typical of the Dejerine-Sottas type of hypertrophic interstitial neuritis. Roentgen myelography reveals thickened nerve roots (Rao, Fitz, and Harwood-Nash, 1974).

**PATHOPHYSIOLOGY.** Limited biochemical studies have suggested a systemic disorder of cerebroside sulfate metabolism (Dyck et al., 1970), a deficiency of fatty acid dehydrogenase, or an abnormality in the choline phosphoglycerides as the cause of hypertrophic interstitial neuritis. A major difficulty in interpreting these biochemical abnormalities is that the changes may be a consequence of the neuropathy rather than the cause. Further studies are clearly indicated. Axonal flow of dopamine-$\beta$-hydroxylase in adrenergic unmyelinated nerves is abnormal (Brimijoin, Capek, and Dyck, 1973).

The nerves are enlarged throughout their course and the primary sensory neurons show degeneration (Dyck and Gomez, 1968). In sural nerve biopsy specimens the transverse diameter is markedly enlarged and the myelinated nerve fibers are decreased in number. Segmental demyelinization is frequent and the myelin sheaths are thin. Microscopically there is concentric lamellar fibrosis around demyelinated axons, giving rise to a typical onion-bulb appearance. Muscle biopsy reveals the presence of neurogenic atrophy.

**GENETICS.** The disease is inherited in an autosomal recessive pattern. Electromyography may be helpful in detecting family members with the disease who are asymptomatic. The dominantly inherited forms of Dejerine-Sottas disease described in the literature may represent milder varieties of peroneal muscular atrophy (Dyck et al., 1970).

### *Congenital hypomyelination neuropathy*

A condition similar to Dejerine-Sottas disease has been described as congenital hypomyelination neuropathy (Kennedy, Sung, and Berry, 1977). Although the clinical features are similar to Dejerine-Sottas disease, the disturbance in myelination was more severe. Clinically the child was inactive and hypotonic at birth. Her motor development was delayed to the extent that she could not walk unaided at 5½ years of age. Examination revealed scoliosis, slender extremities, absent tendon reflexes, and palpably enlarged nerves. There was moderate weakness, greater in the distal muscles. Vibration and position sense were absent distally, but light touch was only minimally impaired. Temperature and pain were intact.

Sural nerve biopsy revealed a total lack of myelin sheaths with preservation of the axon. There were an increased number of Schwann cells, excessive basement membranes, and onion-bulb formations. Biochemical studies revealed low levels of myelin lipid. The condition was thought to be a developmental failure of the peripheral nervous system to form myelin. Electromyography revealed very low motor nerve conduction velocity (2 to 3 m/sec) with prolonged terminal latencies.

### Friedreich's ataxia

CLINICAL FEATURES. Friedreich's ataxia is a hereditary degenerative disease characterized by progressive ataxia (Baker, 1934; Ford, 1966). The symptoms appear insidiously during childhood. Early motor and intellectual development is generally normal, although cases are described in which the motor milestones are attained slowly. The first symptom noted by the parents is the tendency to frequent stumbling and falling. If the child is of school age, difficulty in writing soon becomes apparent. In addition, the child may have ataxia of the arms with difficulty in handling a fork or spoon. Speech becomes indistinct and garbled.

Examination reveals typical skeletal deformities. There is commonly a thoracic scoliosis. The feet show a high arch (pes cavus) and a hammer toe. The hammer toe is characterized by flexion of the distal joint and hyperextension of the proximal joint. Skeletal deformities are often present from a very early age and antedate the ataxia. Cranial nerves are generally normal, although optic atrophy may appear late in the course of the disease. The tendon reflexes are absent. Bilateral Babinski's signs are present. Ataxia of the upper and lower extremities is a striking feature. The patient walks with a broad-based unsteady gait. The Romberg sign is positive. The finger-to-nose and heel-to-knee tests elicit intention tremors and dysmetria in the arms and legs. Examination of the sensory system by precise quantitative means reveals impairment of touch, but pain and temperature are normal. Clinically, position and vibration sense are impaired. Speech is markedly affected and has an explosive, irregular quality. Mental deterioration is common.

The majority of the symptoms and signs of Friedreich's ataxia result from involvement of the spinal cord and cerebellum. This disease represents the classic example of spinocerebellar degeneration. The disease progresses without obvious remissions. The involvement of the peripheral nerve is largely reflected by absent tendon reflexes and decreased or absent sensory nerve action potentials.

In the differential diagnosis of Friedreich's ataxia, peroneal muscular atrophy, hypertrophic interstitial neuritis, Refsum's disease, and abetalipoproteinemia should be considered (Table 4-5).

LABORATORY FINDINGS. The electrocardiogram shows evidence of myocardial involvement in 30% of the patients. Indeed, on rare occasions, involvement of the heart may be the first manifestation of the disease. Electromyography (Dyck and Lambert, 1968b; Dunn, 1973) reveals decreased amplitude of muscle action potentials and low-normal motor conduction velocity. There is a decrease or absence of the digital (sensory) nerve action potential (Oh and Halsey, 1973).

PATHOPHYSIOLOGY. Pathologically the major changes are found in the dorsal columns of the spinal cord, the spinocerebellar tracts, and the pyramidal tracts. These areas of the spinal cord show atrophy and degeneration. Also there is loss of large myelinated fibers in the peripheral nerve and loss of cells in the dorsal root ganglia (Hughes, Brownell, and Hewer, 1968). There is atrophy or degeneration of the nuclei and of the tracts in the lower brain stem. In addition, loss of Purkinje cells of the cerebellum has been described. Pathologic examination of the heart reveals enlargement and pericardial adhesions, with necrosis and degeneration of the muscle fibers caused by interstitial myocarditis.

Biochemical studies of fibroblasts cultured from patients with Friedreich's ataxia have shown decreased pyruvate oxidation resulting from decreased activity of pyruvate and alpha-ketoglutarate dehydrogenase (Blass, Kark, and Menon, 1976). The relationship between these biochemical abnormalities and the disease is unclear.

GENETICS. This disease is usually inherited in an autosomal recessive pattern.

## Neuropathies associated with sensory defects

Several clinical syndromes of an inherited nature have as their outstanding feature the failure to respond in a normal manner to obviously painful stimuli (Table 4-6). The patients have sensory impairment without muscular weakness. The tendon reflexes are absent or decreased because the afferent, or sensory, portion of the reflex arc is interrupted. These hereditary sensory neuropathy (HSN) syndromes are differentiated on the basis of hereditary pattern, sensory loss, and pathologic features, including involvement of the dorsal root ganglia, loss of myelinated fibers, and evidence for progression (Ohta et al., 1973).

### Hereditary sensory radicular neuropathy (HSN I)

Hereditary sensory radicular neuropathy is a familial disease inherited as a mendelian dominant trait (Mandell and Smith, 1960). It may be noted as early as 4 years of age but generally has its onset in the second decade of life. The disease generally begins in the feet, and the child shows delay in attainment of motor milestones with some gait incoordination. Early in the child's development there is an indifference to painful stimuli. Plantar ulceration of the feet, fractures, and destruction of joints develop. In the older individual, numbness and lack of pain sensation are frequent complaints. The sensory deficit progresses to the knees and elbows but rarely involves the trunk. Bladder and bowel sensation remain intact. On examination skin ulceration and skeletal involvement are apparent. There is impairment of all the sensory modalities including pain, temperature, touch, vibration, and position sense. The peripheral loss of pain perception is greater than that of touch or temperature. Motor strength is usually normal with no evidence of fasciculation or atrophy. Peroneal muscle atrophy with pes cavus has been reported

(Dyck et al., 1965). The tendon reflexes are absent in the area of sensory loss. Sensory loss may not be symmetric, but often involves the limbs distally extending up to the knees and elbows. The peripheral nerves are not enlarged to palpation. In vitro studies of sural nerves show decreased amplitudes of the A, AS, and C compound action potentials (Dyck et al., 1971). The basic pathology is degeneration and disappearance of nerve cells in the dorsal root ganglia (Denny-Brown, 1951). Study of a portion of a peripheral nerve removed from an involved area reveals degeneration and a markedly reduced number of unmyelinated and small myelinated fibers. The sporadic occurrence of a disease with the preceding manifestations has been termed "progressive sensory radicular neuropathy."

A dominantly inherited form of HSN with ataxia, scoliosis, and deafness has been described (Robinson, Jan, and Miller, 1977). These patients had clinical features resembling HSN I and II, but loss of pain sensation was minimal and ulcerating acropathy was not present.

### Congenital sensory neuropathy (HSN II)

Congenital sensory neuropathy is a familial disease inherited as an autosomal recessive trait (Winkelmann, Lambert, and Hayles, 1962; Ohta et al., 1973). It has its onset at birth; however, symptoms are not apparent until the second half of the first year. The parents first notice that the infant does not respond normally to painful stimuli. Painless necrotic ulcers of the lips and hands develop. Later in childhood, skeletal fractures occur and are associated with some destruction of joints. Progressive deafness may be noted. The patients may be retarded. Neurologic examination shows impairment of all sensory modalities over the face, extremities, and upper trunk. Light touch is most severely affected, followed by pain sensation and then temperature sensation. There may be some sparing of sensory loss over the lower trunk and about the anus. The tendon

**Table 4-6.** Differentiation of sensory syndromes

| | Hereditary sensory radicular neuropathy (HSN I*) | Congenital sensory neuropathy (HSN II) | Familial dysautonomia (HSN III) | Congenital sensory neuropathy with anhidrosis (HSN IV) | Congenital indifference to pain | Nonprogressive sensory radicular neuropathy | Progressive sensory neuropathy |
|---|---|---|---|---|---|---|---|
| Hereditary | Dominant | Recessive | Recessive | Recessive | — | — | Recessive |
| Onset | Second decade | Birth | Birth | Birth | Birth | Birth | First decade |
| Course | Plantar ulcers, fractures, joint destruction | Skin ulcers, deafness, fractures | Death may occur in infancy, otherwise gradual improvement | High fever, skin ulcers, fractures | Skin ulcers, fractures | Hyptonic at birth, skin ulcers, fractures | Skin ulcers, fractures, loss of digits |
| Mentation | Normal | May be retarded | May be retarded | Retarded | Normal | Normal | Normal |
| Sensory loss Distribution | Distal extremities | Extremities, forehead, trunk | Generalized | Generalized | Generalized | Distal extremities | Distal progressing to trunk |
| Pain | Absent | Absent | Reduced | Absent | Absent | Absent (body insensitive) | Absent |
| Temperature | Absent | Absent | Normal (? reduced) | Reduced | Normal | Absent | Reduced |
| Touch | Absent | Absent | Normal | Absent | Normal | Absent | Absent |
| Tendon reflexes | Absent in involved areas | Absent | Decreased | Decreased | Normal | Absent in involved areas | Absent |
| Sweating | Normal | Normal | Increased | Absent | Normal | Normal | Normal |
| Histamine "flare" | Absent | Absent | Absent | Absent | Present | Normal | Absent |
| Pathology | Loss of ganglion cells and myelinated fibers | Absence of myelinated fibers and skin nerve endings | Demyelinization of posterior column and dorsal root fibers, decrease in unmyelinated fibers | Absence of Lissauer's tract and dorsal root fibers | Normal skin and nerve | Loss of myelinated fibers | Loss of myelinated fibers and increase in fibrous tissue |

*HSN—Hereditary sensory neuropathy

reflexes are absent; sweating is impaired in areas of sensory loss.

Electrodiagnostic studies reveal normal to slightly decreased motor conduction velocity but absent sensory action potentials. There is no flare response to intradermal histamine administration (see Chapter 1). The basic pathology is an absence of myelinated fibers in the sensory nerve, decrease in unmyelinated fibers especially at the ankle, segmental demyelinization and remyelinization, and a lack of nerve end organs in the skin. The patients with congenital sensory neuropathy may have progressive symptoms or the disease may become stationary.

Another form of congenital sensory neuropathy with selective loss of pain perception in the extremities and selective loss of small myelinated fibers has been described (Low, Burke, and McLeod, 1978).

### Familial dysautonomia (Riley-Day syndrome, HSN III)

Familial dysautonomia occurs predominantly but not exclusively in Jewish children and is characterized by feeding difficulty from birth, failure to produce overflow of tears, absent corneal reflexes, hypoactive or absent tendon reflexes, moderate hypotonia, poor motor coordination, postural hypotension, emotional lability, relative indifference to pain, and absence of fungiform papillae on the tongue (Riley and Moore, 1966; Dancis and Smith, 1966).

The fundamental defect in this disease is unknown, but an imbalance between the parasympathetic and sympathetic nervous systems has been suggested. The autonomic symptomatology has been related in part to a deficiency in catecholamine release (Smith and Dancis, 1967). The demonstration of high homovanillic acid and low vanillylmandelic acid excretion is characteristic of the disturbance in catecholamine metabolism.

The absent corneal reflexes and relative indifference to pain, absence of taste buds, and abnormal response to intradermal administration of histamine all point to a peripheral sensory defect. The absent or depressed tendon reflexes and hypotonia can also be explained on the basis of an interruption of the sensory arc of the stretch reflex. Normal motor nerve conduction studies have been reported. Light touch is normal, although uncomfortable sensations are produced by stroking the soles of the feet.

It has been possible to reverse some of these sensory deficits, namely, the abnormal histamine response, absent tendon reflexes, and absent tearing by the intravenous infusion of methacholine. These studies have suggested an insufficiency of acetylcholine as the basic mechanism of the disease (Ziegler, Lake, and Kopin, 1976; Smith and Hui, 1973).

Pathologically, the predominant central nervous system lesion is focal demyelinization of the posterior columns of the spinal cord and myelin degeneration of dorsal root fibers (Fogelson, Rorke, and Kaye, 1967; Pearson, Axelrod, and Dancis, 1974). Sural nerve biopsy has shown a marked decrease in unmyelinated nerves (Aguayo, Nair, and Bray, 1971). These pathologic observations may explain the abnormal sensory findings in these patients. Abnormalities have also been described in the brain stem, which could explain the reflex and tone changes on the basis of alteration in gamma efferent activity (Brown, Beauchemin, and Linde, 1964). In addition, changes in the sympathetic ganglia have been described.

### Congenital sensory neuropathy with anhidrosis (HSN IV)

Congenital sensory neuropathy with anhidrosis is a familial disease inherited as an autosomal recessive trait (Vassella et al., 1968; Pinsky and DiGeorge, 1966). It is present from birth. Symptoms appear after a few months, characterized by unexplained episodes of high fever and a delayed motor development. The child does not respond appropriately to painful stimuli. Skin ulcers and fractures develop. There may be self-mutilation in the form of tongue biting.

On examination a generalized sensory loss of pain and touch is apparent. Temperature sensation is reduced. The tendon reflexes are reduced. There may be generalized hypotonia.

Sweating is absent or markedly reduced. The flare response to intradermal histamine is absent. The pathologic changes consist of an absence of Lissauer's tract and the dorsal root fibers.

### Other sensory syndromes

A nonprogressive sensory radicular neuropathy has been described by Ogden and associates (1959). The infant described was markedly hypotonic (floppy), with considerable difficulty in sucking until 7 months of age. Motor development was very slow. The child did not walk until 4½ years, and then with incoordination. She developed frequent skin ulcerations and skeletal fractures, with destruction and loss of terminal phalanges following osteomyelitis. On examination there was complete loss of all sensation extending from the feet to the knees and from the fingers to the wrists. There was insensitivity to pain over the entire trunk, except for a small area in the lower left abdominal quadrant. The motor strength was normal. The tendon reflexes were absent in the involved areas. The nerve biopsy showed degeneration consistent with involvement of the sensory neurons in the dorsal root ganglia. This particular entity differs from hereditary sensory radicular neuropathy by its earlier onset, widespread distribution, absence of a positive familial history, and lack of progression of symptoms.

Progressive sensory neuropathy has been reported in children and is transmitted as an autosomal recessive disease (Johnson and Spalding, 1964). This condition differs from hereditary sensory radicular neuropathy by a recessive mode of inheritance, early onset, and progressive loss of sensation extending to the trunk. Clinical features are similar to hereditary sensory radicular neuropathy, with involvement of all sensory modalities, loss of tendon reflexes, and progression of the neurologic abnormalities. The loss of sensation and tendon reflexes with preservation

of motor strength and autonomic function localizes the pathology in the dorsal root ganglia. Pathologic examination shows degeneration of the peripheral nerve.

Congenital indifference to pain presents a distinct entity without known pathologic abnormality (Critchley, 1956). In early infancy the parents note that the child does not respond to obviously painful situations. As a result of this lack of appropriate response, the infant may incur mutilating injuries and frequently develops ulcers of the hands and feet. Skeletal fractures without obvious pain occur. On neurologic examination the only sensation impaired is pain. The patient is able to perceive and identify a painful stimulus but does not respond in the usual manner. Touch, temperature, position, and vibration modalities are intact. Strength is normal. The tendon reflexes are normal. The triple response to an intradermal injection of histamine is normal. The nature of the defect in congenital indifference to pain is unknown. There has been no defect found at autopsy in the pathways known or thought to be associated with pain (Magee, 1963). It is important to note that this indifference to pain occurs over the entire body. This condition does not seem to be progressive. It is important in attempting to make this diagnosis that the patient has normal intelligence. Hysteria is excluded by the early onset.

The other conditions considered in the differential diagnosis of sensory syndromes have multiple sensory modalities involved and may show a progressive or nonprogressive course. Syringomyelia characterized by loss of pain and temperature sensations and preservation of touch sensation should be excluded. The differentiating features of the congenital sensory neuropathies are presented in Table 4-6.

### Neuropathies associated with connective tissue diseases

The mesenchymal (collagen) diseases are characterized by involvement of many systems with a spectrum of clinical symptomatology and common pathologic abnormalities of connective tissue. These diseases produce abnormalities in different areas of the nervous system largely through pathologic alteration in the small nutrient arteries' vascular supply (Glaser, 1955). Neurologic symptoms are encountered in polyarteritis nodosa, lupus erythematosus, rheumatoid arthritis, scleroderma, and dermatomyositis.

For a discussion of myositis associated with connective tissue diseases, see Chapter 8.

Polyarteritis nodosa (Ford and Siekert, 1965), a rare childhood disease, is a systemic illness characterized by weight loss, fever, abdominal pain, muscle pain and tenderness, polyserositis, arthritis, congestive heart failure, hypertension, focal indurated skin lesions, and renal involvement. This disease occurs predominantly in males. Neurologic examination reveals peripheral nerve dysfunction in one third to one half of the patients (Lovshin and Kernohan, 1948). Other neurologic manifestations include seizures, cranial nerve involvement, and psychosis. In general, the peripheral neuropathy is widespread and severe. The initial symptoms are pain and paresthesias, followed by weakness and depressed tendon reflexes. Distal weakness is characteristic. Often the clinical picture consists of involvement of several nerves at the same time (mononeuritis multiplex). Involvement of only one nerve has not been observed. The diagnosis is suspected by multiple system involvement and confirmed by the pathologic alterations of blood vessels in muscle, nerve, kidney, or other affected organs (Blackwood, 1963). The primary lesion is subendothelial edema, followed by fibrinoid necrosis of the media, destruction of the internal elastic lamina, and infiltration of all layers of the blood vessel by inflammatory cells. The vessels are often occluded by thrombus formation. Sural nerve biopsy of clinically involved nerves has shown similar arterial changes (Dyck, 1972).

Systemic lupus erythematosus is characterized by fever, rash, arthritis, cardiac enlargement, hepatosplenomegaly, and pneumonia. Renal disease occurs early in systemic lupus erythematosus. This disease occurs predominantly in females. Involvement of the nervous system in adult patients with systemic lupus erythematosus is characterized by seizures, psychosis, hemiplegia, and polyneuropathy (Scheinberg, 1956). In children with systemic lupus erythematosus, these neurologic signs are very uncommon (Peterson, Vernier, and Good, 1963). The diagnosis is suspected by the presence of multiple system manifestations and confirmed by appropriate laboratory tests, including the LE clot test and the determination of antinuclear antibodies.

Rheumatoid arthritis, a common disease in childhood, is characterized by a polyarthritis affecting multiple joints. It is also associated with involvement of liver, spleen, heart, eyes, and nervous system. Both myopathic and neuropathic involvement (Pallis and Scott, 1965) have been described. These are more commonly seen in the adult patient. The presence of a peripheral neuropathy in rheumatoid arthritis in children is exceedingly rare. It is difficult to distinguish between peripheral nerve involvement resulting from pressure and that caused by vasculitis.

Peripheral neuropathy has been described in scleroderma, but is exceedingly rare (Kibler and Rose, 1960). The vascular changes in scleroderma are not as severe as those in the other mesenchymal diseases.

## Neuropathies associated with neoplastic diseases

### Leukemia

Neurologic complications of leukemia appear to be increasing in frequency since effective chemotherapeutic agents have prolonged the life of children with this disease (Hyman et al., 1965; Nieri, Burgert, and Groover, 1968; Sullivan, 1963; Pochedly, 1975; Marshall and Chessells, 1977). There are three types of neuropathology seen in association with leukemia. The most common form is meningeal leukemia, which is characterized by increased intracranial pressure and lack of focal neurologic signs. Leukemic infiltrations or hemorrhage into the brain parenchyma is the second most common form. In the third form, the cranial and peripheral nerves are impaired as a result of leukemic infiltration along the nerve roots. The sciatic and peroneal nerve roots may be involved, causing pain, sensory loss, or motor weakness. The nervous system symptoms frequently occur while the patient's disease is in remission. The diagnosis of leukemia is suspected from the clinical findings of pallor, hepatosplenomegaly, and bone tenderness. It is confirmed by bone marrow aspiration. Radiation and intrathecal injection of methotrexate may produce improvement in the neurologic signs. In the patient who develops peripheral nerve involvement during a remission, the possibility of toxic damage by a chemotherapeutic agent must be considered.

### Hodgkin's disease

Hodgkin's disease may affect the brain, spinal cord, and cranial and peripheral nerves (Hutchinson et al., 1958; Sohn, Valensi, and Miller, 1967). Impairment of spinal cord and spinal roots from leptomeningeal infiltration is the most common nervous system form of Hodgkin's disease. However, local enlargement of lymph nodes may cause peripheral nerve compression. The brachial plexus and lumbar plexus may be involved, with local compression producing paresthesias and weakness. There may be actual invasion of the nerve fibers by neoplastic tissue. An extensive peripheral neuropathy, resembling the Guillain-Barré syndrome, may result from infiltration of the nerve fibers by neoplastic cells. The appearance of neurologic signs in Hodgkin's disease often indicates that the disease may undergo rapid progression. Herpes zoster affecting the cranial nerves is commonly seen in patients with Hodgkin's disease.

### Neurofibromatosis

In neurofibromatosis, the cranial nerves, spinal cord nerve roots, and peripheral nerves may be the site of involvement by tumor formation (Meszaros, Guzzo, and Schorsch, 1966; Russell and Rubenstein, 1963). The clinical symptomatology depends on the nerve affected. Pathologically the affected nerve has an irregular, cylindric shape often termed a "plexiform neurofibroma." The diagnosis of neurofibromatosis is made from the typical manifestation of soft skin nodules associated with areas of pigmentation known as café-au-lait spots. In addition, there are lesions of bone that may be related to tumor formation or an associated mesodermal defect.

### Spinal cord tumors

Spinal cord tumors arising within the spinal cord parenchyma are known as intramedullary tumors. All those outside the spinal cord are called extramedullary tumors. The extramedullary tumors may be either intradural or extradural. The extramedullary tumors produce their initial and predominant symptoms by compression on one or more nerve roots, giving rise to pain, often of a radiating nature. The nerve root compression may also result in weakness and sensory changes. Eventually extramedullary tumors produce compression on the spinal cord, resulting in damage to the corticospinal tract, anterior horn cells, and spinothalamic tracts.

The most common tumors of the spinal cord (Haft, Ransohoff, and Carter, 1959; Lassman and James, 1967) in children are dermoid cysts, teratomas, neurofibromas, neuroblastomas, ganglioneuromas, lipomas, and meningiomas. Most commonly, the spinal cord tumors arise in the cervical and thoracic areas.

The symptoms and signs of a spinal cord tumor depend on its location. Persistent pain, weakness, and either the failure to attain urinary continence or the development of urinary incontinence suggest the possibility of a spinal cord tumor.

The neurologic signs depend on the location of the tumor. Weakness and sensory change localized to the distribution of one or two spinal roots strongly indicate the presence of a tumor. If there has been spinal cord compression, there may be hyperactive reflexes and bilateral Babinski's signs. A sensory level over the trunk may be demonstrated. Lipomas of the lumbosacral region may be strongly suspected if there is a dermal sinus, a soft midline mass in the lumbosacral region, or excessive hair or pigmentation in this area. Lumbosacral lipomas often affect the nerve roots of the cauda equina and produce a variety of signs. There may be weakness and muscle atrophy in the lower extremities, with decreased or absent tendon reflexes. Sensory changes, often difficult to demonstrate in the young child, may be elicited in the older child. Rectal sphincter tone may be decreased. It is especially important to examine for perianal sensation loss.

# REFERENCES

Ackner, B., et al.: Acute porphyria: a neuropsychiatric and biochemical study, J. Psychosom. Res. **6:**1, 1962.

Adler, J. B., and Patterson, R. L.: Erb's palsy: long-term results of treatment in eighty-eight cases, J. Bone Joint Surg. **49A:**1052, 1967.

Adour, K. K., and Wingerd, J.: Idiopathic facial paralysis (Bell's palsy): factors affecting severity and outcome in 446 patients, Neurology **24:**1112, 1974.

Adour, K. K., et al.: Prednisone treatment for idiopathic facial paralysis (Bell's palsy), N. Engl. J. Med. **287:** 1268, 1972.

Aguayo, A. J., Nair, C. P. V., and Bray, G. M.: Peripheral nerve abnormalities in the Riley-Day syndrome, Arch. Neurol. **24:**106, 1971.

Arbus, G. S., et al.: Effect of chronic renal failure, dialysis, and transplantation on motor nerve conduction velocity in children, Can. Med. Assoc. J. **20:**517, 1975.

Aronsson, S., et al.: Long-term dietary treatment of tyrosinosis, J. Pediatr. **72:**620, 1968.

Asbury, A. K., Victor, M., and Adams, R. D.: Uremic polyneuropathy, Arch. Neurol. **8:**413, 1963.

Austin, J., et al.: Abnormal sulfatase activities in two human diseases (metachromatic leucodystrophy and gargoylism) Biochem. J. **93:**15c, 1964.

Austin, J. H.: Observations in metachromatic leucoencephalopathy, Trans. Am. Neurol. Assoc. **83:**149, 1958.

Avram, M. M., Feinfeld, D. A., and Huatuco, A. H.: Search for the uremic toxin, N. Engl. J. Med. **298:** 1000, 1978.

Baker, A. B.: Friedreich's ataxia: a clinical and pathological study, Am. J. Pathol. **10:**113, 1934.

Bale, P. M., et al.: Pathology of Tangier disease, J. Clin. Pathol. **24:**609, 1971.

Barltrop, D.: Acute intermittent porphyria in a child with a note on the glycine loading test, Pediatrics **34:**696, 1964.

Bassen, F. A., and Kornzweig, A. L.: Malformation of the erythrocytes in a case of atypical retinitis pigmentosa, Blood **5:**381, 1950.

Behan, P. O., et al.: Cell-mediated hypersensitivity to neural antigens. Occurrence in human patients and nonhuman primates with neurological diseases, Arch. Neurol. **27:**145, 1972.

Berg, B. O.: Syndrome of infant botulism, Pediatrics **59:**321, 1977.

Berg, B. O., Rosenberg, S. H., and Asbury, A. K.: Giant axonal neuropathy, Pediatrics **49:**894, 1972.

Biehl, J. P., and Vilter, R. W.: Effect of isoniazid on vitamin $B_6$ metabolism; its possible significance in producing isoniazid neuritis, Proc. Soc. Exp. Biol. Med. **85:**389, 1954.

Bischoff, A., and Ulrich, J.: Peripheral neuropathy in globoid cell leukodystrophy (Krabbe's disease). Ultrastructural and histochemical findings, Brain **92:**861, 1969.

Blackwood, W.: Greenfield's neuropathy. ed. 2, Baltimore, 1963, The Williams & Wilkins Co., p. 114.

Blass, J. P., and Gibson, G. E.: Abnormality of a thiamine-requiring enzyme in patients with Wernicke-Korsakoff syndrome, N. Engl. J. Med. **297:**1367, 1977.

Blass, J. P., Pieter Kark, R. A., and Menon, N. K.: Low activities of the pyruvate and oxoglutarate dehydrogenase complexes in five patients with Friedreich's ataxia, N. Engl. J. Med. **295:**62, 1976.

Bleifer, S. B., and Alphas, S. J.: Acute intermittent porphyria: report of a case in an infant aged eight months, with discussion of porphyrin metabolism, J. Pediatr. **46:**552, 1955.

Bleifer, S. B., and Alphas, S. J.: Acute intermittent porphyria: report of a case associated with porphobilingen in the urine of four of five children, N. Engl. J. Med. **260:**978, 1959.

Boder, E., and Sedgwick, R. P.: Ataxia-telangiectasia: a review of 101 cases. In Walsh, G., editor: Cerebellum, posture, and cerebral palsy, Little Club Clin. Dev. Med. **8:**110, 1963.

Bolthauser, E., Bischoff, A., and Isler, W.: Giant axonal neuropathy, J. Neurol. Sci. **31:**269, 1977.

Brimijoin, S., Capek, P., and Dyck, P. J.: Axonal transport of dopamine-beta-hydroxylase by human sural nerves in vitro, Science **180:**1295, 1973.

Brody, I. A., and Wilkins, R. H.: Charcot-Marie-Tooth disease, Arch. Neurol. **17:**552, 1967.

Brown, M. R.: The mechanism involved in polyneuritis as exemplified by post-diphtheritic polyneuritis, Ann. Intern. Med. **36:**786, 1952.

Brown, W. J., Beauchemin, J. A., and Linde, L. M.: A neuropathological study of familial dysautonomia (Riley-Day syndrome) in siblings, J. Neurol. Neurosurg. Psychiatry **27:**131, 1964.

Campbell, E. D. R., et al.: Value of nerve-excitability measurements in prognosis of facial palsy, Br. Med. J. **2:**7, 1962.

Carpenter, S., et al.: Giant axonal neuropathy, Arch. Neurol. **31:**312, 1974.

Casey, E. B., et al.: Vincristine neuropathy: clinical and electrophysiological observation, Brain **96**:69, 1973.

Cavanagh, J. B., and Mellick, R. S.: On the nature of the peripheral nerve lesions associated with acute intermittent porphyria, J. Neurol. Neurosurg. Psychiatry **28**:320, 1965.

Cayler, G. G., Blumenfeld, C. M., and Anderson, R. L.: Further studies of patients with the cardiofacial syndrome, Chest **60**:161, 1971.

Chaco, J.: Subclinical peripheral nerve involvement in unilateral Bell's palsy, Am. J. Phys. Med. **52**:195, 1973.

Cherington, M.: Botulism: ten-year experience, Arch. Neurol. **30**:432, 1974.

Chhuttani, P. N., Chawla, L. S., and Sharma, T. D.: Arsenical neuropathy, Neurology **17**:269, 1967.

Chisholm, J. J.: The use of chelating agents in the treatment of acute and chronic lead intoxication in childhood, J. Pediatr. **73**:1, 1968.

Chisholm, J. J., Jr.: Poisoning due to heavy metals, Pediatr. Clin. North Am. **17**:591, 1970.

Clay, S. A., et al.: Acute infantile motor unit disorder: infantile botulism? Arch. Neurol. **34**:236, 1977.

Collings, H.: Polyneuropathy associated with nitrofuran therapy, Arch. Neurol. **3**:656, 1960.

Craig, W. S., and Clark, J. M. P.: Obturator palsy in the newly born, Arch. Dis. Child. **37**:661, 1962.

Critchley, E. M. R., Clark, D. B., and Wikler, A.: Acanthocytosis and neurological disorder without betalipoproteinemia, Arch. Neurol. **18**:134, 1968.

Critchley, M.: Congenital indifference to pain, Ann. Intern. Med. **45**:737, 1956.

Dancis, J., and Smith, A. A.: Current concepts: familial dysautonomia, N. Engl. J. Med. **274**:207, 1966.

Dayan, A. D., Ogul, E., and Graveson, G. S.: Polyneuritis and herpes zoster, J. Neurol. Neurosurg. Psychiatry **35**:170, 1972.

DeLeon, G. A., Grover, W. D., and Huff, D. S.: Neuropathologic changes in ataxia-telangiectasia, Neurology **26**:947, 1976.

Denny-Brown, D.: Hereditary sensory radicular neuropathy, J. Neurol. Neurosurg. Psychiatry **14**:237, 1951.

Dowell, V. R., Jr.: Infant botulism: new guise for an old disease, Hospital Practice **13**:67, 1978.

Dreyfus, P. M.: Clinical application of blood transketolase determinations, N. Engl. J. Med. **267**:569, 1962.

Dubois, G., Harzer, K., and Baumann, N.: Very low arylsulfatase A and cerebroside sulfatase activities in leukocytes of healthy members of metachromatic leukodystrophy family, Am. J. Hum. Genet. **29**:191, 1977.

Duchenne, G. B.: Selections from the clinical works of Dr. Duchenne. London, 1883, The New Sydenham Society, p. 210.

Dunn, H. G.: Nerve conduction studies in children with Friedreich's ataxia and ataxia-telangiectasia, Dev. Med. Child. Neurol. **15**:324, 1973.

Dunn, H. G., et al.: The neuropathy of Krabbe's infantile cerebral sclerosis (globoid cell leukodystrophy), Brain **92**:329, 1969.

Dyck, P. J.: Inherited neuronal degeneration and atrophy affecting peripheral motor, sensory, and autonomic neurons. In Dyck, P. J., Thomas, P. K., and Lambert, E. H., editors: Peripheral neuropathy, vol. II, Philadelphia, 1975, W. B. Saunders Co., p. 825.

Dyck, P. J., and Gomez, M. R.: Segmental demyelinization in Dejerine-Sottas disease: light, phase-contrast, and electron microscopic studies, Mayo Clin. Proc. **43**:280, 1968.

Dyck, P. J., and Lambert, E. H.: Lower motor and primary sensory neuron diseases with peroneal muscular atrophy. I. Neurologic, genetic, and electrophysiologic findings in hereditary polyneuropathies, Arch. Neurol. **18**:603, 1968a.

Dyck, P. J., and Lambert, E. H.: Lower motor and primary sensory neuron diseases with peroneal muscular atrophy. II. Neurologic, genetic, and electrophysiologic findings in various neuronal degenerations, Arch. Neurol. **18**:619, 1968b.

Dyck, P. J., Conn, D. L., and Okazaki, H.: Necrotizing angiopathic neuropathy: three dimensional morphology of fiber degeneration related to sites of occluded vessels, Mayo Clin. Proc. **47**:461, 1972.

Dyck, P. J., Lais, A. C., and Offord, K. P.: The nature of myelinated nerve fiber degeneration in dominantly inherited hypertrophic neuropathy, Mayo Clin. Proc. **49**:34, 1974.

Dyck, P. J., et al.: A Virginia kinship with hereditary sensory neuropathy: peroneal muscular atrophy and pes cavus, Mayo Clin. Proc. **40**:685, 1965.

Dyck, P. J., et al.: Histologic and lipid studies of sural nerves in inherited hypertrophic neuropathy: preliminary report of a lipid abnormality in nerve and liver in Dejerine-Sottas disease, Mayo Clin. Proc. **45**:286, 1970.

Dyck, P. J., et al.: Segmental demyelination secondary to axonal degeneration in uremic neuropathy, Mayo Clin. Proc. **46**:400, 1971.

Eberle, E., et al.: Early predictors of incomplete recovery in children with Guillain-Barré polyneuritis, J. Pediatr. **86**:356, 1975.

Eeg-Olofsson, O., and Petersen, I.: Childhood diabetic neuropathy, Acta Paediatr. Scand. **55**:163, 1966.

Eisen, A., and Humphreys, P.: The Guillain-Barré syndrome: a clinical and electrodiagnostic study of 25 cases, Arch. Neurol. **30**:438, 1974.

Eng, G. D.: Brachial plexus palsy in newborn infants, Pediatrics **48**:18, 1971.

Engel, W. K., et al.: Neuropathy in Tangier disease, Arch. Neurol. **17**:1, 1967.

Erb, W.: Ueber eine eigenthümliche localization von Lachmungen in Plexus Brachialis, Heidelberg, Ver Naturhist Med Verein **1**:130, 1874.

Fardeau, M., and Engel, W. K.: Ultrastructural study of a peripheral nerve biopsy in Refsum's disease, J. Neuropathol. Exp. Neurol. **28**:278, 1969.

Feldman, G. V.: Radial nerve palsies in the newborn, Arch. Dis. Child. **32**:469, 1957.

Fisher, C. M., and Adams, R. D.: Diphtheritic polyneuritis: a pathological study, J. Neuropathol. Exp. Neurol. **15**:243, 1956.

Fogelson, M. H., Rorke, L. B., and Kaye, R.: Spinal cord changes in familial dysautonomia, Arch. Neurol. **17**:103, 1967.

Ford, F. R.: Diseases of the nervous system: in infancy, childhood and adolescence, ed. 5, Springfield, Ill., 1966, Charles C Thomas, Publisher.

Ford, R. G., and Siekert, R. G.: Central nervous system manifestations of periarteritis nodosa, Neurology **15**:114, 1965.

Freemon, F. R., Parker, R. L., Jr., and Greer, M.: Unusual neurotoxicity of kanamycin, J.A.M.A. **200**:410, 1967.

Friedman, A. P., and Olsen, C. W.: Bilateral paralysis of the facial and masticatory nerves following arsenic poisoning, Bull. Los Angeles Neurol. Soc. **6**:85, 1941.

Gamstorp, I., et al.: Peripheral neuropathy in juvenile diabetes, Diabetes **15**:411, 1966.

Gardner-Thorpe, C., Foster, J. B., and Barwick, D. D.: Unusual manifestations of herpes zoster: a clinical and electrophysiological study, J. Neurol. Sci. **28**:427, 1976.

Gilles, F. H., and French, J. H.: Postinjection sciatic nerve palsies in infants and children, J. Pediatr. **58**:195, 1961.

Glaser, G. H.: Neurologic manifestations in collagen diseases, Neurology **5**:751, 1955.

Gordon, S. L., et al.: Residua of Guillain-Barré polyneuritis in children, J. Bone Joint Surg. **59A**:193, 1977.

Gotto, A. M., et al.: On the protein defect in abetalipoproteinemia, N. Engl. J. Med. **284**:813, 1971.

Greene, H., Hug, G., and Schubert, W. K.: Arylsulfatase A in the urine and metachromatic leukodystrophy, J. Pediatr. **71**:709, 1967.

Haft, H., Ransohoff, J., and Carter, S.: Spinal cord tumors in children, Pediatrics **23**:1152, 1959.

Hansen, R. L., et al.: Immunological studies on an aberrant form of ataxia telangiectasia, Am. J. Dis. Child. **131**:518, 1977.

Hart, M. N., Hanks, D. T., and Mackay, R.: Ultrastructural observations in Guillain-Barré syndrome, Arch. Pathol. **93**:552, 1972.

Haymaker, W., and Kernohan, J. W.: Landry-Guillain-Barré syndrome, Medicine **28**:59, 1949.

Haymaker, W., and Woodhall, B.: Peripheral nerve injuries, ed. 2, Philadelphia, 1962, W. B. Saunders Co.

Heller, G. L., and DeJong, R. N.: Treatment of the Guillain-Barré syndrome, Arch. Neurol. **8**:179, 1963.

Henderson, L. O., et al.: Abnormal concentration and anomalous distribution of apolipoprotein A-1 in Tangier disease, Metabolism **27**:165, 1978.

Hepner, W. R., Jr.: Some observations on facial paresis in the newborn infant: etiology and incidence, Pediatrics **8**:494, 1951.

Herbert, P. N., et al.: Tangier disease, N. Engl. J. Med. **299**:519, 1978.

Heyman, A., et al.: Peripheral neuropathy caused by arsenical intoxication, N. Engl. J. Med. **254**:401, 1956.

Hudson, F. P., McCandless, A., and O'Malley, A. G.: Sciatic paralysis in newborn infants, Br. Med. J. **1**:223, 1950.

Hughes, J. T., and Brownell, B.: Pathology of peroneal muscular atrophy (Charcot-Marie-Tooth disease), J. Neurol. Neurosurg. Psychiatry **35**:648, 1972.

Hughes, J. T., Brownell, B., and Hewer, R. L.: The peripheral sensory pathways in Friedreich's ataxia, Brain **91**:803, 1968.

Hutchinson, E. C., et al.: Neurological complications of the reticuloses, Brain **81**:75, 1958.

Hyman, C. B., et al.: Central nervous system involvement by leukemia in children. I. Relationship to systemic leukemia and description of clinical and laboratory manifestations, Blood **25**:1, 1965.

Jammes, J. L.: The autonomic nervous system in peroneal muscular atrophy, Arch. Neurol. **27**:213, 1972.

Johnson, R. H., and Spalding, J. M. K.: Progressive sensory neuropathy in children, J. Neurol. Neurosurg. Psychiatry **27**:125, 1964.

Jones, W. A., and Jones, G. P.: Peripheral neuropathy due to isoniazid, Lancet **1**:1073, 1953.

Joy, R. J. T., Scalettar, R., and Sodee, D. B.: Optic and peripheral neuritis: probable effect of prolonged chloramphenicol therapy, J.A.M.A. **173**:1731, 1960.

Kayden, H. J.: Abetalipoproteinemia, Ann. Rev. Med. **23**:285, 1972.

Kendall, D.: Motor complications of herpes zoster, Br. Med. J. **2**:616, 1957.

Kennedy, B. H., et al.: Guillain-Barré syndrome, Mayo Clin. Proc. **53**:93, 1978.

Kennedy, W. R., Sung, J. H., and Berry, J. F.: A case of congenital hypomyelination neuropathy, Arch. Neurol. **34**:337, 1977.

Kibler, R. F., and Rose, F. C.: Peripheral neuropathy in the "collagen diseases": a case of scleroderma neuropathy, Br. Med. J. **1**:1781, 1960.

Kilroy, A. W., et al.: Two syndromes following rubella immunization: clinical observations and epidemiological studies, J.A.M.A. **214**:2287, 1970.

Kimura, J., Giron, L. T., and Young, S. M.: Electrophysiological study of Bell Palsy, Arch. Otolaryngol. **102**:140, 1976.

Kimura, J., Rodnitzky, R. L., and Okawara, S-H.: Electrophysiologic analysis of aberrant regeneration after facial nerve paralysis, Neurology **25**:899, 1975.

Knox, J. D. E., Levy, R., and Simpson, J. A.: Herpes zoster and the Landry-Guillain-Barré syndrome, J. Neurol. Neurosurg. Psychiatry **24**:167, 1961.

Kocen, R. S., et al.: Familial α-lipoprotein deficiency (Tangier disease) with neurological abnormalities, Lancet **1**:1341, 1967.

Kocen, R. S., et al.: Nerve biopsy findings in two cases

of Tangier disease, Acta Neuropathol. (Berl.) **26**:317, 1973.

Koch, T., et al.: Giant axonal neuropathy: a childhood disorder of microfilaments, Ann. Neurol. **11**:438, 1977.

Korobkin, R., et al.: Glue-sniffing neuropathy, Arch. Neurol. **32**:158, 1975.

Krabbe, K.: New familial, infantile form of diffuse brain-sclerosis, Brain **39**:74, 1916.

Lake, B. D.: Segmental demyelination of peripheral nerves in Krabbe's disease, Nature **217**:171, 1968.

Lampkin, B. C., and Schubert, W. K.: Pernicious anemia in the second decade of life, J. Pediatr. **72**:387, 1968.

Langworth, E. P., and Taverner, D.: The prognosis in facial palsy, Brain **86**:465, 1963.

Lassman, L. P., and James, C. C. M.: Lumbosacral lipomas: critical survey of 26 cases submitted to laminectomy, J. Neurol. Neurosurg. Psychiatry **30**:174, 1967.

Lawrence, D. G., and Locke, S.: Neuropathy in children with diabetes mellitus, Br. Med. J. **1**:784, 1963.

Layzer, R. B., and Conant, M.: Neuralgia in recurrent herpes simplex, Arch. Neurol. **31**:233, 1974.

Lester, P. D., and McAlister, W. H.: Congenital iliac anomaly with sciatic palsy, Radiology **96**:397, 1970.

Levine, I. M., Estes, J. W., and Looney, J. M.: Hereditary neurological disease with acanthocytosis, Arch. Neurol. **19**:403, 1968.

Lichtenfeld, P.: Autonomic dysfunction in the Guillain-Barré syndrome, Am. J. Med. **50**:772, 1971.

Lin-Fu, J. S.: Vulnerability of children to lead exposure and toxicity, N. Engl. J. Med. **289**:1229, 1973.

Lockman, L. A., Kennedy, W. R., and White, J. G.: The Chédiak-Higashi syndrome: electrophysiological and electron microscopic observations on the peripheral neuropathy, J. Pediatr. **70**:942, 1967.

Lovshin, L. L., and Kernohan, J. W.: Peripheral neuritis in periarteritis nodosa, Arch. Intern. Med. **82**:321, 1948.

Low, N. L., Schneider, J., and Carter, S.: Polyneuritis in children, Pediatrics **22**:972, 1958.

Low, P. A., Burke, W. J., and McLeod, J. G.: Congenital sensory neuropathy with selective loss of small myelinated fibers, Ann. Neurol. **3**:179, 1978.

Lundberg, A., et al.: Heredopathia atactica polyneuritiformis (Refsum's disease): experience of dietary treatment and plasmapheresis, Eur. Neurol. **8**:301, 1972.

Lysaught, J. N., and McCleery, J. M.: Acute intermittent porphyria: report of a case in an infant aged eight months, with discussion of porphyrin metabolism, J. Pediatr. **46**:552, 1955.

Madrid, R., Bradley, W. G., and Davis, C. J. F.: The peroneal muscular atrophy syndrome, J. Neurol. Sci. **32**:91, 1977.

Magee, K.: Congenital indifference to pain, Arch. Neurol. **9**:635, 1963.

Magee, K. R., and DeJong, R. N.: Paralytic brachial neuritis, J.A.M.A. **174**:1258, 1960.

Mandell, A. J., and Smith, C. K.: Hereditary sensory radicular neuropathy, Neurology **10**:627, 1960.

Manning, J. J., and Adour, K. K.: Facial paralysis in children, Pediatrics **49**:102, 1972.

Marshall, W. C., and Chessells, J. M.: Neurological complications of childhood leukaemia, Arch. Dis. Child. **52**:850, 1977.

McDonald, W. I., and Kocen, R. S.: Diphtheritic neuropathy. In Dyck, P. J., Thomas, P. K., and Lambert, E. H., editors: Peripheral neuropathy, vol. 2, Philadelphia, 1975, W. B. Saunders Co., p. 1281.

McFarland, H. R., and Heller, G. L.: Guillain-Barré disease complex, Arch. Neurol. **14**:196, 1966.

McLeod, J. G., and Penny, R.: Vincristine neuropathy: an electrophysiological and histological study, J. Neurol. Neurosurg. Psychiatry **32**:297, 1969.

McNicholl, B., and Egan, B.: Congenital pernicious anemia: effects on growth, brain and absorption of $B_{12}$, Pediatrics **42**:149, 1968.

Mechelse, K., et al.: Bell's palsy: prognostic criteria and evaluation of surgical decompression, Lancet **2**:57, 1971.

Melchior, J. C., and Clausen, J.: Metachromatic leukodystrophy in early childhood: treatment with a diet deficient in vitamin A, Acta Paediatr. Scand. **57**:2, 1968.

Meszaros, W. T., Guzzo, F., and Schorsch, H.: Neurofibromatosis, Am. J. Roentgen. **98**:557, 1966.

Miller, H. G., and Stanton, J. B.: Neurological sequelae of prophylatic inoculation, Q. J. Med. **23**:1, 1954.

Mills, W. G.: A new neonatal syndrome, Br. Med. J. **2**:464, 1949.

Mitchell, P. L., and Meilman, E.: The mechanism of hypertension in the Guillain-Barré syndrome, Am. J. Med. **42**:986, 1967.

Moress, G. R., D'Agostino, A. N., and Jarcho, L. W.: Neuropathy in lymphoblastic leukemia treated with vincristine, Arch. Neurol. **16**:377, 1967.

Muller, D. P., Lloyd, J. K., and Bird, A. C.: Long-term management of abeta-lipoproteinemia: possible role for vitamin E, Arch. Dis. Child. **52**:209, 1977.

Nelson, K. B., and Eng. G. D.: Congenital hypoplasia of the depressor anguli oris muscle: differentiation from congenital facial palsy, J. Pediatr. **81**:16, 1972.

Nieri, R. L., Burgert, E. O., and Groover, R. V.: Central-nervous system complications of leukemia: a review, Mayo Clin. Prac. **43**:70, 1968.

Ochoa, J.: Isoniazid neuropathy in man: quantitative electron microscope study, Brain **93**:831, 1970.

Ogden, T. E., Robert, F., and Carmichael, E. A.: Some sensory syndromes in children: indifference to pain and sensory neuropathy, J. Neurol. Neurosurg. Psychiatry **22**:267, 1959.

Oh, S. J.: Botulism: electrophysiological studies, Ann. Neurol. **1**:481, 1977.

Oh, S. J., and Halsey, J. H.: Abnormality in nerve potentials in Friedreich's ataxia, Neurology **23**:52, 1973.

Ohta, M., et al.: Hereditary sensory neuropathy, type II: clinical, electrophysiologic, histologic, and biochemical studies of a Quebec kinship, Arch. Neurol. **29**:23, 1973.

Osler, L. D., and Sidell, A. D.: The Guillain-Barré syndrome, N. Engl. J. Med. **262**:964, 1960.

Pallis, C. A., and Scott, J. T.: Peripheral neuropathy in rheumatoid arthritis, Br. Med. J. **1**:1141, 1965.

Pearson, H. A., Vinson, R., and Smith, R. T.: Pernicious anemia with neurologic involvement in childhood, J. Pediatr. **65**:334, 1964.

Pearson, J., Axelrod, F., and Dancis, J.: Current concepts of dysautonomia: neuropathological defects, Ann. N. Y. Acad. Sci. **228**:288, 1974.

Pegum, J. S.: Nicotinic acid and burning feet, Lancet **2**:536, 1952.

Peiffer, J., et al.: Generalized giant axonal neuropathy: a filament forming disease of neuronal, endothelial, glial, and Schwann cells in a patient without kinky hair, Acta Neuropathol. **40**:213, 1977.

Peiris, O. A., and Miles, D. W.: Galvanic stimulation of the tongue as a prognostic index in Bell's Palsy, Br. Med. J. **2**:1162, 1965.

Peterman, A. F., et al.: Infectious neuronitis (Guillain-Barré syndrome) in children, Neurology **9**:533, 1959.

Peterson, R. D. A., Vernier, R. L., and Good, R. A.: Lupus erythematosus, Pediatr. Clin. North Am. **10**:941, 1963.

Pickett, J., et al.: Syndrome of botulism in infancy: clinical and electrophysiologic study, N. Engl. J. Med. **295**:770, 1976.

Pinsky, L., and DiGeorge, A. M.: Congenital familial sensory neuropathy with anhidrosis, J. Pediatr. **68**:1, 1966.

Pochedly, C.: Neurologic manifestations in acute leukemia III: peripheral neuropathy and chloroma, N. Y. State J. Med. **75**:878, 1975.

Posner, J. B., et al.: Hyponatremia in acute polyneuropathy, Arch. Neurol. **17**:530, 1967.

Prosser, P. R., and Karam, J. H.: Diabetes mellitus following rodenticide ingestion in man, J.A.M.A. **239**(3):1148, 1978.

Ransford, A. O., and Hughes, S. P. F.: Complete brachial plexus lesions, J. Bone Joint Surg. **59**:417, 1977.

Rao, C. V. G., Fitz, C. R., and Harwood-Nash, D. C.: Dejerine-Sottas syndrome in children (hypertrophic interstitial polyneuritis), Am. J. Roentgenol. **122**:70, 1974.

Refsum, S.: Heredopathia atactica polyneuritiformis: a familial syndrome not hitherto described, Acta Psychiatr. Neurol. (Suppl. 38) 1946.

Refsum, S., Salomonsen, L., and Skatvedt, M.: Heredopathia atactica polyneuritiformis in children, J. Pediatr. **35**:335, 1949.

Richterich, R., Van Mechelen, P., and Rossi, E.: Refsum's disease (heredopathia atactica polyneuritiformis): an inborn error of lipid metabolism with storage of 3, 7, 11, 15-tetramethyl hexadecanoic acid, Am. J. Med. **39**:230, 1965.

Ricker, K., and Hertel, G.: Electrophysiological findings in the syndrome of acute ocular muscle palsy with ataxia (Fisher syndrome), J. Neurol. **214**:35, 1976.

Riley, C. M., and Moore, R. H.: Familial dysautonomia differentiated from related disorders: case reports and discussion of current concepts, Pediatrics **37**:435, 1966.

Robinson, A.: Ataxia-telangiectasia presenting with craniostenosis, Arch. Dis. Child. **37**:652, 1962.

Robinson, G. C., Jan, J. E., and Miller, J. R.: A new variety of hereditary sensory neuropathy, Hum. Genet. **35**:153, 1977.

Rosen, A. D., and Vastola, E. F.: Clinical effects of cyclophosphamide in Guillain-Barré polyneuritis, J. Neurol. Sci. **30**:179, 1976.

Rosenthal, S., and Kaufman, S.: Vincristine neurotoxicity, Ann. Intern. Med. **80**:733, 1974.

Russell, D. S., and Rubinstein, L. J.: Pathology of tumors of the nervous system, ed. 2, Baltimore, 1963, The Williams & Wilkins Co., p. 242.

Saberman, M. N., and Teta, L. T.: The Melkersson-Rosenthal syndrome, Arch. Otolaryng. **84**:292, 1966.

Sahgal, V., and Olsen, W. O.: Heredopathia atactica polyneuritiformis (phytanic acid storage disease), Arch. Intern. Med. **135**:585, 1975.

San Agustin, M., Nitowsky, H. M., and Borden, J. N.: Neonatal sciatic palsy after umbilical vessel injection, J. Pediatr. **60**:408, 1962.

Schaffner, W., et al.: Polyneuropathy following rubella immunization, Am. J. Dis. Child. **127**:684, 1974.

Scheinberg, L.: Polyneuritis in systemic lupus erythematosus, N. Engl. J. Med. **255**:416, 1956.

Schwartz, J. F., et al.: Bassen-Kornzweig syndrome: deficiency of serum beta-lipoprotein, Arch. Neurol. **8**:438, 1963.

Seto, D. S. Y., and Freeman, J. M.: Lead neuropathy in childhood, Am. J. Dis. Child. **197**:337, 1964.

Silbergeld, E. K., and Chisolm, J. J., Jr.: Lead poisoning: altered urinary catecholamine metabolites as indicators of intoxication in mice and children, Science **192**:153, 1976.

Smith, A. A., and Dancis, J.: Catecholamine release in familial dysautonomia, N. Engl. J. Med. **277**:61, 1967.

Smith, A. A., and Hui, F. W.: Unmyelinated nerves in familial dysautonomia, Neurology **23**:8, 1973.

Sobrevilla, L. A., Goodman, M. L., and Kane, C. A.: Demyelinating central nervous system disease, muscular atrophy and acanthocytosis (Bassen-Kornzweig syndrome), Am. J. Med. **37**:821, 1964.

Sohn, D., Valensi, Q., and Miller, S. P.: Neurologic manifestations of Hodgkin's disease, Arch. Neurol. **17**:429, 1967.

Solitare, G. B., and Lopez, V. F.: Louis-Bar's syndrome (ataxia-telangiectasia): neuropathologic observations, Neurology **17**:23, 1967.

Stevens, H.: Melkersson's syndrome, Neurology **15**:263, 1965.

Sullivan, M. P.: Leukemic infiltration of meninges and spinal nerve roots, Pediatrics **32**:63, 1963.

Sunderman, F. W., Jr.: Diethyldithiocarbamate therapy of thallotoxicosis, Am. J. Med. Sci. **253**:209, 1967.

Suzuki, K., and Suzuki, Y.: Globoid cell leucodystrophy (Krabbe's disease): deficiency of galactocerebroside β-galactosidase, Proc. Nat. Acad. Sci. **66**:302, 1970.

Swick, H. M., and McQuillen, M. P.: The use of steroids in the treatment of idiopathic polyneuritis, Neurology **26**:205, 1976.

Taverner, D., Cohen, S. B., and Hutchinson, B. C.: Comparison of corticotropin and prednisolone in treatment of idiopathic facial paralysis (Bell's palsy), Br. Med. J. **4**:20, 1971.

Taverner, D., et al.: Prevention of denervation in Bell's palsy, Br. Med. J. **1**:391, 1966.

Thomas, J. E., and Howard, F. M.: Segmental zoster paresis—a disease profile, Neurology **22**:459, 1972.

Thomas, P. K.: Metabolic neuropathy, J. R. Coll. Physicians Lond. **5**:154, 1973.

Thomas, P. K., and Calne, D. B.: Motor nerve conduction velocity in peroneal muscular atrophy: evidence for genetic heterogeneity, J. Neurol. Neurosurg. Psychiatry **37**:68, 1974.

Thomas, P. K., and Eliasson, J. G.: Diabetic neuropathy. In Dyck, P. J., Thomas, P. K., and Lambert, E. H., editors: Peripheral neuropathy, vol. 2, Philadelphia, 1975, W. B. Saunders Co., p. 956.

Thomas, P. K., and Lascelles, R. G.: The pathology of diabetic neuropathy, Q. J. Med. **35**:489, 1966.

Tschudy, D. P.: Biochemical lesions in porphyria, J.A.M.A. **191**:718, 1965.

Tyler, H. R.: Botulism, Arch. Neurol. **9**:652, 1963.

Van Gelder, D. W., and Darby, F. U.: Congenital and infantile beri-beri, J. Pediatr. **25**:226, 1944.

Varavithya, W., Dhanamitta, S., and Valyasevi, A.: Bilateral ptosis as a sign of thiamine deficiency in childhood, Clin. Pediatr. **14**:1063, 1975.

Vassella, F., et al.: Congenital sensory neuropathy with anhidrosis, Arch. Dis. Child. **43**:124, 1968.

Watson, C. J., and Schwartz, S.: A simple test for urinary porphobilinogen, Proc. Soc. Exp. Biol. Med., **47**:393, 1941.

Weller, T. H., and Witton, H. M.: The etiologic agents of varicella and herpes zoster: serologic studies with the viruses as propagated in vitro, J. Exp. Med. **108**:869, 1958.

Whitaker, J. N., et al.: The ultrastructure of circulating immunocytes in Guillain-Barré syndrome, Neurology **20**:765, 1970.

Windmiller, J., et al.: Vincristine sulfate in the treatment of neuroblastoma in children, Am. J. Dis. Child. **111**:75, 1966.

Winegrad, A. I., and Greene, D. A.: Diabetic polyneuropathy: the importance of insulin deficiency, hyperglycemia and alterations in myoinositol metabolism in its pathogenesis, N. Engl. J. Med. **295**:1416, 1976.

Winkelmann, R. K., Lambert, E. H., and Hayles, A. B.: Congenital absence of pain: report of a case and experimental studies, Arch. Dermatol. **85**:325, 1962.

Wochnik-Dyjas, D., Niewiadomsky, M., and Kostrzewska, E.: Porphyric polyneuropathy and its pathogenesis in the light of electrophysiological investigations, J. Neurol. Sci. **35**:243, 1978.

Wolf, S. M., et al.: Treatment of Bell palsy with prednisone: a prospective randomized study, Neurology **28**:158, 1978.

Wright, E. A., and McQuillen, M. P.: Hypoexcitability of ulnar nerve in patients with normal motor nerve conduction velocities, Neurology **23**:78, 1973.

Yao, J. K., and Dyck, P. J.: Lipid abnormalities in hereditary neuropathy, J. Neurol. Sci. **36**:225, 1978.

Yudell, A., et al.: The neuropathy of sulfatide lipidosis (metachromatic leukodystrophy), Neurology **17**:103, 1967.

Zacks, S. I., Langfitt, T. W., and Elliott, F. A.: Herpetic neuritis, Neurology **14**:744, 1964.

Ziegler, M. G., Lake, C. R., and Kopin, I. J.: Deficient sympathetic nervous response in familial dysautonomia, N. Engl. J. Med. **294**:630, 1976.

# CHAPTER 5

# Diseases of the neuromuscular junction

Through electrochemical reactions, the neuronal cell body generates an electrical impulse, the nerve action potential, which is conducted along the motor axon. In larger myelinated fibers this action potential moves from one node of Ranvier to another by a process termed "saltatory conduction." When the action potential reaches the terminal filaments of the axon, an unexplained mechanism causes vesicles (quanta) of acetylcholine to be released by exocytosis from release sites in the presynaptic region at the axon terminal (Heuser and Reese, 1973). Each vesicle contains approximately 10,000 acetylcholine molecules. After the acetylcholine passes through the release sites in the presynaptic membrane, it traverses the synaptic cleft (Elmqvist, 1965; Katz, 1962; Heuser, Reese, and Landis, 1974). On the postsynaptic membrane (end-plate) of the muscle cell a specific structural unit, the acetylcholine receptor, receives and binds the acetylcholine molecules (Fig. 5-1).

The binding of acetylcholine to receptor sites is associated with alterations in the postsynaptic membrane; the membrane manifests increased permeability to cations, especially sodium, potassium, and calcium. Electrical depolarization ensues. An ionic current is established that results in end-plate depolarization. Spontaneously released vesicles induce only localized end-plate depolarization. When end-plate depolarization exceeds

a certain threshold after a *nerve action potential* reaches the presynaptic area and 100 to 200 vesicles are released simultaneously and traverse the synaptic cleft, an end-plate potential results and a *muscle action potential* is generated. The extent of the depolarization is determined by the number of acetylcholine molecules bound by receptors. At any one time, only a minority of receptors at each neuromuscular junction is involved.

The acetylcholine bound to the receptor sites is rapidly hydrolyzed in the presence of acetylcholinesterase; free acetylcholine is removed by diffusion. Hydrolysis results in the formation of free choline and an acetyl group; the latter is eventually transformed into acetic acid.

The neuromuscular junction area contains the terminal portion of the axon, the synaptic cleft, which is approximately 40 to 50 nm wide, and a number of primary enfoldments (junctional folds) in the muscle membrane (Hubbard, 1973). In the terminal portion of the axon (presynaptic area), there are many small vesicles that contain acetylcholine and larger vesicles containing unknown substances (Engel et al., 1974). Most of the acetylcholine enclosed in the vesicles is synthesized in the cytoplasm of the terminal axon from choline and acetyl-CoA; the synthesis is mediated by choline acetyltransferase. The concentration of choline appears to be rate limiting. The vesicles are formed in an

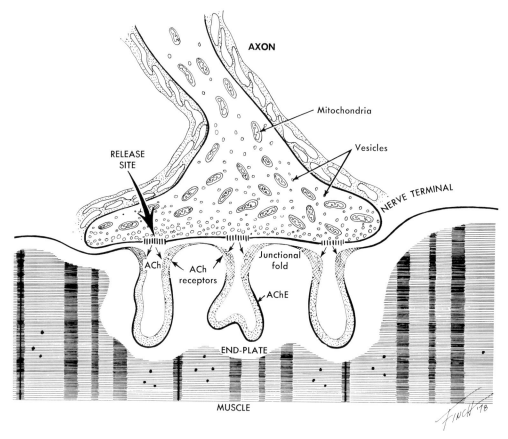

**Fig. 5-1.** This simplified drawing of the neuromuscular junction demonstrates relationship between presynaptic and postsynaptic membranes, junctional folds, and stored acetylcholine-containing vesicles. (Adapted from Drachman, 1978.)

unknown manner and, after gathering along the presynaptic membrane, bind with the membrane before acetylcholine release.

Axoplasmic flow from the cell body probably provides the necessary vesicles, mitochondria, and choline acetyltransferase. The nerve ending releases not only acetylcholine but also adenosine triphosphate and yet-to-be-identified substances including protein (Musik and Hubbard, 1972; Silinsky and Hubbard, 1973).

Although this explanation stresses the role of acetylcholine in neurotransmission, substantial evidence indicates that several substances are stored in the region of the presynaptic membrane, that they may be neurotransmitters, and that the postsynaptic membrane area contains mechanisms for their degradation. Other substances may be synthesized in the neuronal cell body, traverse the axon and then the synaptic cleft, and act as trophic agents in maintaining normal muscle structure and function.

The complexities of synthesis, packaging, storage, and release are compounded by the modifying effects of maturation. As an example, premature infants display posttetanic exhaustion (duration to 35 seconds) after repetitive stimulation of 20 impulses per second. Term infants are more resistant to this phenomenon but have less reserve than adults (Koenigsberger, Patten, and Lovelace, 1973).

On a weight basis, neonates require a

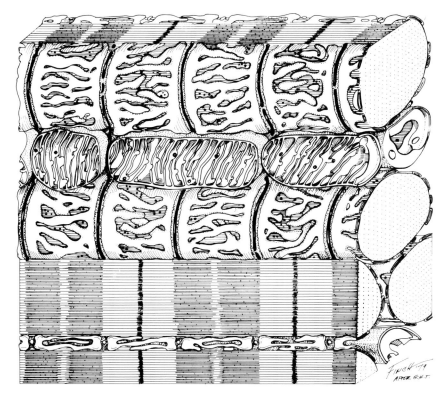

**Fig. 5-2.** Sarcoplasmic reticulum is composed of tubules and sacs that envelop myofibrils and form sac at A-I band junction. Transverse tubular system (T-system) is shown encircling myofibrils and is in juxtaposition to sarcoplasmic reticulum. Several large mitochondria are also depicted. Glycogen particles are between meshes of reticulum. (Modified from Revel, 1962.)

larger dose of depolarizing neuromuscular relaxants (for example, decamethonium or succinylcholine) than adults to manifest equal neuromuscular blockade (Cook and Fischer, 1978).

The potassium ion is the most important ion in maintaining and altering cellular resting potential. The 80 mv potential across the plasma membrane is the result of differences in concentration of ions inside and outside the cell. When the muscle is at rest the charge within the cell is negative in respect to that of the ions outside.

The plasma membrane is modified in the area of the neuromuscular junction to form multiple deep sulci that effectively increase the postsynaptic area. The infolding of the plasma membrane reaches to the A-I band interface and extends inward to form the transverse tubular (T-system) (see Chapter 2) (Porter and Palade, 1957).

The sarcoplasmic reticulum of the muscle is an intricate matrix of tubules and sacs interposed between the myofibrils (Bennett, 1956). The tubules of the sarcoplasmic reticulum surround the myofibrils and form a sac at the A-I band junction. This sac is juxtaposed to the T-system but is not connected. This area of confluence is known as the triad (Fig. 5-2).

The muscle action potential flows along the T-system after depolarization of the tubules and releases calcium ions from the neighboring sacs of the sarcoplasmic reticulum (Hoyle, 1970; Inesi and Malan, 1976; Endo, 1977). Subsequently, calcium ions are taken up and complexed in a troponin-calcium bond; adenosine triphosphatase (ATPase), which is fixed to the myosin cross bridges, hydrolyzes adenosine triphosphate (ATP) and causes release of high-energy phosphate bonds (Ebashi and Endo, 1968). A sequence of events is initiated, during which the actin filaments slide and reduce or obliterate the width of the H band (Figs. 2-3 and 2-4).

In reverse fashion, the muscle relaxes when calcium is taken up by the sarcoplasmic reticulum after the release of high-energy phosphate from ATP by ATPase residing in the sarcotubular system.

### Myasthenia gravis

Myasthenia gravis is a condition characterized by easy fatigability and fluctuating strength in the skeletal muscles, in children most often those subserved by the cranial nerves. The weakness is almost uniformly counteracted by anticholinesterase drugs.

**CLINICAL FEATURES.** Diseases of the neuromuscular junction are unusual in children. Myasthenia gravis is the most prevalent of these diseases; about 1% of all patients with myasthenia gravis are children (Teng and Osserman, 1956). The incidence of myasthenia gravis probably ranges between 0.5 and 3 per 100,000 population (Kurland and Alter, 1961).

Fatigability is the hallmark of myasthenia gravis. Patients weaken rapidly with exercise, and symptoms worsen through the day. The symptoms range in severity from mild ptosis to severe respiratory involvement, sometimes ending fatally despite optimum therapy. Early difficulty often includes unilateral or bilateral ptosis, strabismus, swallowing difficulties, and decrease in tidal volume. Deep tendon reflexes are usually present. Electrodiagnostic studies reflect fatigue on repetitive nerve stimulation and posttetanic exhaustion.

**CLASSIFICATION OF TYPES.** Although many variations occur, childhood myasthenia gravis can be classified in three general categories: (1) neonatal transient, (2) neonatal persistent, and (3) juvenile.

NEONATAL TRANSIENT MYASTHENIA GRAVIS. Neonatal transient myasthenia gravis is found in infants of mothers with myasthenia gravis. Symptoms usually appear in the first few hours after birth but onset may be delayed until the third day (Millichap and Dodge, 1960). Initial symptoms consist of weak suck, diffuse muscle weakness, little spontaneous movement, weak Moro's reflex, respiratory weakness, dysphagia, and ptosis. In rare instances, hypotonia in the newborn can result from myasthenia gravis. Symptoms usually persist for 1 to 4 weeks, although they may persist for months (Branch, Swift, and Dyken, 1978; Desmedt and Borenstein, 1977). The degree of maternal involvement does not foretell the likelihood or severity of transient myasthenia in the newborn. Only 10% to 15% of infants born to myasthenic mothers seem to be affected (Fraser and Turner, 1953; Viets and Brown, 1951; Namba, Brown, and Grob, 1970). Maternal thymectomy before or during pregnancy may not avert the possibility of transient neonatal myasthenia (Geddes and Kidd, 1951).

Transient neonatal myasthenia may be associated with an additional deficit in neuromuscular transmission. In one case, after a child of a myasthenic mother was found to have mild weakness at birth, electromyographic studies revealed a block on repetitive stimulation that responded to neostigmine. Neuromuscular transmission slowly returned to normal after application of multiple trains of stimuli. Post-tetanic facilitation was not observed. As the child matured, the block lessened and the child eventually recovered fully (Wise and McQuillen, 1970). This type of abnormality is common in adult patients with myasthenia gravis.

NEONATAL PERSISTENT MYASTHENIA GRAVIS (CONGENITAL MYASTHENIA GRAVIS). In neonatal persistent myasthenia gravis, the mother does not have myasthenia gravis. Symptoms of this type of myasthenia gravis usually appear on the first day of life but sometimes not until the third or fourth day. They include ptosis, poor cry, and general weakness (Millichap and Dodge, 1960; Namba, Brown, and Grob, 1970). Severe swallowing and respiratory difficulties may necessitate ventilatory assistance and tube feeding. On the other hand, symptoms may be so mild that the condition is not recognized for a year or two. As the disease continues, ptosis, external ophthalmoplegia, and facial weakness usually dominate the clinical picture. At times weakness of the bulbar muscles may be severe (Oberklaid and Hopkins, 1976). The disease is usually mild but is present for life, although occasional spontaneous remissions occur.

Among a number of reported familial cases are pedigrees in which there is no involvement of the extraocular muscles. The clinical symptomatology is dominated by feeding and respiratory impairment in the neonatal period (Greer and Schotland, 1960; Conomy, Levinsohn, and Fanaroff, 1975).

Possibly this condition has a higher than expected incidence of familial occurrence, or there may be a selection of the cases reported. In any event, just over 40% of familial cases appear before the age of 2 (Namba, Brown, and Grob, 1970).

JUVENILE MYASTHENIA GRAVIS. Juvenile myasthenia gravis resembles the adult form of myasthenia gravis. The disease usually develops after age 10. Girls are affected more often than boys, perhaps 6 times as often (Millichap and Dodge, 1960). In older patients, women are affected 3 times as often as men until the age of 40, after which the incidence is equal.

Although ptosis is the most common clinical sign, ophthalmoplegia and facial weakness are frequent. Limb weakness, symmetric or asymmetric, is also common. Weakness fluctuates from day to day and from one part of the day to another, usually being more evident late in the day. The course may be severe, necessitating frequent hospitalizations and mechanical respiratory assistance (Keynes, 1949). Complete or partial remissions occur in 25% of the cases, usually within the first 2 years after onset (Rowland and Layzer, 1971).

Often the disease is localized in the ocular muscles, but it may be diffuse from the beginning. Severity of symptoms varies widely;

symptoms do not include sensory changes or abnormalities of the pupil. Ptosis, strabismus, dysarthria, and dysphagia are evident in fluctuating degrees.

Although uncommon, profound muscle wasting may occur. In severe adult myasthenia gravis, neurogenic atrophy of the muscles of the tongue and other bulbar muscles and associated fatty pseudohypertrophy with proliferation of terminal nerve fibers have been reported. Terminal proliferation of axons may result as the motor fibers compensate for dysfunction of the neuromuscular transmission mechanism (Brownell, Oppenheimer, and Spalding, 1972).

A number of cases with onset in the second decade occurring in two families have been reported. Symptoms included limb-girdle weakness of a continuous nature. Electromyography revealed polyphasic action potentials of short duration, suggestive of a myopathy. Anticholinesterase therapy improved the electromyographic findings. Another case, possibly sporadic, has been reported that responded to thymectomy after failure of anticholinesterase therapy (McQuillen, 1966; Campa, Johns, and Adelman, 1971; Fenichel, 1978). Obviously these patients may not have myasthenia gravis, because both the clinical and electrodiagnostic studies are atypical.

An unusual manifestation of juvenile myasthenia gravis has been reported in a teenage boy with symptoms of 9 months' duration. The degree of weakness varied but was generally worse during the day. Repetitive strength testing induced transient improvement in the proximal muscles followed by progressive fatigability. The findings during electrical stimulation studies were most compatible with myasthenia gravis, but the incremental response to stimulation was similar to that reported in the mysathenic syndrome associated with bronchial neoplasm (Eaton-Lambert syndrome). Treatment with guanidine and neostigmine resulted in good clinical response (Dahl and Sato, 1974).

A puzzling condition, labeled myasthenic myopathy, has been reported (Rowland et

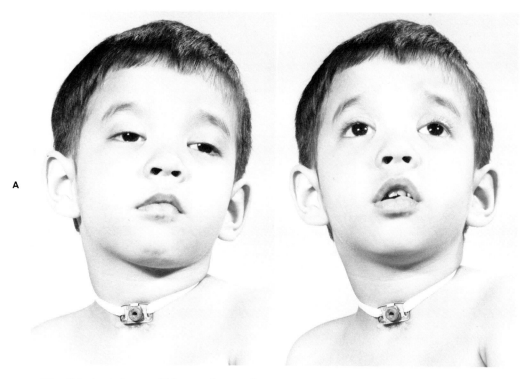

**Fig. 5-3. A,** A 3-year-old boy with myasthenia gravis since age 19 months who underwent thymectomy at 22 months of age. Before administration of edrophonium, ptosis and lack of forehead movement despite great effort are evident. **B,** After administration of edrophonium (Tensilon) he is able to lift his lids and raise his forehead.

al., 1973). In this disorder, associated with thymoma, the distribution of weakness closely resembles myasthenia gravis, but the pharmacologic reactions typical of myasthenia are not present. This condition has not been reported in children.

DIAGNOSIS. The procedure of the diagnostic test for myasthenia gravis is relatively straightforward. The intravenous test dose of edrophonium (Tensilon) for children weighing up to 30 kg is 1 mg; for children weighing more, 2 mg. In infants the recommended dose is 0.5 mg. If necessary, older children may be given up to 0.2 mg/kg, not to exceed a total of 10 mg. Appropriate equipment and personnel for respiratory assistance must be immediately available. Subcutaneous or intramuscular administration is usually unsatisfactory. After intravenous administration,

muscle weakness decreases within a minute or two; the beneficial effects disappear within 5 minutes (Fig. 5-3). Before the edrophonium is given, it is essential to assess the baseline of weakness by administering a placebo in the form of saline. Degree of ptosis, strength of fist closing, and number of repetitive fist closings may be used during this assessment. Neostigmine is occasionally used for diagnostic studies, but the side effects of muscarinic and nicotinic action may prove unpleasant and persist much longer than when edrophonium chloride is given.

Curare testing should not be used to establish the diagnosis unless the physician is experienced with the test and necessary support equipment and personnel are immediately at hand.

Voluntary muscle function decreases within 20 minutes after intravenous infusion of sodium lactate (5 mg/kg of body weight in a 1M solution) in patients with myasthenia but not in normal patients. Because a decrease in extracellular calcium level diminishes the amount of acetylcholine released with each nerve impulse, and because the serum calcium concentration decreases in normal and myasthenic individuals during lactate infusion, the lactate effect may be mediated through calcium changes (Patten, Oliver, and Engel, 1974). This test may prove valuable in the future for diagnostic purposes.

**LABORATORY FINDINGS.** A number of associated laboratory changes are usually demonstrable in myasthenia gravis.

ELECTRODIAGNOSIS. Abnormalities have been described following electrical stimulation of ulnar and median nerves. Among the techniques employed, one utilizes stimulating electrodes (5 mm in diameter) that are applied with a fixed interelectrode distance (for example, 2 or 3 cm) to the ulnar and median nerves at the wrists. Evoked potentials are recorded from the abductor pollicis brevis muscle during median nerve stimulation and the abductor digiti minimi muscle during ulnar nerve stimulation by means of small lead surface electrodes. The active electrode is placed over the motor point and the indifferent electrode over the muscle tendon (Horowitz et al., 1976). Square wave impulses of short duration (for example, 0.15 to 0.20 msec) are delivered at varying frequencies (for example, 1, 3, 5, 8, 10, 15, 20, and 50 Hz). Different criteria may be applied to determine whether myasthenia gravis is present, but a decrement of greater than 7% is usually considered to be abnormal in response to repetitive supramaximal stimulation (Ozdemir and Young, 1971). In one study, if amplitudes of the second through the sixth evoked potentials demonstrated a gradual decrement, and if the decrement of any of the potentials was greater than 10% when compared with the first, the diagnosis was considered established (Horowitz et al., 1976).

The regional curare test is employed in conjunction with electrodiagnostic stimulation tests. In these tests, a blood pressure cuff is utilized to obstruct all blood supply to the arm by raising the inflated pressure to 100 mm Hg above systolic pressure after the arm is elevated for 1 minute. A scalp vein needle, directed distally, is inserted into a superficial forearm vein before the cuff is inflated above systolic pressure.

The arm is lowered and *d*-tubocurarine (in adults, 0.2 mg in 20 ml of 0.9% sodium chloride) is injected. The cuff remains inflated for 6½ minutes.

Thereafter supramaximal stimulation of the median and ulnar nerves is performed as described before. Stimulation at 3 Hz for 15 seconds is applied at 5 and 6 minutes after the injection is begun, while the arm is still ischemic. After 6½ minutes the cuff is deflated, the blood circulates through the arm for 90 seconds, and then the nerves are stimulated (for example, at 3, 5, 10, 15, or 20 Hz) for 15 seconds every 60 to 90 seconds until 11 or 12 minutes have passed. The test is normal unless a decrement of 10% occurs. In the case of an abnormal test, stimulation may be continued at the rate that produces the greatest decrement every 3 to 4 minutes for 20 minutes and every 5 to 10 minutes thereafter until 40 to 45 minutes have passed. By this time improvement should be evident. (Horowitz et al., 1976). This study has not been extensively tested on children, and the dose of curare and saline should be adjusted accordingly.

MORPHOLOGY. In patients with myasthenia gravis, the muscles are small but otherwise normal. Microscopically the muscle tissue may be relatively normal, but muscle fibers are often atrophied. On superficial inspection they appear to be involved singly, but closer inspection may show group lesions of multiple atrophied fibers suggestive of denervation. Electron microscopic study of the postsynaptic area reveals the plasmalemmal folds to be fewer than normal and abnormally shallow, a pattern consistent with denervation atrophy (Bickerstaff, Evans, and Woolf, 1960; Fardeau, 1973).

Histochemical study shows the atrophied muscle fibers to be primarily type II, which are predominantly glycolytic in metabolic activity. In other areas, necrosis of muscle fibers and lymphorrhages are seen. These lymphorrhages, found in the thyroid gland and occasionally in other organs (Wolf, Rowland, and Schotland, 1966), are aggregations of lymphocytes that are primarily perivenous and often abut on areas of muscle necrosis (Engel and McFarlin, 1966). Occasional muscle changes consistent with interstitial polymyositis have been reported (Rowland et al., 1956).

Thymomas occur in about 10% of adult patients with myasthenia gravis but do not appear in children.

**PATHOPHYSIOLOGY.** The defect underlying virtually all cases of myasthenia gravis is the result of an autoimmune mechanism that causes an effective decrease in the number of available acetylcholine receptors on the postsynaptic membrane (Drachman, 1978). The breakthrough in determining this phenomenon occurred when specific toxins from the venoms of elapid snakes that bind to the acetylcholine receptors became available. Particularly, the use of $^{125}$I-labelled $\alpha$-bungarotoxin has been exceedingly valuable (Miledi and Potter, 1971). The material binds irreversibly and specifically to the acetylcholine receptors. Another material, $\alpha$-cobra toxin, binds specifically but is slowly released from the binding sites (Lee, 1972). Studies reveal decreased acetylcholine receptor sites in myasthenic patients (Drachman, 1978).

Other studies demonstrate structural changes, including fewer than expected shallow folds in the postsynaptic membrane and reduction in overall terminal size. Ultramicroscopic studies reveal what appears to be a normal number of normal-sized acetylcholine vesicles in these areas. The injection of $\alpha$-cobra toxin into animals reproduces the clinical and electrodiagnostic features of myasthenia gravis.

The immune mechanism responsible for myasthenia gravis is not completely understood, although immunologic abnormalities have been known for decades (Nastuk and Strauss, 1961). The development of antibodies to acetylcholine receptors and their use in animals demonstrated the induction of typical electrical responses of myasthenia gravis (that is, decremental responses on repetitive nerve stimulation) after use of the material (Patrick and Lindstrom, 1973). The mechanism through which humans become immunized with resultant myasthenia gravis is unknown, but the thymic lymphocytes are probably involved (Vincent et al., 1978). As more sensitive radioimmunoassay techniques have been developed, an increasingly higher percentage of myasthenia gravis patients have been found to have receptor-binding antibodies (Bender et al., 1975; Lindstrom et al., 1976). Nevertheless, there is still a lack of uniform relationship of the antibody titers to the clinical condition of the patients.

Antibodies to acetylcholine receptors may diminish the number of available receptors by at least three different mechanisms: blockage of the active site of the receptor molecule, increased degradation of receptors, or decreased synthesis of receptors (Drachman, 1978). Current evidence suggests that the antibodies cause accelerated degeneration of acetylcholine receptors as well as blockage of the receptors (Kao and Drachman, 1977; Drachman et al., 1977). There is no evidence that acetylcholine receptor synthesis is affected.

In the past, several other theories have been postulated concerning the etiology of myasthenia gravis. One theory hypothesized the secretion of material by the thymus (thymin) that could affect neuromuscular transmission (Goldstein, 1971); yet another theory proposed that myasthenia gravis results from a diffuse abnormality in the lower motor neuron. It is postulated that there is a humoral substance (myasthenin) that positively affects the well-being of the anterior horn cell body, which in turn nurtures the twigs of its axonal tree. As a result of myasthenin failure, susceptible peripheral axonal fiber tips and the muscle fibers they supply malfunction (Engel and Warmolts, 1971; Engel et al., 1974).

Both of these theories appear to have limited applicability at this time.

**GENETIC FINDINGS.** Familial myasthenia gravis is uncommon, accounting for only 3.5% of all cases. Congenital myasthenia constitutes one third of these cases. In monozygotic twins, the disease is present in both sibs roughly one third of the time (Jacob, Clack, and Emery, 1968; McLean and McKone, 1973). The pattern of inheritance is variable (Pirskanen, 1977).

**TREATMENT.** Therapy for the various types of myasthenia will be discussed individually.

NEONATAL TRANSIENT MYASTHENIA GRAVIS. The infant must be treated to maintain ventilation and swallowing abilities for the duration of the transient weakness. If the patient does not have significantly impaired respiration or swallowing mechanisms, drugs should be withheld. If the child's swallowing mechanism is not seriously impaired but medication is required, oral neostigmine may be employed. Pyridostigmine appears to cause fewer muscarinic side effects and can be made into a syrup with 0.1 ml containing 1 mg of drug.

Infants who cannot swallow should receive $\frac{1}{30}$ of the oral dose of pyridostigmine by injection or 0.1 mg of neostigmine methylsulfate 30 minutes before feeding. Dosage adjustment can occur thereafter to allow for efficient swallowing and respiration and minimize untoward side effects. Therapy is rarely necessary for more than 4 to 6 weeks.

NEONATAL PERSISTENT MYASTHENIA GRAVIS. The facial weakness may be so severe that there is impairment of feeding, which is additive to the weakness of the muscles of deglutition. Ophthalmoplegia may be partial. Although symptoms of facial weakness and swallowing difficulty are usually responsive to anticholinesterase therapy, ophthalmoplegia is often refractory to anticholinesterase therapy. The use and value of steroids for the treatment of myasthenic ophthalmoplegia in the newborn have not been well-documented. In the occasional case of marked generalized weakness, thymectomy should be considered. There is insufficient data to

aid the clinician in choosing between thymectomy or steroid therapy, if anticholinesterase therapy does not prove optimal.

JUVENILE MYASTHENIA GRAVIS. A number of factors must be placed into the equation that determines the therapeutic approach. It is most important to separate those patients who have only extraocular weakness from those who have generalized myasthenia. Many of the patients with limited extraocular myasthenia will improve substantially or experience remission; those with generalized myasthenia have a less promising outlook.

Treatment of patients with juvenile myasthenia gravis who have only extraocular involvement should begin with anticholinesterase therapy, preferably pyridostigmine (see Table 5-1).

Those patients with limited involvement who do not respond to pyridostigmine should receive every-other-day prednisone therapy (20 to 30 mg/m²). (The dose for an average 10-year-old will be 20 to 30 mg in the morning every other day.) If improvement does not occur or the effect is not optimal, the dosage should be increased by 5 mg/dose every 2 weeks until optimum strength and stamina are achieved. After several months, it may be possible to adjust the dosage downward while the patient continues to maintain the same performance level.

Evidence suggests that prednisone therapy is better than anticholinesterase therapy in extraocular muscle myasthenia gravis; however, the possible long-term side effects of steroids make anticholinesterase therapy the first choice. More information concerning the anticholinesterase drugs and steroids follows later in this chapter.

For those individuals who have generalized juvenile myasthenia gravis, attempts at control with anticholinesterase drugs, preferably pyridostigmine, should be made. Failure to achieve optimum improvement of symptoms should result in serious consideration of thymectomy. Following thymectomy, the use of anticholinesterase drugs and/or the introduction of prednisone therapy is

**Table 5-1.** Drug therapy of myasthenia gravis (beginning dosages)

| Drug | Infants | Children | Onset of action and duration | Remarks |
|---|---|---|---|---|
| Ambenonium chloride (Mytelase) | 1-2 mg (oral) every 4 hours | 2.5-5 mg (oral) every 4 hours | 20-30 minutes 4-5 hours | Longer duration of effect than pyridostigmine and may accumulate |
| Atropine sulfate | 0.01 mg/kg (subcutaneous) | 0.02-0.04 mg/kg (subcutaneous) | 3-5 minutes 2-3 hours; variable | Used as temporary expedient only; may be repeated in 4 hours if necessary |
| Edrophonium chloride (Tensilon) | 0.15 mg/kg (intravenous, subcutaneous, intramuscular) | 0.2 mg/kg (intravenous, subcutaneous, intramuscular) | 20-30 seconds 3-4 minutes | Caution: concentration is 10 mg/ml (5 kg child receives 0.1 ml); effect occurs within minutes after intravenous administration; use of other drugs for diagnostic purposes is seldom necessary or advised |
| Ephedrine sulfate | 2-3 mg (oral) every 6 hours | 5-10 mg (oral) every 4 hours | 30-40 minutes 4-5 hours | Used as supplementary drug only |
| Neostigmine bromide (Prostigmin) | 1-2 mg (oral) every 4 hours | 7.5-15 mg (oral) every 4 hours | 10-20 minutes 3-4 hours | Caution: If it must be given parenterally, only $1/30$ of oral dose should be given as neostigmine methylsulfate (Prostigmine) |
| Prednisone | 60 mg/m$^2$ every other day, (oral, one dose in A.M.) | 60 mg/m$^2$ every other day, (oral, one dose in A.M.) | Improvement noted in 1 to 6 weeks | Recommended only after anticholinesterase therapy and thymectomy have failed; anticholinesterase drugs should be discontinued and respiration supported mechanically if necessary; must administer antacid and potassium chloride also; need extensive inpatient care (Engel et al., 1974) |
| Pyridostigmine bromide (Mestinon) | 4-10 mg (oral) every 4 hours, syrup form | 30-45 mg (oral) every 4 hours | 10-35 minutes 3½-4½ hours | Caution: If it must be given parenterally, only $1/30$ of oral dose should be given. Slow-release form available (180 mg); chloride form available for patients intolerant of bromide |

usually necessary and advisable. Further information concerning anticholinesterase therapy, steroid therapy, and thymectomy should be sought later in this chapter.

Plasmapheresis in the therapy of myasthenia is undergoing evaluation (Pinching, Peters, and Davis, 1976; Howard and Sanders, 1979).

ANTICHOLINESTERASE DRUGS. Children are usually treated with pyridostigmine bromide or neostigmine. Pyridostigmine bromide causes fewer muscarinic side effects. In adult patients, pyridostigmine bromide exerts a more beneficial effect on bulbar muscles than neostigmine. The pharmacologic effect of a 60 mg pyridostigmine tablet is equivalent to a 15 mg tablet of neostigmine. The injectable form of pyridostigmine bromide is rarely used; it is 30 times as effective as the oral form. The dosage necessary for adequate control of symptoms varies widely (Table 5-1). Undertreatment to a slight degree is preferable to overtreatment.

Persistent weakness can be assessed by a diagnostic test. Edrophonium chloride is injected intravenously at the expected time of maximal benefit of the maintenance drug while the patient's strength is monitored. Increase in strength suggests that a larger dosage of anticholinesterase drug is worthy of clinical trial. Rarely, anticholinesterase drugs may transiently stimulate the end-plate and cause temporary improvement in the presence of chronic anticholinesterase overdosage. Subsequently, overdosage may cause a cholinergic crisis.

Persistence of weakness despite therapy may necessitate tracheotomy, mechanical respiratory assistance, suctioning, antibiotics, and other forms of supportive therapy.

The patient should be hospitalized during initiation of therapy and should not be discharged until the weakness is well regulated with a routine therapeutic regimen. If the child is too young to swallow pills or if the swallowing mechanism is severely compromised, a syrup is available; the syrup contains 60 mg/5 ml of pyridostigmine bromide. The doses should be increased systematically to determine the most beneficial

amount. In older children, pyridostigmine bromide is usually given every 4 hours, beginning with a 30 mg dose. The maximal effect of the drug occurs in an hour, and edrophonium chloride may be given intravenously to determine whether more improvement can be achieved by increasing the dosage of anticholinesterase drug. The slow-release preparation of pyridostigmine bromide may be used in children who can swallow the tablets.

The muscarinic symptoms of intoxication include lacrimation, salivation, vomiting, diarrhea, and bradycardia. Reduction of symptoms can be effected by the use of a small dose of atropine. Subsequent doses of anticholinesterase drugs should be decreased. Atropine usually need not be given routinely.

The muscarinic effects usually precede nicotinic effects, which include weakness, cramps, and muscular fasciculations.

CORTICOTROPIN AND CORTICOSTEROIDS. Corticotropin and corticosteroid therapy are of value in myasthenia gravis (Cape and Utterback, 1972; Namba, 1972; Shapiro, Namba, and Grob, 1971; Warmolts and Engel, 1972). Steroid therapy is probably effective because abnormalities of the immune system appear causal in neuromuscular dysfunction. Increasing evidence suggests that alternate-day therapy with relatively large doses of prednisone is effective in juvenile and adult myasthenia.

Prednisone may not be associated with an initial period of progressive weakness, as has been reported with ACTH therapy (Engel et al., 1974), if anticholinesterase therapy is first discontinued and respiration is mechanically supported as necessary.

Complications of prednisone therapy include cataracts, diabetes mellitus, hypertension, and osteoporosis. The therapist should be thoroughly familiar with the regimen and its dangers before instituting prednisone therapy (Engel et al., 1974).

EXPERIMENTAL DRUGS. Germine monoacetate, a semisynthetic derivative of *Veratrum* alkaloids, has been used experimentally with some promise. The compound generates repetitive electrical activity after a single normal action potential, thus amplifying muscle tension and proportionately increasing neuromuscular transmission (Flacke, 1973). This facilitation mechanism affects the sensory nervous system, resulting in spurious sensations of taste and temperature.

THYMECTOMY. Thymectomy is becoming more important in the treatment of myasthenia gravis. After years of controversy punctuated by transatlantic claims and counterclaims, thymectomy has been accepted as a successful method of therapy (Mulder, Herrmann, and Buckberg, 1974). It has been used particularly in young women without thymoma who have had myasthenia for a short time (Keynes, 1954). Thymectomy has not been used extensively in juvenile myasthenia gravis, but its use is becoming more widespread. Although the efficacy of thymectomy is controversial, the positive results are encouraging (Ryniewicz and Badurska, 1977); success has been achieved in patients with onset of symptoms during the first and second years of life (Clarke and Van de Velde, 1971; Sutin and Hewitson, 1966; Swaiman and Varco, 1972). The patient undergoing thymectomy needs careful monitoring and observation before, during, and after the procedure.

Thymomas rarely occur in juvenile myasthenia gravis, and therefore the removal of thymus tissue because of the possibility of these tumors is unnecessary.

The beneficial effects of thymectomy are not fully explained (Sambrook et al., 1976; Scadding, Thomas, and Havard, 1977). It is likely that the thymus is associated with the formation of antibodies directed at the acetylcholine receptors in the postsynaptic membrane (Twomey et al., 1979).

MYASTHENIC CRISIS VERSUS CHOLINERGIC CRISIS. The patient may be unable to maintain adequate respiration or manage oropharyngeal secretions if drug therapy has not been properly followed; if the drug regimen has included antibiotics, certain central nervous system depressants such as narcotics, barbiturates, tranquilizers, and antiarrhythmic and local anesthetic agents (quinidine, quinine, procainamide, propranolol, lidocaines, and related drugs); or if hypokalemia has been induced. This development of profound weakness is known as a myasthenic crisis and may lead to death rapidly unless appropriate therapy is instituted promptly. Unfortunately, the clinical pattern is similar to that resulting from overdosage of anticholinesterase drugs or so-called cholinergic crisis. At times, cholinergic crisis is associated with increased perspiration and oropharyngeal secretions, vomiting, and diarrhea.

It is critical to determine whether the muscle weakness results from too much or too little medication. The differentiation may be difficult to achieve from the history or examination.

The patient should be hospitalized. Personnel and equipment for providing ventilatory assistance should be immediately at hand.

The child should be given 1 to 2 mg of edrophonium chloride intravenously (Table 5-1) at the time the peak effect of ongoing anticholinesterase therapy is expected or at 30-minute intervals during this period. Improvement usually indicates the presence of a myasthenic crisis and warrants further administration of long-acting anticholinesterase drugs. The most important indicator of improvement is an increase in vital capacity. Edrophonium may not affect limb muscle strength and respiratory muscle strength equally.

A note of caution is necessary. Anticholinesterase drugs can temporarily stimulate the end-plate but may in time produce a neuromuscular block by occupying acetylcholine binding sites. This situation may lead to the transient improvement of muscle function in the presence of a chronic overdosage of anticholinesterase drugs (Flacke, 1973). Occasionally a patient has immediate syncope after injection but usually recovers rapidly without therapy (Engel et al., 1974).

In addition to drug administration, tracheotomy and artificial support of respiration with suctioning of accumulating secretions are important in maintaining the patient through the episode. If edrophonium administration does not appear to improve the condition or the condition deteriorates, a cholinergic crisis is probably present. This situation necessitates tracheotomy and mechanical support of respiration and discontinuance of anticholinesterase therapy. Administration of atropine sulfate may be needed to reduce perspiration, abdominal cramps, diarrhea, and vomiting. Fastidious nursing techniques are necessary (Engel et al., 1974).

It may be difficult to differentiate cholinergic crisis from myasthenic crisis. If so, all drugs should be withheld and mechanical respiration should be employed as necessary for 48 to 72 hours to determine the true nature of the problem.

### Myasthenic syndrome (other conditions associated with myasthenia)

Although most patients with myasthenic syndrome appear to have associated disease processes, some may have primary impairment of the neuromuscular junction apparatus, yet they do not have conventional myasthenia gravis. A boy who began having ptosis at 5 days of age and had continued difficulty with squint and generalized weakness has been reported. The use of anticholinesterase drugs was without effect.

Subsequent studies documented decreased acetylcholine release, small nerve terminals, and impairment of end-plate acetylcholine esterase activity. The pathophysiology of this condition is not certain, and the abnormality could reside in either the presynaptic or postsynaptic area. On the basis of their studies, the investigators postulated an abnormality of acetylcholine esterase action in the postsynaptic membrane area (Engel, Lambert, and Gomez, 1977).

The myasthenic syndrome has accompanied both hyperthyroidism and hypothyroidism. Symptoms in hyperthyroidism include weakness and inability to sustain muscle contraction, with a predilection for muscles of the pelvic girdle and thigh. Greenberg and LaRuffa (1966) reported the case of an 8½-year-old boy with hyperthyroidism and myasthenia gravis. He had ptosis and diffuse weakness. He was initially treated with propylthiouracil but did not improve. The addition of prednisone to the regimen caused mild improvement. The association with myasthenia was noted later when he responded to neostigmine, although he had not previously benefited from edrophonium chloride. The combination of antithyroid and anticholinesterase drugs proved beneficial. Other reports are similar (Schlezinger and Corin, 1968).

Ptosis is not common in hyperthyroidism but impairment of ocular muscle movement occurs frequently. The eyelids are often retracted, resulting in the familiar pattern of proptosis. The presence of ptosis in a patient with hyperthyroidism should suggest coexistent myasthenia gravis. Muscular twitching and tremors may also provide important diagnostic clues.

Patients with coexistent hypothyroidism and myasthenia gravis appear to have an increased requirement for anticholinesterase drugs. Although treatment with thyroxine is of some benefit, the patient also needs anticholinesterase drugs in moderate dosage. Other signs and symptoms of hypothyroidism are usually present, including slow contraction of muscles, stiffness, and occasionally, myotonia. The deep tendon reflexes tend to have a slow relaxation phase.

Myasthenia syndrome occurs in association with small cell carcinoma of the lung (Eaton-Lambert syndrome) in adults, who usually improve after anticholinesterase drug therapy. The disease usually spares the extraocular and facial muscles. The disease can be differentiated from myasthenia gravis by electrodiagnostic procedures. In patients with this form of myasthenic syndrome, muscle action potentials increase in amplitude with continuous muscle stimulation, which contrasts greatly with the decremental response in patients with true myasthenia gravis (Elmqvist and Lambert, 1968; Takamori, 1972). The pathophysiologic error appears to be in the release or size of the vesicles (Lambert and Elmqvist, 1971). Patients generally respond better to guanidine than to anticholinesterase drugs.

In a 10-year-old boy, the myasthenic syndrome preceded acute leukemia (Shapira et al., 1974). The syndrome has also been reported several times in association with lupus erythematosus. In addition to therapy for lupus erythematosus, the patients require anticholinesterase medication (Wolf and Barrows, 1966).

The myasthenic syndrome has been reported in an 18-year-old boy who developed rheumatoid arthritis at age 14. The myasthenic symptoms and signs were reversible with anticholinesterase therapy. The rheumatoid arthritis spontaneously remitted 5 years later (Aarli, Milde, and Thunold, 1975).

One patient, a 3-year-old girl, was found to have myasthenic syndrome and cerebellar ataxia associated with a neuroblastoma. Removal of the neuroblastoma resulted in cessation of ophthalmoplegia, ptosis, facial weakness, and ataxia (Robinson and Howard, 1969).

The myasthenic syndrome has also been associated with the use of trimethadione (Tridione), and in this situation the response to anticholinesterase drugs has been relatively poor. In one case, the patient was symptom-free and within 4 months after discontinuation of the trimethadione did not need pyridostigmine (Peterson, 1966). The relationship between myasthenia gravis and trimethadione is unknown, although trimethadione has induced both the nephrotic syndrome and lupus erythematosus in humans.

Myasthenic syndrome has been associated with wasp sting (Brumlik, 1976), myotonic dystrophy (Schoen, 1977), and penicillamine therapy of rheumatoid arthritis (Bucknell et al., 1975).

### Myasthenic syndrome associated with antibiotics

A relationship between myasthenic symptoms and antibiotic administration was first reported in association with neomycin sulfate (Pridgen, 1956). Subsequently, myasthenic symptoms have been associated with neomycin, streptomycin, dihydrostreptomycin, kanamycin, polymyxin, bacitracin, lincomycin, and colistin. Streptomycin impairs stimulus transmission in myasthenic patients (Hokkanen and Toivakka, 1969). Other drugs that appear to facilitate the development of myasthenic response to antibiotics include ether, succinylcholine, gallamine triethiodide, and tubocurarine.

Myasthenic weakness is most likely to develop postoperatively, and it is usually manifested by respiratory failure, diffuse muscular weakness, and pupillary and visual abnormalities (McQuillen, Cantor, and O'Rourke, 1968). Naturally occurring myasthenia gravis is mimicked, because both peripheral and bulbar muscles are involved. The deep tendon reflexes may be normal, hyporeflexic, or areflexic. Problems of this nature occur at all ages, including the first day of life.

The route of administration of the offending antibiotic is unimportant. The affected muscles do respond to direct electrical stimulation, but the response is decreased from normal.

The nature of the neuromuscular block differs from that occurring with curare. The block is less pronounced with faster rates of stimulation and can often be overcome by administering calcium. The effects suggest that the block is presynaptic, but little more is known about the mechanism (McQuillen, Cantor, and O'Rourke, 1968).

Intravenous administration of calcium is the most efficacious approach, but therapy with neostigmine and edrophonium chloride is beneficial.

### Organophosphate poisoning

Insecticides of the organophosphate type, widely used commercially and domestically, are potent central nervous system antagonists and should be handled with great care (Smith, 1977). Parathion is probably the most commonly used. Other substances in this group are malathion, tetraethylpyrophosphate, and a number of other compounds used as nerve gases in warfare.

**MECHANISMS OF ACTION.** Organophosphates inhibit cholinesterase by a mechanism not completely delineated. Cholinesterases have been divided arbitrarily into two types: acetylcholinesterase, the *true* type, and butyrylcholinesterase, the *pseudo* type. Both types hydrolyze acetylcholine, but acetylcholinesterase is more efficient and faster acting. Butyrylcholinesterase slowly hydrolyzes acetylcholine but quickly hydrolyzes butyrylcholine, which is not a natural neurotransmitter. These two esterases also differ in ability to degrade other compounds. Acetylcholinesterase resides primarily in neurons and at the neuromuscular junction; butyrylcholinesterase resides in glial cells, plasma, liver, and other organs. Organophosphate compounds inhibit both cholinesterases. Reduced butyrylcholinesterase activity in plasma is a helpful indicator in diagnosing organophosphate poisoning, and blood should be drawn for study of this enzyme whenever the diagnosis is suspected.

Although the diagnosis can be confirmed by determining the pseudocholinesterase activity of the red cells, the information may not be available until the patient's clinical crisis has passed. In the case of suspected poisoning, blood studies for pseudocholinesterase activity should be initiated.

**CLINICAL FEATURES.** The patient may be exposed to organophosphates in a number of ways, most often through the respiratory tract or by absorption from the skin. Symptoms result from continuous stimulation of the receptor on the postsynaptic membrane by acetylcholine because of the lack of acetylcholinesterase activity. The symptoms of this continuous postsynaptic membrane stimulation may be conveniently categorized in two groups: muscarinic and nicotinic. The usual early symptoms are muscarinic.

**MUSCARINIC EFFECTS.** Muscarinic symptoms consist of nausea, epigastric and substernal tightness, sweating, and belching. The route of exposure may predetermine the nature of early symptoms. Ingestion results in gastrointestinal distress. After absorption through the skin, sweating and muscular fasciculations are common. Inhalation causes respiratory effects consisting principally of bronchospasm. Regardless of the method of contact, severe exposure results in increased peristaltic activity in the entire gastrointestinal tract, causing vomiting and diarrhea, followed by salivation, lacrimation, profuse sweating, dyspnea, and sometimes wheezing. Overwhelming exposure often causes involuntary urination and defecation and excessive bronchial secretion. Pulmonary edema may become apparent (Durham and Hayes, 1962).

**NICOTINIC EFFECTS.** Nicotinic effects, usually appearing later than the muscarinic effects, consist primarily of fasciculations of muscle and severe muscle cramping, usually with fatigability and weakness. Prolonged exposure often causes severe weakness, including failure of the respiratory muscles.

Toxicity in the form of delayed Guillain-Barré syndrome has been reported following organophosphate poisoning (Fisher, 1977; Eisen and Humphreys, 1974; Doull, 1976).

The peripheral nervous system is not the only segment of the nervous system involved. Symptoms of central dysfunction include headache, anxiety, withdrawal, and coma (Durham and Hayes, 1962). If death occurs, it is usually from respiratory compromise brought on by profuse bronchial secretions, respiratory muscle weakness, bronchoconstriction, and depression of medullary respiratory centers.

Children as young as 8 weeks old have been victims of organophosphate poisoning (Eitzman and Wolfson, 1967; Mackey, 1966). The history of exposure is essential in early diagnosis. The organic solvents used as vehicles in insecticide sprays potentiate the effects of organophosphates. They facilitate rapid skin absorption, and even small amounts can be dangerous to children if their clothes become saturated with the spray. Phenothiazines also potentiate the toxic effects (Arterberry et al., 1962). Major tranquilizers should not be used to counteract the early toxic symptoms of anxiety and restlessness.

**TREATMENT.** The drugs used primarily for organophosphate poisoning are atropine and 2-pyridine aldoxime methiodide (2-PAM) or 2-pyridine aldoxime methylchloride (2-PAM chloride, pralidoxime chloride) (Milby, 1971). Large doses of atropine are needed to prevent or ameliorate the profound muscarinic symptoms and control tachycardia and arrhythmias that may result in death. Administration of atropine to an anoxic patient may of itself result in ventricular tachycardia and fibrillation. Therefore an adequate airway and proper respiration must be established before atropine is administered to an unconscious patient with compromised respiration.

Atropine should be given intravenously if possible, 1 to 2 mg in small children. The patient should improve in 4 minutes and the maximum effect should be gained by 8 minutes. If no improvement is apparent after 8 minutes, intravenous injection of 1 mg should be repeated at 5- to 10-minute intervals unless there are indications of atropine intoxication.

Atropine appears to have little benefit in controlling central nervous system symptoms. Seizures may develop during treatment, and if so, an anticonvulsant drug should be administered. Succinylcholine potentiates anticholinesterase drugs and should not be given to these patients.

Of the specific antidotes to anticholinesterase poisoning, 2-PAM chloride appears to be the most useful (Arterberry et al., 1962; Durham and Hayes, 1962; Quinby and Clappison, 1961). 2-PAM chloride belongs to the chemical group known as oximes. These drugs have relatively few side effects in humans. Since they liberate cyanide in vitro and in vivo, their shelf life is limited, and they should be examined frequently for the presence of free cyanide. The oximes promote three general actions: (1) reactivation

of inhibited cholinesterase, (2) binding and subsequent inactivation of organophosphate, and (3) inhibition of excessive cholinesterase activity. 2-PAM chloride and the other oximes do not appear to effect cholinesterase activity in the brain or pass the blood-brain barrier. However, there is some controversy on this matter (Rosenberg, 1960).

The dosage of 2-PAM chloride is 20 to 40 mg/kg of body weight, injected intravenously over 30 minutes; this dosage may be repeated in 1 hour if necessary (Milby, 1971; Zavon, 1971).

## REFERENCES

Aarli, J. A., Milde, E. J., and Thunold, S.: Arthritis in myasthenia gravis, J. Neurol. Neurosurg. Psychiatry **38:**1048, 1975.

Arterberry, J. D., et al.: Potentiation of phosphorus insecticides by phenothiazine derivatives, J.A.M.A. **182:**848, 1962.

Bender, A. N., et al.: Myasthenia gravis: a serum factor blocking acetylcholine receptors of the human neuromuscular junction, Lancet **1:**607, 1975.

Bennett, H. S.: The sarcoplasmic reticulum of striped muscle, J. Biophys. Biochem. Cytol. **2:**171, 1956.

Bickerstaff, E. R., Evans, J. V., and Woolf, A. L.: The ultrastructure of human myasthenic and nonmyasthenic motor end plates, Brain **83:**638, 1960.

Brownell, B., Oppenheimer, D. R., and Spalding, J. N. K.: Neurogenic muscle atrophy in myasthenia gravis, J. Neurol. Neurosurg. Psychiatry **35:**311, 1972.

Brumlik, J.: Myasthenia gravis associated with wasp sting, J.A.M.A. **235:**2120, 1976.

Bucknell, R. C. et al.: Myasthenia gravis associated with penicillamine treatment of rheumatoid arthritis, Br. Med. J. **1:**600, 1975.

Campa, J. F., Johns, T. R., and Adelman, L. S.: Familial myasthenia with "tubular aggregates," Neurology **21:**449, 1971.

Cape, C. A., and Utterback, R. A.: Maintenance adrenocorticotropic hormone (ACTH) treatment in myasthenia gravis, Neurology **22:**1160, 1972.

Clarke, R. R., and Van de Velde, R. L.: Congenital myasthenia gravis: a case report with thymectomy and electron microscopic study of resected thymus, Am. J. Dis. Child. **122:**356, 1971.

Conomy, J. P., Levinsohn, M., and Fanaroff, A.: Familial infantile myasthenia gravis: a cause of sudden death in young children, J. Pediatr. **87:**428, 1975.

Cook, D., and Fischer, C.: Characteristics of succinylcholine neuromuscular blockade in neonates, Anesth. & Analg. **57:**63, 1978.

Dahl, D. S., and Sato, S.: Unusual myasthenic state in a teen-age boy, Neurology 24:897, 1974.

Desmedt, J. E., and Borenstein, S.: Time course of neonatal myasthenia gravis and unsuspectedly long duration of neuromuscular block in distal muscles (letter), N. Engl. J. Med. 296:633, 1977.

Doull, J.: Pesticide-induced delayed neurotoxicity: poison control or medical aspects. In Proceedings of a conference on pesticide-induced neurotoxicity, Environmental Protection Agency, 1976.

Drachman, D.: Myasthenia gravis, N. Engl. J. Med. 298:136, 1978.

Drachman, D. B., et al.: Effect of myasthenic immunoglobulin on acetylcholine receptors of cultured muscle, Ann. Neurol. 1:504, 1977.

Durham, W. F., and Hayes, W. J., Jr.: Organic phosphorus poisoning and its therapy, Arch. Environ. Health 5:21, 1962.

Ebashi, S., and Endo, M.: Calcium ion and muscle contraction, Prog. Biophys. Mol. Biol. 18:128, 1968.

Eisen, A., and Humphreys, P.: The Guillain-Barré syndrome: a clinical and electrodiagnostic study of 25 cases, Arch. Neurol. 30:438, 1974.

Eitzman, D. V., and Wolfson, S. L.: Acute parathion poisoning in children, Am. J. Dis. Child. 114:397, 1967.

Elmqvist, D.: Potassium induced release of transmitter at the human neuromuscular junction, Acta Physiol. Scand. 64:340, 1965.

Elmqvist, D., and Lambert, E. H.: Detailed analysis of neuromuscular transmission in a patient with the myasthenic syndrome sometimes associated with bronchogenic carcinoma, Mayo Clin. Proc. 43:689, 1968.

Engel, A. G., Lambert, E. H., and Howard, F. M.: Immune complexes (IgG and C3) at the motor endplate in myasthenia gravis, Mayo Clin. Proc. 52:267, 1977.

Engel, W. K., and McFarlin, D. E.: Muscle lesions in myasthenia gravis: discussion, Ann. N.Y. Acad. Sci. 165:68, 1966.

Engel, W. K., and Warmolts, J. R.: Myasthenia gravis: a new hypothesis of the pathogenesis and a new form of treatment, Ann. N.Y. Acad. Sci. 183:72, 1971.

Engel, W. K., et al.: Myasthenia gravis, Ann. Intern. Med. 81:225, 1974.

Fardeau, M.: Normal ultrastructural aspects of human motor end-plate and its pathological modifications. In Pearson, C. M., editor: The striated muscle, Baltimore, 1973, The Williams & Wilkins Co., p. 342.

Fenichel, G. M.: Clinical syndromes of myasthenia in infancy and childhood, Arch. Neurol. 35:97, 1978.

Fisher, J. R.: Guillain-Barré syndrome following organophosphate poisoning, J.A.M.A. 238:1950, 1977.

Flacke, W.: Drug therapy: treatment of myasthenia gravis, N. Engl. J. Med. 288:27, 1973.

Fraser, D., and Turner, J. W.: Myasthenia gravis and pregnancy, Lancet 2:417, 1953.

Geddes, A. K., and Kidd, H. M.: Myasthenia gravis of the newborn, Can. Med. Assoc. J. 64:152, 1951.

Goldstein, G.: Myasthenia gravis and the thymus, Annu. Rev. Med. 22:119, 1971.

Greenberg, S. R., and LaRuffa, P. J.: Myasthenia gravis in uncontrolled juvenile hyperthyroidism, J. Pediatr. 69:289, 1966.

Greer, M., and Schotland, M.: Myasthenia gravis in the newborn, Pediatrics 26:101, 1960.

Heuser, J. E., and Reese, T. S.: Evidence for recycling of synaptic vesicle membrane during transmitter release at the frog neuromuscular junction, J. Cell. Biol. 57:315, 1973.

Heuser, J. E., Reese, T. S., and Landis, D. M. D.: Functional changes in frog neuromuscular junctions studied with freeze-fracture, J. Neurocytol. 3:109, 1974.

Hokkanen, E., and Toivakka, E.: Streptomycin-induced neuromuscular fatigue in myasthenia gravis, Ann. Clin. Res. 1:220, 1969.

Horowitz, S. H., et al.: Electrophysiologic diagnosis of myasthenia gravis and the regional curare test, Neurology 26:410, 1976.

Howard, J. F., and Sanders, D. B.: Plasma exchange in the treatment of myasthenia gravis, Arch. Neurol. 36:251, 1979.

Hubbard, J. I.: Microphysiology of vertebrate neuromuscular transmission, Physiol. Rev. 53:674, 1973.

Jacob, A., Clack, E. R., and Emery, A. E. H.: Genetic study of sample of 70 patients with myasthenia gravis, J. Med. Genet. 5:257, 1968.

Kao, I., and Drachman, D. B.: Myasthenic immunoglobulin accelerates acetylcholine receptor degradation, Science 196:527, 1977.

Katz, B.: The transmission of impulses from nerve to muscle, and the subcellular unit of synaptic action, Proc. R. Soc. Biol. 155:455, 1962.

Keynes, G.: The results of thymectomy in myasthenia gravis, Br. Med. J. 2:611, 1949.

Keynes, G.: Surgery of the thymus gland: second (and third) thoughts, Lancet 1:1197, 1954.

Koenigsberger, M. R., Patten, B., and Lovelace, R. E.: Studies of neuromuscular function in the newborn. I. A comparison of myoneural function in the full term and the premature infant, Neuropädiatrie 4:350, 1973.

Kurland, L. T., and Alter, M.: Current status of the epidemiology and genetics of myasthenia gravis. In Viets, H. R., editor: Myasthenia gravis, Springfield, Ill., 1961, Charles C Thomas, Publisher, p. 307.

Lambert, E. H., and Elmqvist, D.: Quantal components of end-plate potentials in the myasthenic syndrome, Ann. N.Y. Acad. Sci. 183:183, 1971.

Lee, C. Y.: Chemistry and pharmacology of polypeptide toxins in snake venom, Ann. Rev. Pharmacol. 12:265, 1972.

Lindstrom, J. M., et al.: Antibody to acetylcholine receptor in myasthenia gravis: prevalence, clinical correlates, and diagnostic value, Neurology 26:1054, 1976.

Mackey, R. W.: Parathion poisoning in a young infant, Am. J. Dis. Child. **111:**321, 1966.

McLean, W. T., and McKone, R. C.: Congenital myasthenia gravis in twins, Arch. Neurol. **29:**223, 1973.

McQuillen, M. P.: Familial limb-girdle myasthenia, Brain **89:**121, 1966.

McQuillen, M. P., Cantor, H. E., and O'Rourke, J. R.: Myasthenic syndrome associated with antibiotics, Arch. Neurol. **18:**402, 1968.

Milby, T. H.: Prevention and management of organophosphate poisoning, J.A.M.A. **216:**2131, 1971.

Miledi, R., and Potter, L. T.: Acetylcholine receptors in muscle fibres, Nature **233:**599, 1971.

Millichap, J. G., and Dodge, P. R.: Diagnosis and treatment of myasthenia gravis in infancy, childhood, and adolescence, Neurology **10:**1007, 1960.

Mulder, D. G., Herrmann, C., and Buckberg, G. D.: Effect of thymectomy in patients with myasthenia gravis: a sixteen year experience, Am. J. Surg. **128:**202, 1974.

Musik, J., and Hubbard, J. I.: Release of protein from mouse motor nerve terminals, Nature **237:**279, 1972.

Namba, T.: Corticotropin therapy in patients with myasthenia gravis, Arch. Neurol. **26:**144, 1972.

Namba, T., Brown, S. B., and Grob, D.: Neonatal myasthenia gravis: report of two cases and review of the literature, Pediatrics **45:**488, 1970.

Nastuk, W. L., and Strauss, A. J.: Further developments in the search for a neuromuscular blocking agent in the blood of patients with myasthenia gravis. In Viets, H. R., editor: Myasthenia gravis, Proceedings of 2nd International Symposium, Springfield, Ill., 1961, Charles C Thomas, Publisher, p. 229.

Oberklaid, F., and Hopkins, I. J.: "Juvenile" myasthenia gravis in early infancy, Arch. Dis. Child. **51:**719, 1976.

Ozdemir, C., and Young, R. R.: Electrical testing in myasthenia gravis, Ann. N.Y. Acad. Sci. **183:**287, 1971.

Patrick, J., and Lindstrom, J.: Autoimmune response to acetylcholine receptor, Science **180:**871, 1973.

Patten, B. M., Oliver, K. L., and Engel, W. K.: Effect of lactate infusions on patients with myasthenia gravis, Neurology **24:**996, 1974.

Peterson, H. D.: Association of trimethadione therapy and myasthenia gravis, N. Engl. J. Med. **274:**506, 1966.

Pinching, A. J., Peters, D. K., and Davis, J. N.: Remission of myasthenia gravis following plasma-exchange, Lancet **2:**1373, 1976.

Pirskanen, R.: Genetic aspects in myasthenia gravis, Acta Neurol. Scand. **56:**365, 1977.

Porter, E. R., and Palade, G. E.: Studies on the endoplasmic reticulum: III. Its form and distribution in striated muscle cells, J. Biophys. Biochem. Cytol. **3:**269, 1957.

Pridgen, J. E.: Respiratory arrest thought to be due to intraperitoneal neomycin, Surgery **40:**571, 1956.

Quinby, G. E., and Clappison, G. B.: Parathion poisoning: near-fatal pediatric case treated with 2-pyridine aldoxime methiodide (2-PAM), Arch. Environ. Health **3:**538, 1961.

Richman, D. P., Patrick, J., and Arnason, B. G. W.: Cellular immunity in myasthenia gravis, N. Engl. J. Med. **294:**694, 1976.

Robinson, M. J., and Howard, R. N.: Neuroblastoma presenting as myasthenia gravis in a child age 3 years, Pediatrics **43:**111, 1969.

Rosenberg, P.: *In vivo* reactivation by PAM of brain cholinesterase inhibited by paroaoxon, Biochem. Pharmacol. **3:**212, 1960.

Rowland, L. P., and Layzer, R. B.: Muscular dystrophies, atrophies, and related diseases. In Baker, A. B., and Baker, L. H., editors: Clinical neurology, New York, 1971, Harper & Row, Publishers, chap. 37.

Rowland, L. P., et al.: Fatalities in myasthenia gravis: a review of thirty-nine cases with twenty-six autopsies, Neurology **6:**307, 1956.

Rowland, L. P., et al.: Myasthenic myopathy and thymoma, Neurology **23:**282, 1973.

Ryniewicz, B., and Badurska, B.: Follow-up study of myasthenic children after thymectomy, J. Neurol. **217:**133, 1977.

Sambrook, M. A., et al.: Myasthenia gravis: clinical and histological features in relation to thymectomy, J. Neurol. Neurosurg. Psychiatry **39:**38, 1976.

Scadding, G. K., Thomas, H. C., and Havard, C. W. H.: Myasthenia gravis: acetylcholine-receptor antibody titres after thymectomy, Br. Med. J. **1:**1512, 1977.

Schlezinger, N. S., and Corin, M. S.: Myasthenia gravis associated with hyperthyrodism in childhood, Neurology **18:**1217, 1968.

Schoen, R. T.: Myasthenia gravis and myotonic dystrophy in a 13-year-old girl, Neurology **27:**546, 1977.

Shapira, Y., et al.: A myasthenic syndrome in childhood leukemia, Dev. Med. Child. Neurol. **16:**668, 1974.

Shapiro, M. S., Namba, T., and Grob, D.: Corticotropin therapy and thymectomy in management of myasthenia gravis, Arch. Neurol. **24:**65, 1971.

Silinsky, E. M., and Hubbard, J. I.: Release of ATP from rat motor nerve terminals, Nature **243:**404, 1973.

Smith, D. M.: Organophosphorus poisoning from emergency use of handsprayer, Practitioner **218:**877, 1977.

Sutin, G. J., and Hewitson, R. P.: Myasthenia gravis in a 2-year-old treated by thymectomy, S. Afr. Med. J. **40:**1002, 1966.

Swaiman, K. F., and Varco. R. L.: Thymectomy: in fulminating myasthenia gravis of childhood, Minn. Med. **55:**809, 1972.

Takamori, M.: Caffeine, calcium, and Eaton-Lambert syndrome, Arch. Neurol. **27:**285, 1972.

Tens, P., and Osserman, K. E.: Studies in myasthenia gravis: neonatal and juvenile types: a report of 21 and a review of 88 cases, J. Mt. Sinai Hosp. N.Y. **23:**711, 1956.

Twomey, J. J. et al.: Myasthenia gravis: thymectomy and serum thymic hormone activity, Am. J. Med. **66:** 639, 1979.

Viets, H. R., and Brown, M. R.: Medical progress: diseases of muscles, N. Engl. J. Med. **245:**647, 1951.

Vincent, A., et al.: In-vitro synthesis of anti-acetylcholine-receptor antibody by thymic lymphocytes in myasthenia gravis, Lancet **1:**3105, 1978.

Warmolts, J. R., and Engel, W. K.: Benefit from alternate-day prednisone in myasthenia gravis, N. Engl. J. Med. **286:**17, 1972.

Wise, G. A., and McQuillen, M. T.: Transient neonatal myasthenia: clinical and electromyographic studies, Arch. Neurol. **22:**556, 1970.

Wolf, S. M., and Barrows, H. S.: Myasthenia gravis and systemic lupus erythematosus, Arch. Neurol. **14:**254, 1966.

Wolf, S. M., Rowland, L. P., and Schotland, D. L.: Myasthenia as an autoimmune disease: clinical aspects, Ann. N.Y. Acad. Sci. **135:**517, 1966.

Zavon, M. R.: Treatment of organophosphorus and chlorinated hydrocarbon insecticide intoxication, Mod. Treat. **8:**503, 1971.

# CHAPTER 6

# Progressive muscular dystrophies

The relationship of dystrophies to other muscle diseases is somewhat difficult to establish because the criteria employed for classification are imprecise.

Myopathies are primary diseases of striated muscle in which biochemical, morphologic, or neurophysiologic changes occur singly or in combination. These alterations are not the result of dysfunction of the neuromuscular junction, peripheral nerve, anterior horn cells, or central nervous system. This definition may require modification in the future when new basic information accrues.

Dystrophies are hereditary myopathies that are characterized by progressive muscle degeneration and weakness. Although they have been grouped together historically and clinically, they cannot be precisely delineated or classified, because little is known of the specific biochemical, physiologic, or morphologic defects.

The following conditions are customarily grouped as the muscular dystrophies:

1. Duchenne muscular dystrophy
   a. Early onset, X-linked
   b. Early onset, autosomal recessive
2. Late onset, X-linked muscular dystrophy
3. Limb-girdle muscular dystrophy
4. Facioscapulohumeral muscular dystrophy
5. Ocular muscular dystrophy
6. Myotonic dystrophy
   a. Classic type
   b. Myotonic chondrodystrophy
7. Congenital muscular dystrophy
8. Distal muscular dystrophy

It is increasingly evident that multiple clinical entities are subsumed under many of these titles, for example, limb-girdle muscular dystrophy. A profusion of names has been given to these conditions over the years (Table 6-1).

**Table 6-1.** Common terms employed to classify the muscular dystrophies

| Duchenne muscular dystrophy | Late onset, X-linked dystrophy | Facioscapulo-humeral dystrophy | Limb-girdle muscular dystrophy | Myotonic dystrophy |
|---|---|---|---|---|
| Aran-Duchenne dystrophy<br>Progressive muscular dystrophy<br>Pseudohypertrophic muscular dystrophy | Becker's dystrophy | Landouzy-Dejerine dystrophy | Erb's dystrophy<br>Erb's limb-girdle dystrophy<br>Juvenile dystrophy of Erb<br>Leyden-Möbius' pelvic atrophic dystrophy | Steinert's disease<br>Steinert's dystrophy |

## Duchenne muscular dystrophy

The French neurologist G. B. A. Duchenne, a student of electrical stimulation of muscle, described pseudohypertrophic muscular paralysis in 1868, noting in addition to the pseudohypertrophy the presence of large amounts of fat and connective tissue. In his article, Duchenne described for the first time an instrument to procure muscle biopsy material.

CLINICAL FEATURES. The child may walk later than expected, but abnormality of gait often is not evident until age 3 or 4. Frequent falling may occur while the child learns to walk. The initial symptoms are weakness of the hip girdle and later of the shoulder girdle. The patient has progressive impairment, rocking from side to side with a waddling gait and lumbar lordosis, and initially manifests difficulty in climbing stairs and rising from the floor. Mild to moderate weakness of the shoulder girdle is demonstrable. Distal muscles of the arms and legs are not affected early in the disease. Intermittent calf pain may occur during the early stages of the disease.

Difficulty rising from the floor is attended by a maneuver known as Gowers' sign (Fig. 6-1). The patient rises by "pushing off" from the floor, literally pushing the trunk erect by bracing the arm against the front of the thigh. This maneuver results because of the profound weakness of the muscles of the hip, especially the gluteus maximus. These symptoms are almost always present by age 5 or 6 and not later than age 8 (Shaw and Dreifuss, 1969).

Muscle mass is lost in the pectoral, peroneal, and anterior tibial muscles. The patellar tendon reflex is usually extinguished early in the course, but the Achilles tendon reflex persists late into the first decade of life. The patient begins to walk on the toes because of the fixed equinovarus position and falls frequently. Locking of the knees with resultant genu recurvatum posture is common. Immobilization because of intercurrent disease or surgery often accelerates deterioration in strength and balance. Enlargement of the muscles is usually noted in the area of the calves, but the quadriceps, infraspinatus, deltoid, and, less frequently, the gluteus, triceps, and masseter muscles may be involved (Fig. 6-2). Contractures develop and limit dorsiflexion of the foot and extension of the knees and elbows. Patients almost uniformly need a wheelchair after the age of 12, and virtually all are unable to walk by age 16.

Teenage patients have increasing weakness and cannot perform routine daily living functions with arms and fingers. The muscles of the neck become weak, and the head is bent forward. In the terminal stages, lower facial muscles may be involved. The patients die early, often before their twentieth year, from pneumonia. Almost all are dead by age 32 (Shaw and Dreifuss, 1969). Pulmonary function is greatly compromised because of the presence of marked kyphoscoliosis, usually developing after the patient is wheelchair-bound.

Another common complication in dystrophic diseases is cardiomyopathy. In one series of 19 patients, 84% had demonstrable cardiac disease at autopsy (Leth and Wuelff, 1976). Published data have set the incidence of cardiac involvement in Duchenne muscular dystrophy as high as 95%. Chronic heart failure may occur in 50% of affected patients (Gilroy et al., 1963; Wahi, Bhargava, and Mohindra, 1971).

Although not inevitably present, there may be abnormally deep limb and left precordial Q waves and abnormally tall right precordial R waves on electrocardiography (Perloff et al., 1967).

Vectorcardiographic findings in 34 patients with early onset Duchenne muscular dystrophy demonstrated that the characteristic electrocardiographic changes are in the QRS complex. The electrophysiologic abnormality is not readily explainable, and it may be the result of a genetically determined disorder of electrical activity arising from a particular area of the left ventricular myocardium. The abnormalities in the QRS pattern include tall right precordial R waves, increased R-S am-

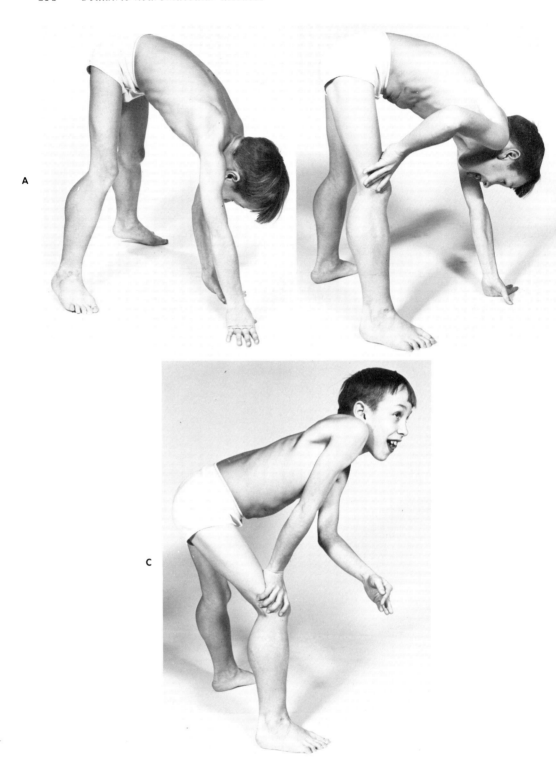

**Fig. 6-1. A,** This patient with Duchenne muscular dystrophy demonstrates the classic Gowers' sign. **B,** He maneuvers into position so that he is supported by both his arms and legs; subsequently, he pushes off floor and rests his hand on his knee. **C,** He then pushes himself upright.

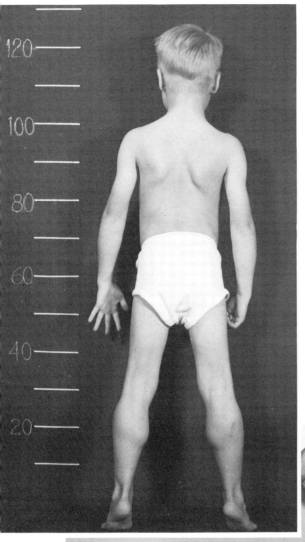

**Fig. 6-2.** The pseudohypertrophy of the gastrocnemius muscles is evident in both photographs. Patients almost invariably have limitation of dorsiflexion of the feet and eventually develop equinovarus deformities. The patient is forced to walk on his toes, further endangering his precarious balance.

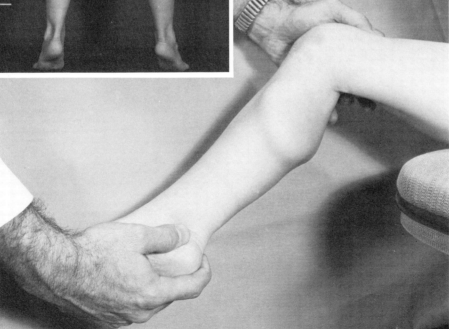

plitude ratios, and deep limb lead and lateral precordial Q waves (Ronan et al., 1972).

Patients with Duchenne dystrophy tend to be mentally subnormal (Prosser, Murphy, and Thompson, 1969; Worden and Vignos, 1962; Vignos, 1977). One study of the brains of such patients has shown pachygyria, distortion of cortical architecture, and low brain weight; microscopic findings include heterotopias (Rosman, 1970). However, another study revealed no changes (Dubowitz and Crome, 1969).

Other intercurrent problems may involve the gastrointestinal tract because of smooth-muscle dysfunction. Megacolon, volvulus, cramping abdominal pain, and malabsorption have been described (Simpson and Khilnani, 1975).

### LABORATORY FINDINGS

MORPHOLOGY. The pathologic findings common in Duchenne muscular dystrophy are indistinguishable from those in other muscular dystrophies and indeed from most other myopathies. Gross muscle bulk diminishes, and in later stages a predominant pink or yellowish pink replaces the dark red of normal muscle. In muscles severely involved, interstitial connective tissue and fat often replace these fibers.

Microscopic changes usually include a decrease in the numbers of fibers and necrosis of the fibers, with associated phagocytosis (Fig. 6-3). Frequently, small fibers are present, apparently the result of regeneration processes; they contain basophilic cytoplasm and relatively large vesicular nuclei. Some enlarged fibers tend to have central nuclei. Overall changes include increase of endomysial connective tissue and fat, loss of striations, and concomitant hyaline, granular, and fatty degeneration of fibers.

In rapidly progressive Duchenne dystrophy, necrosis and phagocytosis are likely to dominate; numerous small fibers with basophilic cytoplasm are evidence of regeneration phenomena. Controlled studies of muscle fibers in Duchenne muscular dystrophy have shown that endomysial stroma increases in young patients as the disease progresses.

Loss of the myofascicular margins by proliferation of the endomysial stroma contributes to the increase in perimysial stroma late in the disease. Disorganization of myotendinous insertions is associated with fat accumulation in these areas (Bell and Conen, 1968). The central nuclei are not localized near tendinous insertions in contrast to normal tissue.

Ultramicroscopic observations of muscle from patients with Duchenne dystrophy demonstrate segmental changes consisting of supercontraction of myofibrils before they fuse and are then disrupted. Regenerative changes are found in many fibers, especially in younger patients (Fig. 6-3, *A*).

Regenerating fibers from younger patients contain large, irregularly shaped nuclei having a large, densely stained nucleolus and a dispersed chromatin pattern. The nuclei are often located peripherally in the fibers. Many aggregates of ribosomal-like particles are present throughout the nuclei. The myofibrils are often poorly oriented, with focal abnormalities such as widening or absence of the Z band and disorganization of myofilaments. Occasionally the fibrillar arrangement is completely disorganized. Large numbers of ribosomes are present in regenerating fibers, predominantly in the paranuclear area and surrounding developing myofibrils (Mastaglia, Papdimitriou, and Kakulas, 1970).

In the substances of the fiber are cells inside the basement membrane that are separated by their own placma membrane (Wakayama, 1976). These cells have been designated as satellite cells (Fig. 2-6, *B*). In normal fibers they are thin, oval, or arcuate, and 5 to 8 $\mu$ in diameter. They have a single nucleus, oval or elongated, with clumped chromatin; surrounding the nucleus is a thin rim of cytoplasm containing a few mitochondria, small vesicles, and ribosomes. In regenerating fibers of Duchenne muscular dystrophy, patients' cells are often larger, contain enlarged irregular nuclei, and manifest dispersed chromatin and a prominent nucleolus. Increased cytoplasm, usually large mitochon-

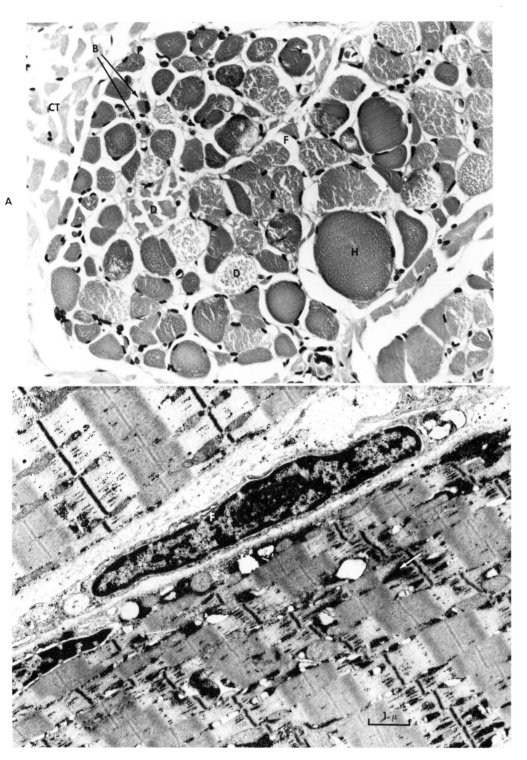

**Fig. 6-3.** Sample of gastrocnemius muscle from a 5-year-old boy with Duchenne muscular dystrophy. **A,** Cross-section demonstrates variation in fiber size, degenerating fibers (*D*), hypertrophic fibers (*H*), increased perimysial connective tissue (*CT*), increased amounts of fat (*F*), and basophilic, regenerating fibers (*B*). (H & E; ×330.) **B,** Ultrastructural appearance of a longitudinal section. Upper fiber appears normal. A prominent fibroblast (*F*) is located in center. Also evident are mitochondrial swelling, numerous vacuoles, Z band streaming (white arrow), and early sarcomere disruption (×12,500). (Courtesy Dr. Stephen A. Smith.)

dria, and occasional thin filaments surrounded by ribosomal aggregates are also present; all are characteristic of regenerating fibers.

ENZYME CHANGES. The basic biochemical abnormalities in Duchenne muscular dystrophy are unknown. Most abnormalities are probably secondary effects and have not contributed to knowledge of the underlying mechanisms.

In Duchenne muscular dystrophy, many enzymes are lost from the sarcoplasm of muscle into the circulation. Elevation of serum aldolase activity in these patients was first reported in 1949 (Sibley and Lehninger). Since then a number of other enzymes have been reported to manifest increased serum activity in Duchenne and other dystrophies. These enzymes include glutamic-oxaloacetic transaminase (GOT), lactic dehydrogenase (LDH), glutamic-pyruvic transaminase (GPT), glucose-phosphate isomerase, phosphoglucomutase, and creatine phosphokinase (CPK). These enzymes reach maximum levels of serum activity in Duchenne muscular dystrophy but are elevated to a lesser extent in limb-girdle dystrophy, facioscapulohumeral muscular dystrophy, polymyositis, severe muscle anoxia, acute myocardial infarction, thyroiditis, and extensive muscle injury.

Of all these enzymes, serum CPK appears to be the most valuable as a diagnostic indicator. In Duchenne muscular dystrophy, its activity increases greatly. It acts primarily in skeletal muscle, smooth muscle, thyroid, and brain, with little action in liver and red blood cells. Serum enzyme activity, especially CPK activity, is relatively increased in infants, and the activity declines with age (Zellweger and Antonik, 1975).

Increased CPK activity is associated with primary myopathic conditions, although slight elevations may be present in neurogenic conditions. In Duchenne dystrophy, the serum activity decreases to a great extent as muscle mass shrinks. As patients become less active and are eventually confined to a wheelchair, serum enzyme activity continues to revert to normal. However, CPK activity may remain abnormally high until the patient is in the late teens.

Because CPK isoenzymes are composed of a dimer, only three types exist: muscle type (MM), brain type (BB), and an intermediate type (MB). Electrophoretic techniques allow differentiation between brain type and that present in skeletal muscle or heart (Goto, 1974). Type MM is the only isoenzyme in skeletal muscle. Heart contains both MM and MB isoenzymes (Dawson and Fine, 1967). Fortunately the problem of differentiation between brain and muscle disease can usually be resolved clinically.

Studies of CPK isoenzymes reveal a significant difference in the MB isoenzyme activity among patients with Duchenne muscular dystrophy and those with other myopathies, including Becker's dystrophy, limb-girdle dystrophy, myotonic dystrophy, facioscapulohumeral dystrophy, and noninflammatory late-onset myopathies. MB isoenzyme abnormalities do not correlate with clinical cardiomyopathy; indeed, MB isoenzymes are increased early in the course of Duchenne muscular dystrophy, while cardiac abnormality is more common late in the disease (Silverman et al., 1976). MB and BB isoenzymes are increased in muscle of over half the patients (Somer, Dubowitz, and Donner, 1976).

Other studies involving calcium uptake and adenosinetriphosphatase (ATPase) determinations performed on fragmented sarcoplasmic reticulum from Duchenne dystrophy muscle revealed a decrease in both the initial and total calcium uptake, with accompanying low ATPase activity. The phase of the disease appears to be unimportant. The data suggest that both basic fiber types are involved in Duchenne muscular dystrophy. The only correlation of these findings with clinical manifestations of Duchenne dystrophy is that the earlier the disease appears, the lower is the ATPase activity of the fragmented sarcoplasmic reticulum (Samaha and Gergely, 1969).

Abnormalities in Duchenne muscular dystrophy also include a substrate-specific endogenous protein kinase alteration, in which proteins of molecular weight 220,000 daltons in the red cell membrane are phosphorylated to a greater degree in patients and carriers than in normal persons (Roses, Herbstreith, and Appel, 1975; Roses et al., 1976).

ATPase activity in Duchenne muscular dystrophy red cell membranes is less inhibited by ouabain than in normal red cell membranes in studies utilizing assay systems with high or low salt content. Epinephrine and cyclic AMP increase total activity in all samples, and epinephrine causes ouabain sensitivity to appear in previously insensitive Duchenne muscular dystrophy red cell membranes (Mawatari, Schonberg, and Olarte, 1976).

Other studies of red cell membranes from Duchenne muscular dystrophy patients have revealed reduced deformability, as measured by the negative pressure required to aspirate an erythrocyte into a micropipette with an internal diameter of 1 to 2 $\mu$m (Percy and Miller, 1975).

Lymphocyte capping is decreased in Duchenne muscular dystrophy as well as other genetically distinct forms of proximal muscular dystrophy (Packard et al., 1978).

Although abnormal forms of myoglobin have been described in Duchenne muscular dystrophy, their relationship to the underlying mechanism is unknown (Miyoshi et al., 1968; Rowland et al., 1968).

PLASMA AMINO ACIDS. The elevation of serum enzyme activity in Duchenne muscular dystrophy is thought to be secondary to a defect of the muscle membrane. If so, amino acids, which are relatively small molecules, could also appear in the plasma and a generalized aminoaciduria could occur. Concentrations of 33 amino acids were determined in the plasma and urine of 20 boys with early onset Duchenne dystrophy and 20 control boys. Taurine excretion in the urine increased, but no other consistent abnormality of urinary amino acid excretion was detected. It has not been demonstrated that the taurine excess in urine is due to an overflow phenomenon. Study of an additional

18 patients with myotonic, limb-girdle, and facioscapulohumeral dystrophy uncovered no abnormality (Bank, Rowland, and Ipsen, 1971).

AMINO ACID INCORPORATION STUDIES. Studies of polyribosomes from muscle extracts of patients with Duchenne muscular dystrophy revealed four to fivefold more collagen produced than in identical control fractions. When soluble enzymes from normal patients were added, the rate of collagen synthesis was restored to normal. These studies suggest that a substance or substances in the soluble fraction of muscle extracts of normal individuals may have the potential for arresting or inhibiting the synthesis of abnormal amounts of connective tissue in patients with Duchenne muscular dystrophy (Ionasescu, 1975; Ionasescu, Zellweger, and Conway, 1971).

In vitro radioactive amino acid incorporation by polyribosomes from muscle biopsy material was studied further in 63 suspected carriers of Duchenne muscular dystrophy and in 20 normal females. A significant increase in amino acid incorporation by the total polyribosomes was found in 42 of the suspected carriers. Serum CPK activity levels were increased in 24, and histologic changes suggestive of dystrophy were found in only eight. Increased collagen synthesis was also found in 20 of the 28 suspected carriers below 30 years of age, but only five of 14 carriers over the age of 30 showed abnormal collagen synthesis (Ionasescu et al., 1973).

MITOCHONDRIAL OXIDATION. Because some cases are associated with a definite family history of Duchenne muscular dystrophy and others appear to develop sporadically, attempts have been made to differentiate the two types.

Palmitate oxidation by mitochondria from skeletal muscle is sharply reduced in the familiar form but normal in the sporadic cases. Reduced rates of oxidation are also noted in established female carriers of the X-linked dystrophic gene (Lin, Hudson, and Strickland, 1972).

Another study involving energy metabolism of muscular dystrophic muscle, including muscle from patients with early onset Duchenne muscular dystrophy, revealed greater than anticipated conversion of radioactive glucose to fructose in both dystrophic patients and female carriers of the disease when matched with normal, fetal, neurogenic, muscular atrophy, and polymyositis comparison groups. These studies suggest that the route of fructose formation in these tissues is from glucose via glucitol. Fructose is readily metabolized by dystrophic muscle (Ellis, Strickland, and Eccleston, 1973). The basis for the observed high rate of conversion of glucose to fructose may be related to an alteration in muscle hexokinase isoenzyme II (Strickland and Ellis, 1975).

**PATHOPHYSIOLOGY.** Although there has been extensive research activity, the mechanism by which the lesions of Duchenne muscular dystrophy are produced is unknown (Appenzeller and Ogin, 1975). Study of fetuses at risk for Duchenne muscular dystrophy revealed that muscular nuclear size was significantly greater in the at risk patients of comparable gestational age. The condition is therefore clearly manifest by the second trimester of pregnancy (Vassilopoulos and Emery, 1977).

The general areas of investigation and sources of theoretical formulation include (1) a neurogenic basis, related primarily to abnormal motor neurons, (2) a vascular abnormality in which malformations or physiologic incompetence result in poor small-vessel perfusion, with or without associated aberration in biogenic amine metabolism, and (3) an intrinsic abnormality within the muscle fiber, possibly related to formation of inappropriate amounts of connective tissue, abnormality in enzyme metabolism, or structural defects.

**NEUROGENIC BASIS.** A few authorities have suggested that a neurogenic process causes Duchenne muscular dystrophy. Electrophysiologic studies demonstrated that isometric twitches of dystrophic muscles developed less tension and were usually slower than those in control persons. There appeared to be a reduction in the number of functioning motor units, although the size of the surviving units appeared to be normal. This led to the concept of the sick motor neuron in dystrophy (McComas, Sica, and Campbell, 1971). Furthermore, a decrease in the velocity of nerve conduction in the distal portion of the axon in comparison with the proximal portion was also noted (McComas, Sica, and Campbell, 1971). The investigators further found that the motor neurons cannot maintain satisfactory synaptic connections with the muscle fibers, a difficulty mirrored by a defect in neuromuscular transmission during repetitive stimulation of nerve or maximal effort (McComas, Sica, and Currie, 1971).

These findings have been criticized (Scarpalezos and Panayiotopoulos, 1973) on the basis of new data derived from more sensitive techniques (Ballantyne and Hansen, 1974). Furthermore, it has been argued that it is not justifiable to draw conclusions from studies of a muscle (the extensor digitorum brevis) that is not usually affected until late in the disease (Emery and Gosden, 1974). On the other hand, the possibliity that muscles could be affected by an abnormal motor neuron is reasonable in view of the known axoplasmic transport of trophic substances necessary to prevent denervation (Hofmann and Thesleff, 1972).

**VASCULAR ABNORMALITY.** In one set of experiments with rabbits, early and midstage histologic lesions reminiscent of Duchenne muscular dystrophy were induced through embolization of intramuscular arteries and arterioles by the single or repeated injection of 20 to 80 $\mu$ dextran particles (Hathaway, Engel, and Zellweger, 1970). Further studies were performed with a subthreshold amount of vasoactive 5-hydroxytryptamine (serotonin) in a single intraperitoneal dose after aortic ligation. As part of the same experiment, other animals were subjected to ligation alone, intraperitoneal injection of serotonin alone, and perfusion of the hind limb with serotonin alone.

The early change in Duchenne muscular

dystrophy as reported by these workers "is a small group of muscle fibers all in about the same state of necrosis or regeneration surrounded by a field of normal fibers" (Mendell, Engel, and Derrer, 1971). These workers go on to state: "The midstage lesions is characterized by a disproportionately large increase of endomysial connective tissue between muscle fibers that are small, enlarged, and sometimes with internal nuclei; often there is but sparse evidence of active muscle fiber necrosis or regeneration in the region." The rats subjected to ligation of the abdominal aorta and then given serotonin had muscle lesions similar to the intramuscular artery and arteriolar lesions induced by embolization (Hathaway, Engel, and Zellweger, 1970). These workers suggested that the two experiments supported the possibility that ischemia is a predominant feature in the disease process. The morphologic lesions were identical to those seen in early and midstage Duchenne muscular dystrophy (Mendell, Engel, and Derrer, 1971). Subsequent studies have demonstrated the ability of phenoxybenzamine or chlorpromazine to prevent the lesions of the ligation-serotonin experiments (Engel and Derrer, 1975).

Imipramine coupled with serotonin injection also causes focal muscle necrosis (Parker and Mendell, 1974). By inhibiting phosphodiesterase, imipramine blocks platelet uptake of biogenic amines and also elevation of cyclic AMP concentration. To pursue the ligation-serotonin studies, further experiments determined the concentrations of catecholamines and indoleamines in the urine and spinal fluid of patients with Duchenne muscular dystrophy. Neither catecholamines nor indoleamines were increased (Mendell, Roelofs, and Engel, 1972). In Duchenne muscular dystrophy muscle, fluorescent histochemical techniques demonstrated biogenic amines in groups of fibers that otherwise appera normal under light microscopy (Fenichel, 1975). Pargyline, a monamine oxidase inhibitor, produces similar lesions in rats (Yu et al., 1974).

Morphometric findings indicate an in-crease of capillary size and a normal number of capillaries per unit of muscle fiber area in this disease (Jerusalem, Engel, and Gomez, 1975). Xenon injection in patients with Duchenne dystrophy reveals no abnormality of blood flow at rest or following exercise (Paulson, Engel, and Gomez, 1974). No evidence of abnormal perfusion or microcirculation substantiates this contention.

INTRINSIC MUSCLE DISEASE. A number of studies of possible abnormalities in synthesis of cell proteins have been performed; some of them are mentioned earlier. Many abnormalities of enzyme function have been reported in Duchenne muscular dystrophy but virtually all of them appear to be of a secondary nature. As mentioned, the sarcoplasmic reticulum in patients with Duchenne muscular dystrophy may function abnormally in its ability to bind calcium. The protein and lipid concentration of the sarcoplasmic reticulum is normal.

Cultured muscle cells from patients with Duchenne muscular dystrophy revealed higher basal activity of adenyl cyclase of myotubes; the activity was not stimulated significantly by epinephrine or isoproterenol as it was in fused control cells. This finding led the investigators to believe that the genetic defect may be an abnormality of the surface membrane of muscle (Mawatari, Miranda, and Rowland, 1976).

The possibility that there are alterations in the internal molecular structure of the membrane in Duchenne muscular dystrophy was further enhanced by freeze fracture studies from eight patients that demonstrated nonuniform distribution and depletion of particles on both protoplasmic and extracellular surfaces of the muscle plasma membrane (Schotland, Bonilla, and Van Meter, 1977).

No overall cohesive theory linking the histologic and biochemical findings has been forthcoming. Nevertheless the complexities and importance of the muscle enzymes, contractile proteins, and collagen provide many possibilities for functional incompetence to result in disease. Studies of carriers tend to support an intrinsic muscle defect hypothesis (Thomson, Sweetin, and Elton, 1974).

Each of the proposed hypotheses of causation has enjoyed a period of ascendancy. Each has proponents with vast research experience and knowledge. The answer or answers remain unknown.

**GENETIC FINDINGS.** The most common form of Duchenne muscular dystrophy is the early onset X-linked type. It is transmitted by the mother to her sons through the abnormal genetic material of the X chromosome. On the basis of this mode of inheritance, 50% of the female carrier's daughters will also be carriers and 50% of her sons will be affected.

Duchenne muscular dystrophy has been estimated to have an incidence of approximately 30 cases per 100,000 male births on the basis of study of CPK activity in newborns (Zellweger and Antonik, 1975).

Laboratory studies of newborn and young brothers of boys with the disorder are helpful in confirming the presence of the disease. CPK studies are particularly helpful, although morphologic changes are present (Hudgson, Pearce, and Walton, 1967; Pearson, 1962).

Because study of cell cultures from amniotic fluid now allows sex determination of the fetus, therapeutic abortion for a pregnancy leading to a male birth may be considered. Studies of fetal blood obtained at 18 and 20 weeks of pregnancy may reveal elevation of CPK activity. Examination of fetal muscle by light and electron microscopy demonstrates the features of Duchenne muscular dystrophy (Mahoney et al., 1977; Emery et al., 1979).

Attempts have been made through enzyme studies, particularly serum CPK determinations and morphologic and electromyographic studies, to determine the carrier state in female relatives with varying degrees of success. As an example, 20% of women known to be carriers have normal serum CPK enzyme activity (Milhorat and Goldstone, 1965). Spontaneous mutations appear to account for 30% of the patients with Duchenne muscular dystrophy (Haldane, 1955).

In another investigation, four definite, one probable, and four possible female carriers were studied by electron microscopy, light microscopy, and serum CPK determinations. Ultrastructural changes were seen in all nine and were considered to be unequivocally abnormal in five. In two of these five, CPK activity was normal and only minimal change was observed on light microscopy. No consistently positive correlation between elevation of serum CPK activity and changes on light or electron microscopy occurred. Because 20% of definite carriers have a normal CPK level, light and electron microscopic studies of muscle biopsy material may be particularly valuable in identifying potential carriers with normal enzyme levels (Roy and Dubowitz, 1970). Despite initial reports, pyruvate kinase activity appears to be of less value than CPK activity in the delineation of the carrier state (Yamuna et al., 1977).

In another investigation, serum CPK activity was by far the best index of the presence of the carrier state. Electromyographic assessment was of little use in genetic counseling. In this investigation, only light microscopy studies were reported (Gardner-Medwin, Pennington, and Walton, 1971).

In yet another study LDH isoenzyme 5 activity proved to be more sensitive than CPK activity for detection of the carrier state (Roses et al., 1977).

Normal enzyme activities should not deter the clinician from further investigation of a suspected carrier. If available, the red cell membrane protein kinase studies discussed earlier (Roses and Appel, 1975; Roses et al., 1976) or the ribosomal studies discussed here could be employed; unfortunately, the wide variability in the results makes interpretation in many individual cases difficult.

Study of muscle polyribosomes from known carriers of Duchenne muscular dystrophy utilizing radioactive amino acid uptake techniques revealed a significant increase in specific activity of monomeric ribosomes, total polyribosomes, and collagen synthesis in 98% of known carriers and 54% of possible carriers of Duchenne muscular dystrophy. At the same time serum CPK was increased in 64% of the known carrier group (Ionasescu, Zellweger, and Burmeister, 1976).

Lymphocyte capping was reduced in female carriers of Duchenne muscular dystrophy. Decreased capping was present even when serum enzyme activities were normal (Packard, 1978).

The scattered focal nature of muscle abnormalities noted in these studies and others supports the likelihood that the differences in X chromosome content as postulated by Lyon may be the definitive factor in the diagnosis of the carrier state in female relatives (Lyon, 1962; Moser and Emery, 1974). In essence, one of the two X chromosomes of each cell in a human female is thought to be inactive. The inactive chromosome is determined by chance. Carriers with a predominant number of muscle cells under the influence of normal X chromosomes are difficult to identify with present laboratory techniques.

In attempts to determine the presence of the carrier state in women by use of electromyographic techniques, Gardner-Medwin (1968) concluded that the techniques are not sufficiently sensitive to detect myopathic changes in carriers of the gene for Duchenne muscular dystrophy. All mothers of affected sons should be considered genetic carriers unless there is proof to the contrary (Roses et al., 1976).

The cases of two girls with both Duchenne muscular dystrophy and Turner's syndrome have been reported (Ferrier, Bamatter, and Klein, 1965; Walton, 1956). Undoubtedly the single X chromosome in these girls carried the gene for the X-linked dystrophy.

It is increasingly apparent that in a number of cases of Duchenne dystrophy, transmission is on an autosomal recessive basis, with the disease affecting both boys and girls in one family (Milhorat and Goldstone, 1965). In these situations, serum CPK activity may be elevated in patients and both parents. The few reports suggest that the autosomal recessive form tends to be more slowly progressive than the early onset X-linked type, but other clinical characteristics are generally the same.

### THERAPY

PATIENT AND FAMILY KNOWLEDGE. The physician should systematically, and with appropriate detail to assure understanding, inform the parent of the Duchenne muscular dystrophy patient about the signs, symptoms, and expected clinical course. It should be made clear that the child will be wheelchair-ridden sometime between the ages of 10 and 12 years. It must be explained that the child will be capable of ongoing involvement in most formal educational activities and many conventional social activities. Sufficient time should be set aside to encourage a frank discussion of the cause of symptoms, treatment (including lack of definitive treatment), and eventual course of the disease. The discussion of expected disability and life expectancy probably is best held in the absence of the child.

The X-linked recessive inheritance pattern of Duchenne muscular dystrophy should be explained fully. One-third or more patients do not report a family history; these cases are thought to issue from mutations. The availability of techniques to detect the carrier state in female siblings of the mother and affected children in classic Duchenne muscular dystrophy must be explained. Furthermore, parents should be told that although there is no generally available technique of prenatal diagnosis, prenatal determination of sex allows for abortion of a male fetus (Hutton and Thompson, 1976). It is probable that study of fetal blood for increased enzyme activity will become widespread and permit prenatal diagnosis (Mahoney et al., 1977).

It must be stated clearly that the carrier state cannot be detected with absolute certainty. The presence of abnormal studies is virtual assurance that a female is a carrier; however, if results of all studies are normal, females cannot be assured that they are not carriers.

WEAKNESS. Unfortunately no medication or combination of medications appears to uniformly retard progression of the disease (Enomoto and Bradley, 1977). In one report, 14 patients with Duchenne muscular dystrophy received prednisone for as long as 28 months. Of these patients, 13 improved and eight retained their gains during the 28 months of the study. No associated change in CPK activity occurred (Drachman, Toyka, and Myer, 1974). It is noteworthy that many other studies of corticosteroids and androgens have not curtailed the relentless course of the disease.

Active exercise should be maintained whenever possible. If children who are confined to bed because of surgery, illness, or injuries are not provided a physical therapy program of continued ambulation and range-of-motion exercises, they may not resume walking. Fracture of the legs should be treated with walking casts as soon as feasible (Vignos, 1968).

Approximately 3 hours of daily walking to maintain strength and reduce contracture formation should be promoted (Ziter and Allsop, 1976). Quality and quantity of advisable activity should be modulated so that there is absence of fatigue after a night's sleep (Zundel and Tyler, 1965).

Strenuous efforts may be necessary to prevent or combat obesity. Decreased activity, boredom, and depression may potentiate weight gain. Obesity may shorten the duration of ambulation, facilitate scoliosis, and contribute to respiratory and cardiac insufficiency.

CONTRACTURES. Contractures of the hip flexors and Achilles tendons commonly occur. Active exercise may thwart for years formation of the contractures of the Achilles tendons. A standing board should be used for 20 minutes twice a day to provide constant stretch of the Achilles tendons.

Subcutaneous tenotomy of the Achilles tendons should be considered in the presence of severe contractures. Local anesthesia is employed. The child should be ambulated on the day of surgery, following application of a light walking cast. Bracing is essential to success after tenotomy operations.

Flexion contractures of the hip should be released surgically before application of a long leg brace. Although bracing is beneficial to some patients, it is not beneficial for all. Long leg braces are employed with a knee spring lock and adjustable ankle stop (Spencer and Vignos, 1962). Braces should not be prescribed for children who continue to ambulate reasonably well; nevertheless, bracing should not be put off until the patient is not ambulatory because lost function is infrequently regained. When the duration of daily walking has declined to less than 1 hour and the child requires external support while walking, bracing should be employed (Ziter and Allsop, 1976).

SCOLIOSIS. The development of scoliosis is difficult to postpone or arrest. Wheelchairs should be fitted with a hard seat in place of the customary sling seat (Taft, 1973). A tightly fitting jacket made of plastic or fiberglass is usually best (Dubowitz, 1964). Both these approaches support the vertebral column in the absence of adequate muscle strength. For the most part, immobilization required for surgical correction of scoliosis will have a detrimental effect on the patient's strength, and under most circumstances it should be avoided. Appliances for support of the head often become necessary.

RESPIRATORY COMPROMISE. Death is often the result of pneumonia. Children become more susceptible to pneumonia as strength recedes. Reduced vital capacity results because of a combination of weakened diaphragmatic muscle, weakened abdominal and chest muscles, scoliosis, and eventual episodes of pulmonary scarring and atelectasis. Treatment of pulmonary involvement and compromise utilizing postural drainage, intermittent positive-pressure techniques, and vigorous antibiotic therapy is necessary.

CARDIAC COMPLICATIONS. During the early years of Duchenne muscular dystrophy cardiac problems are infrequent. Occasionally, cardiac arrhythmias are manifest. Certainly cardiac myopathy has been well documented by pathologic studies. Furthermore, electrocardiographic changes are often demonstrable. Congestive heart failure is the most common clinical difficulty and arises in the later stages of the disease. The customary medical approaches to the treatment of congestive heart failure are of value.

The occasional patient who develops cardiac failure during earlier stages of Duchenne muscular dystrophy may require therapy with digitalis derivatives and diuretics for a number of years.

DRUG PRECAUTIONS. Muscle tone is decreased by anticholinergic drugs and ganglionic blocking agents, and they should be avoided. General anesthesia should be undertaken with great caution. Cardiotoxic drugs, such as halothane, should not be used.

EMOTIONAL AND BEHAVIORAL ABNORMALITIES. Psychosis is uncommon in Duchenne muscular dystrophy (Schecter, 1961). Nevertheless, many Duchenne muscular dystrophy patients and their families require counseling because of the child's preoccupation with self and subsequent withdrawal. These symptoms are often manifestations of depression. The frequently associated intellectual limitation may enhance low tolerance for frustration and potentiate other manifestations of emotional immaturity. The juxtaposition of a progressive condition and increasing dependency on parents and siblings effects a situation that favors manipulative behavior. Parental overprotection can foster improper interpersonal relationships, promote dependence, and retard reality testing. At some time the child realizes that the disease will continue, that there is no satisfactory treatment, and that premature death will ensue. Intervention by the physician or a skilled social worker or clinical psychologist to help the parents encourage the child, discourage overprotection, and prevent withdrawal from society is necessary.

Ambivalence among siblings and sometimes in parents may result from the burden of care imposed on the family as the disease progresses. The parents' reluctance to discipline handicapped children may promote jealousy and confusion in siblings.

From time to time it is necessary to provide special psychic support for the mother and help her deal with her guilt feelings when the disease is clearly transmitted through her.

The mechanism of various behavior patterns must be detailed to the parents and to siblings. The family must set limits on behavior that is untenable despite the progression of the disease.

The problems of children with Duchenne muscular dystrophy, or any such chronic disease, may strike at the integrity of the family. Therapy should be directed toward preventing family deterioration and encouraging the child to achieve maximal levels of development.

### Late onset X-linked muscular dystrophy (Becker's muscular dystrophy)

Late onset X-linked muscular dystrophy, reported by Becker (1955), resembles Duchenne muscular dystrophy but differs primarily in its clinical characteristics. Onset is later and progression is much slower.

Onset is usually during the second decade, but symptoms may be present in the first few years of life or as late as the third decade. The age of onset is consistent within an affected family. The pseudohypertrophy, proximal hip weakness resulting in Gowers' sign, tendency toward intellectual retardation, and electrocardiographic abnormalities are common to this condition and Duchenne muscular dystrophy (Fig. 6-4). The likelihood of intellectual retardation is less than that in Duchenne dystrophy. The severity of the disease appears to be constant within one family (Shaw and Dreifuss, 1969). Unlike most patients with Duchenne dystrophy, almost all patients can still walk at age 15; however, many are no longer walking late in the third decade. Only 50% survive to age 40 (Zellweger and Hanson, 1967). The condition is X-linked. A family history revealing maternal uncles or male siblings who are mildly affected may be the only clinical clue to differentiate this form of dystrophy from Duchenne muscular dystrophy.

Muscle enzyme activity is rarely elevated

to the same degree as in Duchenne muscular dystrophy. Muscle biopsy reveals subtle changes from Duchenne muscular dystrophy. In the Becker form, type II B fibers are normal, whereas in Duchenne muscular dystrophy there is a relative paucity of type II B fibers (Dubowitz and Brooke, 1973). Serum CPK activity is elevated in approximately 60% of women who are known carriers of Becker's muscular dystrophy (Skinner et al., 1975). Virtually all therapeutic suggestions appropriate to Duchenne muscular dystrophy are appropriate for Becker's dystrophy.

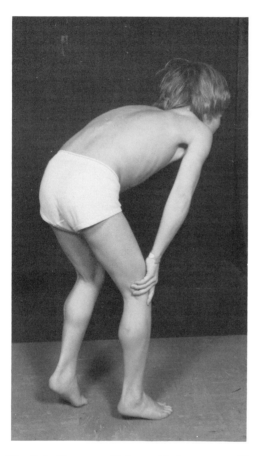

**Fig. 6-4.** Ten-year-old boy with late onset, X-linked (Becker's) muscular dystrophy is in process of executing Gowers' maneuver. Note hypertrophied calves and contractures of Achilles tendons.

### Limb-girdle muscular dystrophy

Limb-girdle muscular dystrophy is not a single disease entity but comprises a group of dystrophies and myopathies. These conditions affect the hip and shoulder girdles and most have an autosomal recessive mode of inheritance.

CLINICAL FEATURES. The first symptoms usually appear during the second decade. Weakness of the shoulder girdle or hip girdle progresses at a slower rate than that in Duchenne muscular dystrophy. Early weakness of the hip girdle often leads to difficulty in climbing stairs and rising from the floor; Gowers' sign is present. Early in the course of the disease, the gluteus maximus, gluteus medius, gluteus minimus, and iliopsoas muscles are involved. Low back pain may be the source of bitter complaint.

After a time, the anterior tibial and peroneal muscles are also compromised. Pseudohypertrophy, sometimes present, usually affects the calf muscles and occasionally the deltoid muscles. Talipes equinovarus develops secondary to contracture of the Achilles tendon (Walton and Gardner-Medwin, 1969). The rate of progression varies from pedigree to pedigree, but many patients cannot walk by age 30.

The facial muscles are rarely involved to any notable degree. Weakness of the neck flexor and extensor muscles is uniformly present. The pectoral muscles are often wasted, and there is loss of strength and mass of the deltoid and biceps muscles; in fact, the biceps may be severely atrophied. The deep tendon reflexes are difficult to elicit. The patients are usually of normal intelligence.

A few patients, some familial, with nonepisodic weakness in the limb-girdle distribution have been found to suffer from myasthenia gravis (McQuillen, 1966; Campa, Johns, and Adelman, 1971).

Some girls described as having Duchenne muscular dystrophy may actually have limb-girdle muscular dystrophy (Penn, Lisak, and Rowland, 1970).

**LABORATORY FINDINGS.** Histologic studies resemble those of Duchenne muscular dystrophy. Increased serum enzyme activity is common but not invariably present. Serum CPK activity is important in determining the preclinical state and to some extent is influenced by the rate of progression. The electromyogram is typical of those found in the myopathies.

Electrocardiographic abnormalities are unusual, but occasionally a patient has low T waves and high-voltage QRS complexes in the precordial leads (Jackson and Carey, 1961).

GENETIC FINDINGS. Although many cases are sporadic, limb-girdle dystrophy appears to be transmitted as an autosomal recessive trait in most pedigrees. In 37 patients with limb-girdle dystrophy from a large group of Amish kindred, shoulder-girdle weakness was noted, and pseudohypertrophy of the calf muscles was present in many (Jackson and Strehler, 1968). The age of onset and rate of progress remain uniform within a kindred.

THERAPY. The therapy of limb-girdle dystrophy is restricted to the physiatric and surgical procedures that retard and correct the contractures (see therapy of Duchenne muscular dystrophy).

### Facioscapulohumeral dystrophy (Landouzy-Dejerine dystrophy)

Landouzy and Dejerine (1885) described facioscapulohumeral dystrophy. Erb had published a report that described essential-

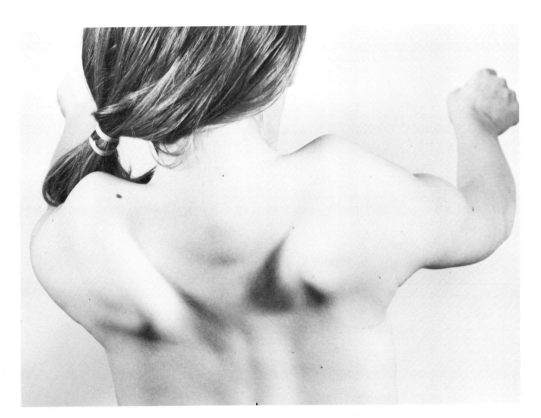

**Fig. 6-5.** Patient with facioscapulohumeral dystrophy. There is profound wasting of muscles associated with scapula. When patient leans forward against a wall with arms extended, instability of scapular fixation because of serratus anterior muscle weakness is apparent.

ly the same condition at about the same time (1884). Both of these reports emphasized the extreme degree of loss of muscle mass.

**CLINICAL FEATURES.** Although symptoms of the disease usually begin in the second decade, they may appear as early as age 5 and as late as age 25. Weakness is usually first apparent in the shoulder girdle, particularly the scapular muscles, and results in elevation and winging of the scapulae and impaired ability to raise the arms (Fig. 6-5). On rare occasions, facioscapulohumeral dystrophy has been associated with Möbius' syndrome. Onset is within the first 2 years of life with rapidly evolving severe weakness of the face, including the extraocular muscles. Progressive weakness of the shoulder and hip girdle muscles continues through the first

decade (Hanson and Rowland, 1971). A diagnosis of isolated Möbius' syndrome may be made in the newborn period. As the child grows older, involvement of other muscles should suggest the correct diagnosis. The trapezius, serratus anterior, and pectoral muscles are usually affected. Asymmetry of involvement is common.

Weakness without extraocular muscle involvement is most common; it may appear in the second year of life, with weakness of the facial muscles preceding all other types. The patient cannot close the eyes, whistle forcefully, or retain air within the cheeks when they are struck lightly (Fig. 6-6). The eyes may not close completely during sleep. The face and forehead are unlined (Fig. 6-7). When attempting a broad smile or grimace,

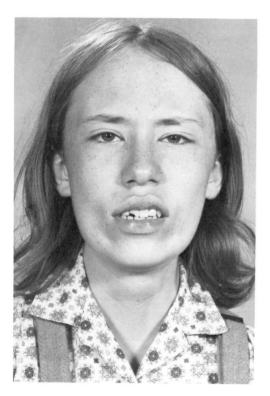

**Fig. 6-6.** Girl with facioscapulohumeral dystrophy is attempting to whistle forcibly. There is pursing of lips and inability to blow out cheeks.

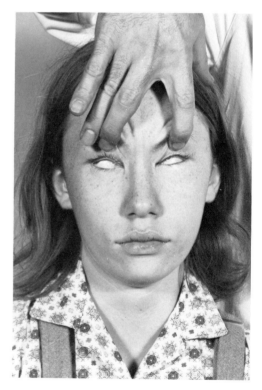

**Fig. 6-7.** Marked weakness of upper facial muscles in patient with facioscapulohumeral dystrophy is evident. Patient cannot close her eyelids tightly and cannot resist relatively modest efforts by examiner to elevate her lids.

the patient has faint movements of the corners of the mouth, which are usually turned slightly downward with accompanying eversion of the lips. Contractures and pseudohypertrophy are extremely rare.

The clavicles are more prominent than usual and incline downward or lie horizontally to accompany the drooping shoulders. During abduction of the arms, the scapulae migrate upwards and promote a curious picture as their superior edges clearly rise above the remainder of the shoulder girdle (Fig. 6-5). The inferior portions of the scapulae protrude posteriorly during this maneuver. It is noteworthy that the deltoid muscles may remain of near normal strength despite the devastation of the neighboring muscles.

Facioscapulohumeral muscular dystrophy may initially show wrist and finger weakness. The weakness may be isolated or limited to the dorsal interosseous, the palmaris interosseous, and the long extensor muscles of the index and middle fingers (Siegl, 1972). If weakness of the forearm muscles occurs, usually the wrist flexors remain intact while there is marked deterioration of the wrist extensors. Wristdrop can be demonstrated when the patient extends the arms with the palms down.

At times in profoundly affected patients, weakness develops in the anterior tibial and peroneal muscles, accompanied by footdrop. Severe weakness of the muscles of the hip girdle results in kyphoscoliosis and lumbar lordosis.

Manifestations may be extremely subtle in relatives of patients. The course is usually very long and insidious. Variations in degree of involvement occur in individuals in one family and from one family to the next (Tyler and Wintrobe, 1950). Most of these patients live a normal life span and are of normal intelligence.

*Facioscapulohumeral neurogenic muscular atrophy* that closely resembles facioscapulohumeral dystrophy because of weakness and loss of muscle bulk in the same distribution has been reported (Fenichel, Emer, and Hunt, 1967).

Myositis in a facioscapulohumeral distribution has been reported on several occasions (see Chapter 8).

**LABORATORY FINDINGS.** Over half of the patients with facioscapulohumeral dystrophy have serum CPK levels within the normal range (Thomsom, Leyburn, and Walton, 1960). Serum CPK activity is most commonly elevated during the first 10 to 15 symptomatic years. Other studies reveal elevated CPK activity in four of six females and 13 of 16 males. These results indicate that serum CPK is usually elevated in subjects up to the age of 50 years but may then return to normal (Hughes, 1971).

Polyribosomes of noncollagenous protein incorporate radioactive amino acids at an increased rate in the early stages of the disease but at low or normal rates in advanced stages. The ribosome content and distribution on sucrose density gradients of polyribosomes from muscle extracts were normal in seven of eight patients with inherited facioscapulohumeral muscular dystrophy (Ionasescu et al., 1972).

Electromyographic and other diagnostic studies in four patients with facioscapulohumeral dystrophy revealed all to have potentials in the vastus lateralis muscle suggestive of myopathy. Electromyography of the extensor digitorum brevis muscle revealed normal findings in two patients, suggestion of neuropathy in one, and suggestion of myopathy in another (Sica and McComas, 1971).

**GENETIC FINDINGS.** Facioscapulohumeral dystrophy is transmitted as an autosomal dominant trait, and the spectrum of involvement in both sexes is wide. The presence of almost imperceptible signs and symptoms in parents may go unnoticed unless diligently sought.

**TREATMENT.** The therapeutic program described for Duchenne muscular dystrophy is applicable to those patients with the severe form that profoundly affects the hip girdle and legs. Severe kyphoscoliosis may require surgical correction. If footdrop is a major handicap, subcutaneous tenotomy may be of value in correcting the contractures of the Achilles tendons.

Reconstructive surgery has been of value for the facial disfiguration secondary to weakness of the expressive muscles. A satisfactory cosmetic result may be achieved with a fascia lata graft attached to the zygomatic muscle and to the zygomatic head of the quadratus labiae superioris muscle (Cocke and Davis, 1971).

Although it may retard contracture formation, exercise does not appear to help the patients retain or regain strength or stamina.

### Scapuloperoneal dystrophy

Several pedigrees have been reported with combined wasting of the scapular and peroneal muscles, both myopathic and neurogenic forms (Emery, Fenichel, and Eng, 1968; Feigenbaum and Munsat, 1970). (See also Chapter 3.) At times it has been difficult to distinguish scapuloperoneal neurogenic atrophy from scapuloperoneal dystrophy despite intensive investigation (Thomas, Calne, and Elliott, 1972).

Onset of the myopathic form begins during the second to fourth decade, frequently with gait impairment caused by weakness of the peroneal and anterior tibial muscles. The calf muscles are of normal bulk and strength. There is wasting of the scapular and deltoid muscles, with discernible, definite but less severe loss of muscle bulk in the biceps and triceps muscles. The muscles of the wrists and fingers may be mildly involved. Facial involvement is unusual; its absence helps to distinguish the condition from facioscapulohumeral dystrophy. The condition is relatively benign, and many patients are only moderately handicapped past middle age. Pseudohypertrophy is uncommon, occurring in the calf muscles, and probably is a relative rather than a true manifestation (Ricker and Mertens, 1968). Both the neurogenic and myopathic forms of scapuloperoneal muscle syndromes have been X-linked in their genetic transmission (Mawatari and Katayama, 1973; Thomas, Calne, and Elliott, 1972).

Electrocardiographic abnormalities suggesting a selective disorder of the conduction system have been reported (Mawatari and Katayama, 1973).

### Myotonic dystrophy

Myotonia is characterized by abnormal persistence of induced or voluntary muscular contraction. The child cannot relax a contracted muscle quickly or release a gripped object rapidly. Myotonia affects predominantly the limb muscles but also the extraocular and facial muscles. Fatigue and cold facilitate myotonia. Among the many inherited clinical entities commonly associated with myotonia are myotonic dystrophy, myotonic chondrodystrophy, paramyotonia congenita, and myotonia congenita. Myotonia may also be associated with periodic paralysis, hypothyroidism, polymyositis, and, on rare occasions, chronic denervation.

CLINICAL FEATURES. Manifestations vary widely. Myotonic dystrophy may develop in the neonatal period or may be so mild as to go unnoticed in elderly patients (Dodge et al., 1965). Women with myotonic dystrophy develop more severe symptoms during pregnancy (Gardy, 1963; Sarnat, O'Connor, and Byrne, 1976). There is a high rate of fetal loss caused by prematurity, spontaneous abortion, and neonatal complications. Many neonates are asymptomatic; however, neonatal symptoms are not correlated with the severity of the maternal illness.

Problems in the neonatal period consist of impaired swallowing and sucking, facial diplegia, and arthrogryposis (see Chapter 3). Associated unilateral or bilateral ptosis is common. The facial diplegia may be erroneously diagnosed as Möbius' syndrome, which includes agenesis of the facial nerve (cranial nerve VII) nuclei (Evans, 1955). Sucking and swallowing difficulties tend to relent with maturation.

During the second year, the child may develop weakness of the proximal hip muscles, which results in gait difficulties and Gowers' sign. The facial diplegia remains (Fig. 6-8),

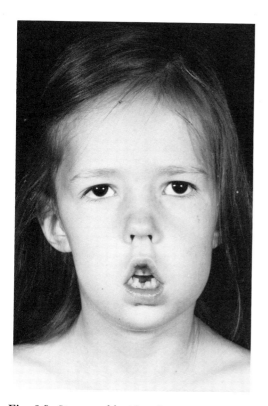

**Fig. 6-8.** Six-year-old girl with myotonic dystrophy demonstrates mild ptosis, facial diplegia, and a characteristic tenting of upper lip. All are common in this condition.

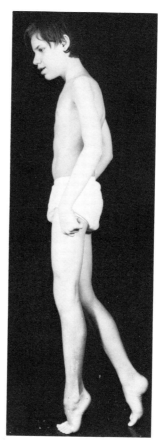

**Fig. 6-9.** Fifteen-year-old boy with myotonic dystrophy has marked wasting of distal muscles of foot, pes cavus deformity, and contractures of Achilles tendons.

and accompanying loss of muscle bulk often causes hollowing of the temporal areas. Progressive weakness and atrophy of distal limb muscles occurs (Fig. 6-9). As the child grows older, other common manifestations of myotonic dystrophy, including cataracts, baldness, and later, gonadal atrophy, often develop. Gonadal atrophy may not occur until the third decade or later. The incidence of intellectual retardation in these children exceeds that in the general population.

Myotonia in the form of "stiffness" is often the primary symptom in children with myotonic dystrophy. Percussion of selected sites, including the deltoid muscle, thenar eminence, and tongue, may reveal evidence of myotonia. Extraocular involvement may be demonstrated by asking the patient to open the eyes suddenly after closing them forcefully for several seconds. The eyelids relax normally, but there is transient residual contraction of the elevators of the globes, and for 1 or 2 seconds after the eyes are opened, the globes involuntarily turn upward (Dyken, 1966). Cataracts may not appear until the middle of the second decade, but they can be detected in younger children by use of slit-lamp examination.

Other ophthalmologic abnormalities include blepharitis with or without keratitis, decreased tear production, and slow pupillary responses on pupillography. The electroretinogram is usually abnormal, with low amplitude of the b wave and decreased light sensitivity of the rods.

An often used method of eliciting evidence of myotonia is to ask the patient to stretch the arms forward and rapidly open and tightly close the fists repetitively. At first, the patient has great difficulty in opening the fists. The fingers unclench and open in a slow-motion pattern. The patient can also be asked to grasp a rod and then suddenly release it. He or she will experience persistence of grip; the degree of myotonia decreases with repetitive trials. Myotonia is often aggravated by cold (see paramyotonia congenita, Chapter 7).

Although older children may have a history of normal infancy and development, close questioning can usually ascertain that the disease has been present since the first decade of life. In addition to hollowing of the cheeks and temples and peripheral myotonia, older children may have prominent ptosis. Speech difficulties may be present because of myotonia of the facial, tongue, and pharyngeal muscles. Associated language difficulties may result from intellectual retardation (Calderon, 1966).

The degree and distribution of clinical involvement vary greatly from individual to individual. Some have overt involvement of the face, neck, and forearms for many years without evidence of spread; others complain of diffuse stiffness caused by myotonia but little weakness.

When the signs and symptoms are well developed, the disease is readily recognizable. Partial ptosis, usually bilateral, and marked loss of bulk in the temporal and masseter muscles, with the resultant "hatchet-face" vapid expression, are striking. The lower lip is often everted and the jaw slack. Men are usually bald. The muscles of the neck are often very weak. The weakness of the extensor muscles of the cervical spine results in cervical kyphosis, and flexion of the head on the neck causes a swanlike configuration. Deep tendon reflexes are often difficult to elicit at a time when evaluation of muscle strength is normal.

Congenital malformations, chiefly talipes equinovarus, are associated with myotonic dystrophy. Increased thickness of the skull has occasionally been reported. Skull films may reveal a small sella turcica, a high-arched narrow palate, and enlarged paranasal sinuses.

Although there are exceptions, serum CPK activity is usually moderately elevated, especially in younger children in whom progression is fairly rapid. Electromyographic findings in these patients are typical of those in myotonia. The usual electromyographic finding is a high-frequency, repetitive discharge in which increases and decreases in both amplitude and frequency occur in a period of seconds and produce a "dive-bomber" effect when the potentials are transformed into sound (see Chapter 2).

Many patients with myotonic dystrophy have abnormal electrocardiograms, and a number of patients have died from cardiac arrhythmias (Payne and Greenfield, 1963; Welsh, Haase, and Bynum, 1964). The most common electrocardiographic abnormalities include a prolonged P-R interval, delayed intraventricular conduction time, and arrhythmias. There is no positive correlation between the degree of skeletal muscle and cardiac muscle involvement. A few patients have pulmonary difficulties, such as carbon dioxide retention and cyanosis. Lethargy and pulmonary hypertension may also be present. Decreased serum IgG levels and increased breakdown of IgG have been reported (Jensen, Jensen, and Jarnum, 1971; Wochner et al., 1966). Although almost all men have testicular atrophy, impaired reproduction is uncommon (Drucker et al., 1961).

Thyroid function is normal in these patients, but a subnormal metabolic rate has been reported in many. The metabolic change is unexplained (Drucker et al., 1961).

Intravenous and oral loads of glucose lead to abnormally high glucose tolerance curves. Hyperinsulinism is commonly present in myotonic dystrophy and is associated with some degree of insulin resistance. Furthermore, the measurement of plasma insulin during oral glucose tolerance testing may be an effective means of detecting clinically unaffected heterozygotes (Barbosa et al., 1974; Nuttall, Barbosa, and Gannon, 1974). Tolbutamide administration may also lead to an abnormally large secretion of insulin in this condition (Huff and Lebovitz, 1968; Mendelsohn et al., 1969).

## LABORATORY FINDINGS

MORPHOLOGY. The commonly described abnormalities in dystrophic processes are found: decrease in fiber numbers, variations of fiber size, necrosis, and replacement of normal fibers by collagen and fat. The changes apparent on light microscopy that are associated more frequently with myotonic dystrophy include a pattern in which nuclei are aligned in central chains (Fig. 6-10), and circularly arranged myofibrils form bands and subsarcolemmal and sarcoplasmic masses (Klinkerfuss, 1967). Proliferation of

the intrafusal fibers of muscle spindles has also been reported (Daniel and Strich, 1964).

Observations of infantile myotonic dystrophy reveal type I muscle fiber hypertrophy, mild increase in the number of centrally located muscle nuclei, and a few sarcoplasmic masses and ring fibers. In patients under 4 years of age, positive acid phosphatase sites are present in both the extrafusal and intrafusal muscle fibers. Similar sites are seen only rarely in adult patients. Electron microscopy reveals dense core tubules that are probably the ultrastructural equivalent of the positive acid phosphatase sites. They are located at the edges of nuclei and are associated with disoriented myofilaments on the periphery of the muscle fiber; their significance is unknown (Karpati et al., 1973).

The myofibril rings are oriented in a plane at right angles to the long axis of the muscle fiber on electron microscopic examination.

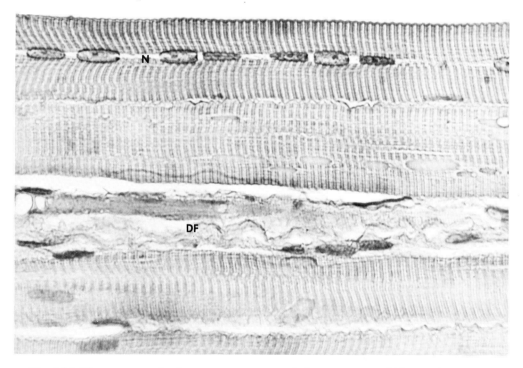

**Fig. 6-10.** Photomicrograph of a gastrocnemius muscle from a 10-year-old boy with myotonic dystrophy. A chain of internal nuclei (*N*) and a degenerating fiber (*DF*) are easily seen. The "lining up" of nuclei is common in myotonic dystrophy, but the configuration is not pathognomonic. (H & E; ×1,050.) (Courtesy Dr. Stephen A. Smith.)

The nuclei of the muscles are often adjacent to the ring myofibrils (Schotland, Spiro, and Carmel, 1966). The ring myofibrils manifest band patterns typical of contracted muscle; therefore it appears that ring myofibrils are either preexisting myofibrils that have been altered and coiled around the long axis of the muscle fiber, or that they are newly formed when the pathologic process involves the existing muscle.

Electron microscopic studies also reveal fine granular chromatin and convoluted nuclear membranes of centronuclear fibers. There are dilated transverse tubules, poorly formed Z bands, many satellite cells, and simple mitochondria. These findings suggest an arrest in fetal muscle maturation owing to sarcolemmal membrane defect, which renders the muscle refractory to normal trophic influences (Sarnat and Silbert, 1976).

Brains of patients with myotonic dystrophy contain moderate numbers of heterotopias (Rosman and Rebeiz, 1967). Pneumoencephalographic studies have revealed progressive ventricular dilation in myotonic dystrophy patients (Refsum et al., 1967).

Calcium uptake is initially high during ATPase studies of fragmented sarcoplasmic reticulum from patients with myotonic dystrophy, but total calcium uptake is normal. Normal or higher than expected efficiency of calcium uptake based on the ratio of calcium uptake to ATPase activity was present. The data suggest that involvement in myotonic dystrophy is primarily in type I fibers. No gross evidence of a positive correlation was found between the biochemical abnormalities and the clinical stages of disease (Samaha and Gergely, 1969). Red cells from patients with myotonic dystrophy also accumulate calcium at a higher than expected rate (Plishker, Gitelman, and Appel, 1978).

Because many organ systems are involved, a generalized defect that transcends muscle must be responsible. A generalized membrane defect has been postulated (Rowland, 1976). Myotonia can be demonstrated in normal muscle fibers by decreasing the chloride content of the incubating fluid (Rüdel and Senges, 1972). Furthermore, the internalized surface membrane, in the form of the transverse tubular system, must function normally to prevent myotonia (Adrian and Bryant, 1974).

Membrane-bound protein kinase has been demonstrated to be decreased in both erythrocytes (Roses and Appel, 1973) and muscle membranes (Roses and Appel, 1974) of affected patients. Electron spin resonance spectroscopy also substantiates the presence of a membrane defect in myotonic erythrocytes (Butterfield et al., 1976).

The nature of the membrane defect is not fully understood. The muscle membrane has a normal resting potential, but there is a marked increase in resting-membrane resistance. These characteristics have been demonstrated in both humans and myotonic goats (Lipicky, Bryant, and Salmon, 1971; Bryant, 1969).

Myotonia can be demonstrated in muscle after electrical stimulation or by percussion, even in the presence of denervation; therefore it is unlikely that a neurogenic process is primary.

Accordingly there is a lack of support for the hypothesis that the defect in myotonic dystrophy is neurogenic (Drachman and Fambrough, 1976). No abnormalities of peripheral nerve morphology have been demonstrated (Pollock and Dyck, 1976).

**GENETIC FINDINGS.** The disease incidence has been reported to be between 2.4 and 4.9 per 100,000 persons (Rowland and Layzer, 1971).

Myotonic dystrophy is transmitted as an autosomal dominant trait. It may be very mild in the parents, and they should be closely studied when the diagnosis is sought in offspring. Studies of other family members should include electromyographic and slit-lamp examinations. Studies clarifying the association of the alleles of myotonic dystrophy with other autosomal marker loci (ABH secretor) can now permit determination of whether an embryo will result in an affected child (Polgar et al., 1972; Renwick et al., 1971).

**TREATMENT.** The myotonic phenomenon is probably the result of instability of the muscle membrane (Norris, 1962; Roses and Appel, 1975). Myotonia can be induced in humans by the hypocholesterolemic agent diazocholesterol (Somers and Winer, 1966). Drugs that are thought to stabilize membrane potentials include quinine, quinidine, procainamide, and phenytoin (Geschwind and Simpson, 1955; Munsat, 1967). Phenytoin appears to be the most useful of these and may be the drug of choice for treatment of myotonia. It has been shown to "normalize" membrane fluidity (Roses et al., 1976). The mechanism of action may be through stabilization of sodium conductance or stimulation of the $Na^+-K^+$ ATPase system.

Comprehensive medical care includes vigilance for the appearance of cataracts, diabetes mellitus, and cardiac arrhythmias. Speech therapy is of questionable value. Hypogonadism and impotency may pose psychologic problems, requiring appropriate intervention. Rarely, cardiac arrhythmias may necessitate medical therapy.

Progressive weakness, rather than myotonia, is the difficulty that usually disturbs the patient. The use of physical therapy, and at times surgery, to relieve contractures, along with proper braces to alleviate footdrop associated with anterior compartment weakness of the legs, may be beneficial.

Myotonic dystrophy patients are susceptible to anesthetic difficulties and must be fully evaluated and monitored during surgery (Ravin, Newmark, and Saviello, 1975).

### Myotonic chondrodystrophy (Schwartz-Jampel syndrome)

Myotonic chondrodystrophy begins in early childhood and consists of generalized myotonia, muscle hypertrophy, unusual facies, short stature, and bone and joint abnormalities consistent with chondrodystrophy (Aberfield, Hinterbuchner, and Schneider, 1965; Schwartz and Jampel,

1962; Cao et al., 1978). There is progressive limitation of joint mobility in adults. Malignant hyperpyrexia has been associated with this condition (Seay and Ziter, 1978).

Serum CPK level is mildly elevated. Electromyography reveals bizarre high-frequency potentials (prolonged and persistent), and electrical silence is not present at rest, during general anesthesia, and after generalized curarization (Taylor et al., 1972). Muscle biopsy findings are consistent with a myopathy (Brown, Garcia-Mullin, and Murai, 1975; Huttenlocher et al., 1969).

Treatment with phenytoin has been of value in increasing ambulation and reducing limitation of joint mobility. The disease is transmitted as an autosomal recessive trait.

### Ocular muscular dystrophy

Muscular dystrophy often localized to the extraocular muscles and on occasion affecting the muscles of swallowing is an unusual condition in children, although common in adults (Drachman, 1968). Some patients have associated weakness of the limb muscles (Drachman, 1968; Victor, Hayes, and Adams, 1962).

Symptoms in childhood include diplopia, ptosis, strabismus, and rarely, retinitis pigmentosa (Erdbrink, 1957). Accompanying weakness of the facial muscles, particularly those of the upper face, is common (Victor, Hayes, and Adams, 1962). Older patients complain of difficulty in swallowing because of the involvement of the esophagus and pharynx.

The disease is compatible with relatively normal longevity, but severe dysphagia may result in aspiration and recurrent pneumonitis. Microscopic study of pharyngeal and esophageal tissue shows the dystrophic process in the striated pharyngeal muscle but not in the smooth muscle (Drachman, 1968).

A number of pedigrees have been reported with this condition, which is commonly transmitted as an autosomal dominant trait (Victor, Hayes, and Adams, 1962). A late onset form of the disease is prevalent in French

Canadians (Lewis, 1966). Involvement is sporadic, particularly in children.

In patients with limb involvement, the distribution of weakness may confuse the differential diagnosis of this condition and myotonic dystrophy (Schotland and Rowland, 1964). The extraocular muscle involvement distinguishes this disease from facioscapulohumeral dystrophy.

Normal serum CPK activity is usually present. Electromyographic examination demonstrates myopathic potentials in the involved peripheral muscles. Biopsy of these muscles demonstrates some degree of myopathic change consistent with a diagnosis of a dystrophic process.

## REFERENCES

Aberfield, A., Hinterbuchner, L., and Schneider, M.: Myotonia, dwarfism, diffuse bone disease, and unusual ocular and facial abnormalities (a new syndrome), Brain **88**:313, 1965.

Adrian, R. H., and Bryant, S. H.: Repetitive discharge in myotonic muscle fibers, J. Physiol. **240**:505, 1974.

Appenzeller, O., and Ogin, G.: Pathogenesis of muscular dystrophies, Arch. Neurol. **32**:2, 1975.

Ballantyne, J. P., and Hansen, S.: Myopathies: the neurogenic hypothesis? Lancet **1**:1060, 1974.

Bank, W. J., Rowland, L. P., and Ipsen, J.: Amino acids of plasma and urine in diseases of muscle, Arch. Neurol. **24**:176, 1971.

Barbosa, J., et al.: Plasma insulin in patients with myotonic dystrophy and their relatives, Medicine **53**:307, 1974.

Becker, P. E.: Eine neue X-chromosomale Muskeldystrophie, Arch. Psychiatr. Nervenkr. **193**:427, 1955.

Bell, C. D., and Conen, P. E.: Histopathological changes in Duchenne muscular dystrophy, J. Neurol. Sci. **7**:529, 1968.

Brown, S., Garcia-Mullin, R., and Murai, Y.: The Schwartz-Jampel syndrome (myotonic chondrodystrophy) in the adult, Neurology **25**:365, 1975.

Bryant, S. H.: Cable properties of external intercostal muscle fibers from myotonic and nonmyotonic goats, J. Physiol. (Lond.) **204**:539, 1969.

Butterfield, D. A., et al.: Spin label study of erythrocyte membrane fluidity in myotonic and Duchenne muscular dystrophy and congenital myotonia, Nature **263**:159, 1976.

Calderon, R.: Myotonic dystrophy: a neglected cause of mental retardation, J. Pediatr. **68**:423, 1966.

Campa, J. F., Johns, T. R., and Adelman, L. S.: Familial myasthenia with "tubular aggregates," Neurology **21**:449, 1971.

Cao, A., et al.: Schwartz-Jampel syndrome: clinical, electrophysiological and histopathological study of a severe variant, J. Neurol. Sci. **35**:175, 1978.

Cocke, W. M., and Davis, W. G.: Reconstruction in Landouzy-Dejerine progressive muscular dystrophy, Plast. Reconstr. Surg. **48**:77, 1971.

Daniel, P. M., and Strich, S. J.: Abnormalities in the muscle spindles in dystrophia myotonia, Neurology **14**:310, 1964.

Dawson, D. M., and Fine, I. H.: Creatine kinase in human tissues, Arch. Neurol. **16**:175, 1967, p. 438.

Dodge, P. R., et al.: Myotonic dystrophy in infancy and childhood, Pediatrics **35**:3, 1965.

Drachman, D., and Fambrough, D.: Are muscle fibers denervated in myotonic dystrophy? Arch. Neurol. **33**:485, 1976.

Drachman, D. B., Toyka, K. V., and Myer, E.: Prednisone in Duchenne muscular dystrophy, Lancet **2**:1409, 1974.

Drachman, D. H.: Ophthalmoplegia plus, Arch. Neurol. **18**:654, 1968.

Drucker, W. D., et al.: On the function of the endocrine glands in myotonic muscular dystrophy, Am. J. Med. **31**:941, 1961.

Dubowitz, V.: Progressive muscular dystrophy: prevention of deformities, Clin. Pediatr. **3**:323, 1964.

Dubowitz, V., and Brooke, M.: Muscle biopsy: a modern approach, Philadelphia, 1973, W. B. Saunders Co., p. 184.

Dubowitz, V., and Crome, L.: The central nervous system in Duchenne muscular dystrophy, Brain **92**:805, 1969.

Dyken, P. R.: Extraocular myotonia in families with dystrophia myotonia, Neurology **16**:738, 1966.

Ellis, D. A., Strickland, J. M., and Eccleston, J. F.: The direct interconversion of glucose and fructose in human skeletal muscle with special reference to childhood muscular dystrophy, Clin. Sci. **44**:321, 1973.

Emery, A. E., et al.: Antenatal diagnosis of Duchenne muscular dystrophy, Lancet **1**:847, 1979.

Emery, A. E., and Gosden, C.: A neurogenic component in muscular dystrophy, J. Med. Genet. **11**:76, 1974.

Emery, E. S., Fenichel, G. M., and Eng, G.: A spinal muscular atrophy with scapuloperoneal distribution, Arch. Neurol. **18**:129, 1968.

Engel, W. K., and Derrer, E. C.: Drugs blocking the muscle-damaging effects of 5-HT and noradrenaline in aorta-ligatured rats, Nature **254**:151, 1975.

Enomoto, A., and Bradley, W.: Therapeutic trials in muscular dystrophy, Arch. Neurol. **34**:771, 1977.

Erb, W. H.: Ueber die "juvenile Form" der progressiven Muskelatrophie ihre Beziehungen zur sogenannter Pseudohypertrophie der Muskeln, Deutsch Arch. Klin Med. **34**:467, 1884, p. 462.

Erdbrink, W. L.: Ocular myopathy associated with retinitis pigmentosa, Arch. Ophthalmol. **57**:335, 1957.

Evans, P. R.: Nuclear agenesis: Moebius syndrome: the congenital facial diplegia syndrome, Arch. Dis. Child. **30**:237, 1955.

Feigenbaum, J. A., and Munsat, T. L.: A neuromuscular syndrome of scapulo-peroneal distribution, Bull. Los Angeles Neurol. Soc. **35**:47, 1970.

Fenichel, G. M.: On the pathogenesis of Duchenne muscular dystrophy, Dev. Med. Child. Neurol. **17**:527, 1975.

Fenichel, G. M., Emery, E. S., and Hunt, P.: Neurogenic atrophy stimulating facioscapulohumeral dystrophy, Arch. Neurol. **17**:257, 1967.

Ferrier, P., Bamatter, F., and Klein, D.: Muscular dystrophy (Duchenne) in a girl with Turner's syndrome, J. Med. Genet. **2**:38, 1965.

Gardner-Medwin, D.: Studies of the carrier state in the Duchenne type of muscular dystrophy, J. Neurol. Neurosurg. Psychiatry **31**:124, 1968.

Gardner-Medwin, D., Pennington, R. J., and Walton, J. N.: The detection of carriers of X-linked muscular dystrophy genes, J. Neurol. Sci. **13**:459, 1971.

Gardy, H.: Dystrophia myotonica in pregnancy, Obstet. Gynecol. **21**:441, 1963.

Geschwind, N., and Simpson, J. A.: Procaine amide in the treatment of myotonia, Brain **78**:81, 1955.

Gilroy, J., et al.: Cardiac and pulmonary complications in Duchenne's progressive muscular dystrophy, Circulation **27**:484, 1963.

Goto, K.: Creatine phosphokinase isoenzymes in neuromuscular disorders, Arch. Neurol. **31**:116, 1974.

Haldane, J. B. S.: Mutation in the sex-linked recessive type of muscular dystrophy: a possible sex difference, Ann. Hum. Genet. **20**:344, 1955.

Hanson, P. A., and Rowland, L. P.: Möbius syndrome and facioscapulohumeral muscular dystrophy, Arch. Neurol. **24**:31, 1971.

Hathaway, P. W., Engel, W. K., and Zellweger, H.: Experimental myopathy after microarterial embolization: comparison with childhood X-linked pseudohypertrophic muscular dystrophy, Arch. Neurol. **22**:365, 1970.

Hofmann, W. W., and Thesleff, S.: Studies on the dystrophic influence of nerve on skeletal muscle, Europ. J. Pharmacol. **20**:256, 1972.

Hudgson, P., Pearce, G. W., and Walton, J. N.: Preclinical muscular dystrophy: histopathological changes observed in muscle biopsy, Brain **90**:565, 1967.

Huff, T. A., and Lebovitz, H. E.: Dynamics of insulin secretion in myotonic dystrophy, J. Clin. Endocrinol. **28**:992, 1968.

Hughes, B. P.: Creatine phosphokinase in facioscapulohumeral muscular dystrophy, Br. Med. J. **3**:464, 1971.

Huttenlocher, P. R., et al.: Osteo-chondro-muscular dystrophy; a new disorder manifested by multiple skeletal deformities, myotonia, and dystrophic changes in muscle, Pediatrics **44**:945, 1969.

Hutton, E. M., and Thompson, M. W.: Carrier detection and genetic counselling in Duchenne muscular dystrophy: a follow-up study, Can. Med. Assoc. J. **115**:749, 1976.

Ionasescu, V.: Distinction between Duchenne and other muscular dystrophies by ribosomal protein synthesis, J. Med. Genet. **12**:49, 1975.

Ionasescu, V., Zellweger, H., and Burmeister, L.: Detection of carriers and genetic counseling in Duchenne muscular dystrophy by ribosomal protein synthesis, Acta Neurol. Scand. **54**:442, 1976.

Ionasescu, V., Zellweger, H., and Conway, T. W.: Ribosomal protein synthesis in Duchenne-muscular dystrophy, Arch. Biochem. Biophys. **144**:51, 1971.

Ionasescu, V., et al.: Abnormal protein synthesis in facioscapulohumeral muscular dystrophy, Neurology **22**:1286, 1972, p. 463.

Ionasescu, V., et al.: Identification of carriers of Duchenne muscular dystrophy by muscle protein synthesis, Neurology **23**:497, 1973.

Jackson, C. E., and Carey, J. H.: Progressive muscular dystrophy: autosomal recessive type, Pediatrics **28**:77, 1961.

Jackson, C. E., and Strehler, D. A.: Limb-girdle muscular dystrophy: clinical manifestations and detection of preclinical disease, Pediatrics **41**:495, 1968.

Jensen, H., Jensen, K. B., and Jarnum, S.: Turnover of IgG and IgM in myotonic dystrophy, Neurology **21**:68, 1971.

Jerusalem, F., Engel, A. G., and Gomez, M. R.: Duchenne dystrophy. I. Morphometric study of the muscle microvasculature, Brain **97**:115, 1975.

Karpati, G., et al.: Infantile myotonic dystrophy: histochemical and electron microscopic features in skeletal muscle, Neurology **23**:1066, 1973.

Klinkerfuss, G. H.: An electron microscopic study of myotonic dystrophy, Arch. Neurol. **16**:181, 1967.

Landouzy, L., and Déjerine, J.: De la myopathie atrophique progressive; myopathie sans neuropathie, débutant d'ordinaire dans l'enfance, par la face, Rev. Med. **5**:81, 253, 1885.

Leth, A., and Wuelff, K.: Myocardiopathy in Duchenne's progressive muscular dystrophy, Acta Paediatr. Scand. **65**:28, 1976.

Lewis, I.: Late-onset muscle dystrophy: oculopharyngoesophageal variety, Can. Med. Assoc. J. **95**:146, 1966.

Lin, C. H., Hudson, A. J., and Strickland, K. P.: Fatty acid oxidation by skeletal muscle mitochondria in Duchenne muscular dystrophy, Life Sci. **11**:355, 1972.

Lipicky, R., Bryant, S., and Salmon, J.: Cable parameters, sodium, potassium, chloride, and water content, and potassium efflux in isolated external intercostal muscle of normal volunteers and patients with myotonia congenita, J. Clin. Invest. **50**:2091, 1971.

Lyon, M. F.: Sex chromatin and gene action in the mammalian X-chromosome, Am. J. Hum. Genet. **14**:135, 1962.

Mahoney, M. J., et al.: Prenatal diagnosis of Duchenne's muscular dystrophy, N. Engl. J. Med. **97**:968, 1977.

Mastaglia, F. L., Papadimitriou, J. M., and Kakulas, B. A.: Regeneration of muscle in Duchenne muscular dystrophy: an electron microscope study, J. Neurol. Sci. **11**:425, 1970.

Mawatari, S., and Katayama, K.: Scapuloperoneal muscular atrophy with cardiopathy, Arch. Neurol. **28**:55, 1973.

Mawatari, S., Miranda, A., and Rowland, L. P.: Adenyl cyclase abnormality in Duchenne muscular dystrophy: muscle cells in culture, Neurology **26**:1021, 1976.

Mawatari, S., Schonberg, M., and Olarte, M.: Biochemical abnormalities of erythrocyte membranes in Duchenne dystrophy, Arch. Neurol. **33**:489, 1976.

McComas, A. J., Sica, R. E., and Campbell, M. J.: "Sick" motoneurons: a unifying concept of muscle disease, Lancet **1**:321, 1971.

McComas, A. J., Sica, R. E. P., and Currie, S.: An electrophysiological study of Duchenne dystrophy, J. Neurol. Neurosurg. Psychiatry **34**:461, 1971.

McQuillen, M. P.: Familial limb-girdle myasthenia, Brain **89**:121, 1966.

Mendell, J. R., Engel, W. K., and Derrer, E. C.: Duchenne muscular dystrophy: functional ischemia reproduces its characteristic lesions, Science **172**:1143, 1971.

Mendell, J. R., Roelofs, R. I., and Engel, W. K.: Ultrastructural development of explanted human skeletal muscle in tissue culture, J. Neuropathol. Exp. Neurol. **31**:433, 1972.

Mendelsohn, L. V., et al.: Insulin responses in myotonia dystrophica, Metabolism **18**:764, 1969.

Milhorat, A. T., and Goldstone, L.: The carrier state in muscular dystrophy of the Duchenne type, J.A.M.A. **194**:131, 1965.

Miyoshi, K., et al.: Myoglobin subfractions: abnormality in Duchenne-type of progressive muscular dystrophy, Science **159**:736, 1968.

Moser, H., and Emery, A. E. H.: The manifesting carrier in Duchenne muscular dystrophy, Clin. Genet. **5**:271, 1974.

Munsat, T. L.: Therapy of myotonia: a double-blind evaluation of diphenylhydantoin, procainamide and placebo, Neurology **17**:359, 1967.

Norris, F. H., Jr.: Unstable membrane potential in human myotonic muscle, Electroencephalogr. Clin. Neurophysiol. **14**:197, 1962.

Nuttall, F. Q., Barbosa, J., and Gannon, M. C.: The glycogen synthase system in skeletal muscle of normal humans and patients with myotonic dystrophy: effect of glucose and insulin administration, Metabolism **23**:561, 1974.

Packard, N., et al.: Systemic membrane defect in the proximal muscular dystrophies, N. Engl. J. Med. **299**:841, 1978.

Parker, J. M., and Mendell, J. R.: Proximal myopathy induced by 5-HT-imipramine simulates Duchenne dystrophy, Nature **247**:103, 1974.

Paulson, O. B., Engel, A. G., and Gomez, M. R.: Muscle blood flow in Duchenne type muscular dystrophy, limb-girdle dystrophy, polymyositis, and in normal controls, J. Neurol. Neurosurg. Psychiatry **37**:685, 1974.

Payne, C. A., and Greenfield, J. C., Jr.: Electrocardiographic abnormalities associated with myotonic dystrophy, Am. Heart J. **65**:436, 1963.

Pearson, C. M.: Histopathological features of muscle in the preclinical stages of muscular dystrophy, Brain **85**:109, 1962.

Penn, A. S., Lisak, R. P., and Rowland, L. P.: Muscular dystrophy in young girls, Neurology **20**:147, 1970.

Percy, A. K., and Miller, M. E.: Reduced deformability of erythrocyte membranes from patients with Duchenne muscular dystrophy, Nature **258**:147, 1975.

Perloff, J. K., et al.: The distinctive electrocardiogram of Duchenne's progressive muscular dystrophy, Am. J. Med. **42**:179, 1967.

Plishker, G. A., Gitelman, H. J., and Appel, S. H.: Myotonic muscular dystrophy: altered calcium transport in erythrocytes, Science **200**:323, 1978.

Polgar, J. G., et al.: The early detection of dystrophia myotonica, Brain **95**:761, 1972.

Pollock, M., and Dyck, P. J.: Peripheral nerve morphometry in myotonic dystrophy, Arch. Neurol. **33**:33, 1976.

Prosser, E. J., Murphy, E. G., and Thompson, M. W.: Intelligence and the gene for Duchenne muscular dystrophy, Arch. Dis. Child. **44**:221, 1969.

Ravin, M., Newmark, Z., and Saviello, G.: Myotonia dystrophica—an anesthetic hazard: two case reports, Anesth. Analg. **54**:216, 1975.

Refsum, S., et al.: Dystrophia myotonica: repeated pneumoencephalographic studies in ten patients, Neurology **17**:345, 1967.

Renwick, J. H., et al.: Confirmation of linkage of the loci for myotonic dystrophy and ABH secretion, J. Med. Genet. **8**:407, 1971.

Ricker, K., and Mertens, H. G.: The differential diagnosis of the myogenic (facio)-scapulo-peroneal syndrome, Europ. Neurol. **1**:275, 1968.

Ronan, G. A., et al.: The vector cardiogram in Duchenne's progressive muscular dystrophy, Am. Heart J. **84**:588, 1972.

Roses, A. D., and Appel, S. H.: Protein kinase activity in erythrocyte ghosts of patients with myotonic muscular dystrophy, Proc. Natl. Acad. Sci. U.S.A. **70**:1855, 1973.

Roses, A. D., and Appel, S. H.: Muscle membrane protein kinase in myotonic muscular dystrophy, Nature **250**:245, 1974.

Roses, A. D., and Appel, S. H.: Phosphorylation of component a of the human erythrocyte membrane in myotonic muscular dystrophy, J. Membr. Biol. **20**:51, 1975.

Roses, A. D., Herbstreith, M. H., and Appel, S. H.: Membrane protein kinase alteration in Duchenne muscular dystrophy, Nature **254**:350, 1975.

Roses, A. D., et al.: Carrier detection in Duchenne muscular dystrophy, N. Engl. J. Med. **294**:193, 1976.

Roses, A. D., et al.: Lactate dehydrogenase isoenzyme

5 in detecting carriers of Duchenne muscular dystrophy, Neurology **27**:414, 1977.

Rosman, N. P.: The cerebral defect and myopathy in Duchenne muscular dystrophy: a comparative clinicopathological study, Neurology **20**:329, 1970.

Rosman, N. P., and Rebeiz, J. J.: The cerebral defect and myopathy in myotonic dystrophy: a comparative clinicopathological study, Neurology **17**:1106, 1967.

Rowland, L. P.: Pathogenesis of muscular dystrophies, Arch. Neurol. **33**:315, 1976.

Rowland, L. P., and Layzer, R. B.: Muscular dystrophies, atrophies, and related diseases. In Baker, A. B., and Baker, L. H., editors: Clinical neurology, New York, 1971, Harper & Row, Publishers, chap. 37.

Rowland, L. P., et al.: Myoglobin and muscular dystrophy: electrophoretic and immunochemical study, Arch. Neurol. **18**:141, 1968.

Roy, S., and Dubowitz, V.: Carrier detection in Duchenne muscular dystrophy, J. Neurol. Sci. **11**:65, 1970.

Rüdel, R., and Senges, J.: Mammalian skeletal muscle: reduced chloride conductance in drug-induced myotonia and induction of myotonia by low-chloride solution, Nauyn-Schmiedebergs Arch. Pharmakol. Exp. Pathol. **274**:337, 1972.

Samaha, F. J., and Gergely, J.: Biochemical abnormalities of the sarcoplasmic reticulum in muscular dystrophy, N. Engl. J. Med. **280**:184, 1969.

Sarnat, H., and Silbert, S.: Maturational arrest of fetal muscle in neonatal myotonic dystrophy, Arch. Neurol. **33**:466, 1976.

Sarnat, H., O'Connor, T., and Byrne, P.: Clinical effects of myotonic dystrophy on pregnancy and the neonate, Arch. Neurol. **33**:459, 1976.

Scarpalezos, S., and Panayiotopoulos, C. P.: Duchenne muscular dystrophy—reservations to the neurogenic hypothesis, Lancet **2**:458, 1973, p. 444.

Schechter, M. D.: The orthopedically handicapped child, Arch. Gen. Psychiatry **53**:247, 1961.

Schotland, D. L., and Rowland, L. P.: Muscular dystrophy: features of ocular myopathy, distal myopathy and myotonic dystrophy, Arch. Neurol. **10**:433, 1964.

Schotland, D. L., Bonilla, E., and Van Meter, M.: Duchenne dystrophy: alteration in muscle plasma membrane structure, Science **196**:1005, 1977.

Schotland, D. L., Spiro, D., and Carmel, P.: Ultrastructural studies of ring fibers in human muscle disease, J. Neuropathol. Exp. Neurol. **25**:431, 1966.

Schwartz, O., and Jampel, R. S.: Congenital blepharophimosis associated with a unique generalized myopathy, Arch. Ophthalmol. **68**:52, 1962.

Seay, A., and Ziter, F.: Malignant hyperpyrexia in a patient with Schwartz-Jampel syndrome, J. Pediatr. **93**:83, 1978.

Shaw, R. F., and Dreifuss, F. E.: Mild and severe forms of X-linked muscular dystrophy, Arch. Neurol. **20**:451, 1969.

Sibley, J. A., and Lehninger, A. L.: Determination of aldolase in animal tissues, J. Biol. Chem. **177**:859, 1949.

Sica, R. E. P., and McComas, A. J.: An electrophysiological investigation of limb-girdle and facioscapulohumeral dystrophy, J. Neurol. Neurosurg. Psychiatry **34**:469, 1971.

Siegl, I. M.: Early signs of Landouzy-Dejerine disease: wrist and finger weakness, J.A.M.A. **221**:302, 1972.

Silverman, L. M., et al.: Significance of creatine phosphokinase isoenzymes in Duchenne dystrophy, Neurology **26**:561, 1976.

Simpson, A. J., and Khilnani, M. T.: Gastrointestinal manifestations of the muscle dystrophies, Am. J. Roentgenol. Radium Ther. Nucl. Med. **125**:948, 1975.

Skinner, R., et al.: The detection of carriers of benign (Becker-type) X-linked muscular dystrophy, J. Med. Genet. **12**:131, 1975.

Somer, H., Dubowitz, V., and Donner, M.: Creatine kinase isoenzymes in neuromuscular diseases, J. Neurol. Sci. **29**:129, 1976.

Somers, J. E., and Winer, N.: Reversible myopathy and myotonia following administration of a hypocholesterolemic agent, Neurology **16**:761, 1966.

Spencer, G. E., and Vignos, P. J.: Bracing for ambulation in childhood progressive muscular dystrophy, J. Bone Joint Surg. **44A**:234, 1962.

Strickland, J. M., and Ellis, D. A.: Isoenzymes of hexokinase in human muscular dystrophy, Nature **253**:464, 1975.

Taft, L. T.: The care and management of the child with muscular dystrophy, Dev. Med. Child. Neurol. **15**:510, 1973.

Taylor, R. G., et al.: Continuous muscle fiber activity in the Schwartz-Jampel syndrome, Electroencephalogr. Clin. Neurophysiol. **33**:497, 1972.

Thomas, P. K., Calne, B. D., and Elliott, C. F.: X-linked scapuloperoneal syndrome, J. Neurol. Neurosurg. Psychiatry **35**:208, 1972.

Thomson, W. H., Leyburn, P., and Walton, J. N.: Serum enzyme activity in muscular dystrophy, Br. Med. J. **2**:1276, 1960.

Thomson, W. H., Sweetin, J. C., and Elton, R. A.: The neurogenic and myogenic hypotheses in human (Duchenne) muscular dystrophy, Nature **249**:151, 1974.

Tyler, F. H., and Wintrobe, M. M.: Studies in disorders of muscle. I. The problem of progressive muscular dystrophy, Ann. Intern. Med. **32**:72, 1950.

Vassilopoulos, D., and Emery, A. E. H.: Muscle nuclear changes in fetuses at risk for Duchenne muscular dystrophy, J. Med. Genet. **14**:13, 1977.

Victor, M., Hayes, R., and Adams, R. D.: Oculopharyngeal muscular dystrophy, N. Engl. J. Med., **267**:1267, 1962.

Vignos, P. J., Jr.: Rehabilitation in progressive muscular dystrophy. In Licht, S., editor, Rehabilitation and medicine, Baltimore, 1968, The Williams & Wilkins Co.

Vignos, P. J., Jr.: Intellectual function and educational achievement in Duchenne muscular dystrophy, Isr. J. Med. Sci. **13**:215, 1977.

Wahi, P. L., Bhargava, K. C., and Mohindra, S.: Cardiorespiratory changes in progressive muscular dystrophy, Br. Heart J. **33**:533, 1971.

Wakayama, Y.: Electron microscopic study on satellite cell in muscle of Duchenne muscular dystrophy, J. Neuropathol. Exp. Neurol. **35**:532, 1976.

Walton, J. N.: The inheritance of muscular dystrophy: further observations, Ann. Hum. Genet. **21**:40, 1956.

Walton, J. N., and Gardner-Medwin, D.: Progressive muscular dystrophy and the myotonic disorders. In Walton, J. N., editor: Disorders of voluntary muscle, ed. 2, Boston, 1969, Little, Brown & Co., p. 470.

Welsh, J. D., Haase, G. R., and Bynum, T. E.: Myotonic muscular dystrophy: systemic manifestations, Arch. Intern. Med. **114**:669, 1964.

Wochner, R. D., et al.: Accelerated breakdown of immunoglobulin G (IgG) in myotonic dystrophy: a hereditary error of immunoglobulin catabolism, J. Clin. Invest. **45**:321, 1966.

Worden, K. D., and Vignos, P. J., Jr.: Intellectual function in childhood progressive muscular dystrophy, Pediatrics **29**:968, 1962.

Yamuna, S., et al.: Serum pyruvate kinase in carriers of Duchenne muscular dystrophy, Clin. Chim. Acta **79**:277, 1977.

Yu, M. K., et al.: Pargyline-induced myopathy with histochemical characteristics of Duchenne muscular dystrophy, Neurology **24**:237, 1974.

Zellweger, H., and Antonik, A.: Newborn screening for Duchenne muscular dystrophy, Pediatrics **55**:30, 1975.

Zellweger, H., and Hanson, J. W.: Slowly progressive X-linked recessive muscular dystrophy (type IIIb), Arch. Intern. Med. **120**:525, 1967.

Ziter, F. A., and Allsop, K. G.: The diagnosis and management of childhood muscular dystrophy, Clin. Pediatr. **15**:540, 1976.

Zundel, W. S., and Tyler, F. H.: The muscular dystrophies, N. Engl. J. Med. **273**:537, 1965.

# CHAPTER 7

# Unusual myopathies and congenital defects of muscle

A myopathy is a disease in which there are morphologic, neurophysiologic, and biochemical changes in the muscle fiber or its membrane. These changes are not due to abnormalities of the central nervous system, anterior horn cell, peripheral nerve, or neuromuscular junction. A clinically useful differential diagnostic approach to the classifica-

**Table 7-1.** Unusual myopathies

| |
|---|
| Congenital |
|    Central core disease* |
|    Multicore disease* |
|    Nemaline myopathy* |
|    Fiber type disproportion* |
|    Myotubular (centronuclear) myopathy* |
|    Type I fiber hypotrophy and central nuclei* |
|    Lysis of myofibrils* |
|    Fingerprint-body myopathy* |
|    Sarcotubular myopathy |
|    Reducing body myopathy* |
|    Lipid myopathies |
|    Mitochondrial myopathies* |
|    Myoadenylate deaminase deficiency |
|    Congenital muscular dystrophy* |
|    Myotonia congenita* |
|    Monomelic myopathy |
|    Distal myopathy |
| Glycogen storage diseases |
| Periodic paralyses |
| Endocrine myopathies |
| Myoglobinuria |

*Hypotonia present at birth.

tion of the unusual myopathies of infancy and childhood (Table 7-1) is based on the characteristic clinical, pathologic, or chemical features. The muscular dystrophies of childhood and myositis are discussed in Chapters 6 and 8.

The general approach to the clinical evaluation of the patient in whom weakness is the predominating symptom is discussed in Chapter 1. When myopathy is the cause, such weakness is usually proximal, occurring especially in the hip and shoulder girdle muscles. Tendon reflexes are usually, but not always, reduced in proportion to the degree of weakness, and fasciculations are not seen. Sensation is normal. Exceptions to these features will be apparent when the individual disease entities are considered.

## CONGENITAL MYOPATHIES

The congenital myopathies consist of diseases associated with characteristic pathologic abnormalities of muscle cell structure or diseases with less well-defined pathologic changes but typical clinical features. The pathogenesis is generally unknown. However, in the lipid storage diseases and mitochondrial myopathies, extensive biochemical investigations have defined some aspects of the basic abnormalities.

The congenital myopathies are usually present at birth with symptoms of weakness and hypotonia. However, several exist in a

**181**

form with onset later in childhood. Variations in onset may reflect either a disease spectrum of a single genetic abnormality or distinct disease processes.

Several disorders without evidence of involvement of the neuromuscular system cause hypotonia and delayed acquisition of motor milestones. These disorders are rarely associated with significant weakness. The most common group of disorders are those associated with involvement of the central nervous system (see Chapter 1). In addition, connective tissue disorders, Prader-Willi syndrome, and benign congenital hypotonia need to be considered in a differential diagnosis of hypotonia. Connective tissue disorders exhibiting hypotonia because of the laxity of joint ligaments include Ehlers-Danlos syndrome, congenital laxity of ligaments, and osteogenesis imperfecta. The Prader-Willi syndrome is characterized by short stature, developmental delay, cryptorchidism, marked hypotonia, and feeding difficulty in the newborn period. The hypotonia and feeding difficulty improve. Hyperphagia develops and the children become grossly obese.

The differential diagnosis of a specific congenital myopathy is difficult because of the common symptoms of weakness and hypotonia often present at birth. The following general statements may prove useful in distinguishing among the various congenital myopathies.

A dominant inheritance pattern is found in central core disease, congenital fiber disproportion, distal myopathy, myotubular myopathy, myotonia congenita, and nemaline myopathy. The remaining congenital myopathies discussed in this section either result from a recessive inheritance or there is insufficient data to make a judgment concerning the mode of inheritance. Some diseases, such as myotubular myopathy and myotonia congenita, have been described with different forms of inheritance.

The majority of congenital myopathies are nonprogressive. In those conditions in which a nonprogressive course generally occurs, an occasional patient may show evidence for progression. Congenital myopathies that are definitely progressive in nature are carnitine deficiency, congenital mitochondrial myopathies, the severe form of congenital muscular dystrophy, myotubular myopathy, and reducing body myopathy.

Proximal weakness characterizes most congenital myopathies. However, distal weakness is encountered in distal myopathy and myotonia congenita. In nemaline myopathy, the upper extremities may be more involved than the lower. In contrast, central core disease and congenital fiber type disproportion are characterized by greater weakness in the lower extremities than in the upper extremities.

Involvement of the muscles subserved by the cranial nerves differentiates several myopathies. Extraocular muscle involvement is observed in congenital muscular dystrophy, mitochondrial myopathy, multicore disease, myotubular myopathy, oculocraniosomatic disease, and reducing body myopathy. Significant involvement of the facial muscles is seen in carnitine deficiency, myotubular myopathy, nemaline myopathy, and reducing body myopathy. Carnitine deficiency may also involve the muscles innervated by cranial nerves V and XII.

A cardiomyopathy has been described in carnitine deficiency, megaconial myopathy, multicore disease (septal defects), myotubular myopathy, and oculocraniosomatic disease. In myotonic dystrophy and Duchenne muscular dystrophy, the heart is also involved.

Skeletal anomalies are found in several of the congenital myopathies, including central core disease, congenital fiber type disproportion, congenital mitochondrial myopathy, and nemaline myopathy. Contractures in the newborn period are seen in congenital fiber type disproportion, congenital muscular dystrophy, and arthrogryposis multiplex congenita.

Pathologically, the congenital myopathies most often involve the type I fibers. However, several diseases are characterized by predominant type II fiber involvement, including congenital fiber type disproportion, myotonia congenita, sarcotubular myopathy, and steroid myopathy. However, selective atrophy of type II fibers may result from any disease producing weakness, including disuse atrophy (Dubowitz and Brooke, 1973).

### Central core disease

CLINICAL FEATURES. Central core disease was described as a nonprogressive congenital myopathy in 1956 (Shy and Magee, 1956). The presenting features are hypotonia and weakness at birth or in early infancy. The family history is often positive for similar disease, indicating a dominant inheritance. Diminished fetal movements have been described. Patients have normal intellectual development but strikingly delayed motor development, especially rolling over and sitting up; they often do not walk until 4 years of age. Progression of the disease is generally not apparent, although weakness persists into adult life and patients continue to have difficulty climbing stairs, rising from a lying or sitting position, and performing vigorous exercise. Slow progression of the disease may be evident in later life (Isaacs, Heffron, and Badenhorst, 1975).

Weakness is primarily proximal in distribution and affects the lower extremities to a greater degree than the upper extremities. Footdrop may be present. All muscles can be moved against gravity. The children are often able to assume unusual positions. Muscles subserved by the cranial nerves are not involved, with the possible exception of mild weakness of the facial and sternocleidomastoid muscles. Tendon reflexes may be normal, decreased, or absent. There are no sensory changes. Muscular atrophy is not evident, and myotonia is not clinically detectable. Skeletal anomalies, such as congenital hip dislocation, kyphoscoliosis, lordosis, funnel chest, mandibular hypoplasia, flexion deformity of the fifth finger, short neck, and flatfeet may be present (Telerman-Toppet, Gerard, and Coërs, 1973).

Serum enzyme levels are normal. General-ly there are a nonspecific increase in urinary creatine and a decrease in urinary creatinine levels. Electromyography shows myopathic potentials characterized by short duration, decreased amplitude, and polyphasia. There are no denervation or myotonic potentials. Motor nerve conduction velocity is normal.

Central core disease is one of the congenital myopathies associated with *malignant hyperpyrexia* (Denborough, Dennett, and Anderson, 1973; Engel et al., 1978). Malignant hyperpyrexia is a rare but often fatal condition characterized by fulminating rise in temperature (greater than 2° C per hour), muscle contracture leading to rigidity, tachycardia and tachypnea, and metabolic and respiratory acidosis. In susceptible individuals this disease follows the use of inhalation anesthetics and muscle relaxants. The condition, inherited in a dominant pattern, is thought to result from a defect in the sarcoplasmic reticulum with an aberration in calcium metabolism. Malignant hyperpyrexia also occurs in individuals with myotonia congenita and other nonspecific myopathies (King, Denborough, and Zapf, 1972). A susceptible individual may be detected by clinical evidence of myopathy, including weakness and contractures, by elevated serum creatine phosphokinase (CPK) level (Isaacs and Barlow, 1974), and by an in vitro study of halothane-induced muscle contraction (Ellis et al., 1972).

PATHOLOGY. The muscle biopsy specimen shows a characteristic alteration in type I muscle fiber that consists of a central core of aberrant fibrillary material (Fig. 7-1). In preparing the biopsy specimen, it is important to use more than one fixative, for example, normal saline and Bouin's fluid (Engel et al., 1961), because the central cores may not be apparent if fixed only in 10% formalin. The noncore areas of muscle appear normal. Pathologic changes seen with routine hematoxylin and eosin staining are accentuated with a Gomori's trichrome stain. Cytochemically the central core is devoid of oxidative enzymes and phosphorylase activity (Dubowitz and Pearse, 1960; Gonatas et al., 1965).

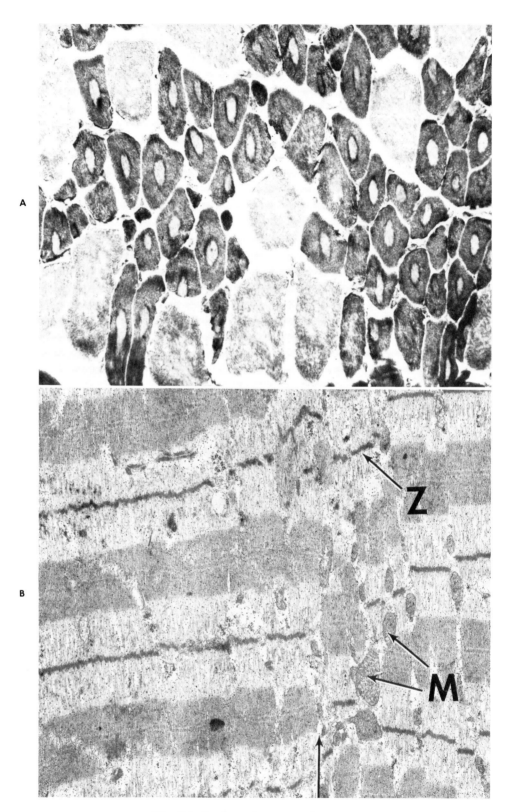

**Fig. 7-1.** For legend see opposite page.

Two types of central core abnormalities have been termed "structured" and "unstructured" (Neville and Brooke, 1973). Electron microscopic study of structured cores reveals identifiable A, I, and Z bands across the core, shortened sarcomere length, absent or rare mitochondria, and widened or irregular Z bands. Histochemically these cores are strongly reactive for myofibrillar ATPase. Unstructured cores contain loosely arranged myofilaments in which the A and I band patterns are absent and the Z band material is blurred and has a streaming appearance. Remnants of the transverse tubules and sarcoplasmic reticulum are present. Mitochondria are not found.

**BIOCHEMISTRY.** Succinic acid dehydrogenase activity and phosphorylase activity are reduced. Actomyosin magnesium-activated ATPase activity and calcium-dependent ATPase activity of the sarcoplasmic reticulum are also reduced. Reduction in the rate and extent of calcium uptake indicates atrophy of the sarcoplasmic reticulum (Isaacs, Heffron, and Badenhorst, 1975).

**TREATMENT.** The orthopedic abnormalities may need surgical correction. Before surgical intervention is undertaken, however, susceptibility to malignant hyperpyrexia should be considered.

*Multicore disease*

Multicore disease is a nonprogressive, congenital myopathy (Engel and Gomez, 1966) manifested by generalized weakness and hypotonia in infancy. Most patients are males. Achievement of motor milestones is delayed, but intelligence is normal. Torticollis has been described at birth in identical male twins (Heffner et al., 1976). Examination reveals dolichocephaly; tall, slender habitus (Engel, Gomez, and Groover, 1971); and generalized weakness, most predominant in proximal muscles. Tendon reflexes are decreased. The muscles subserved by the cranial nerves are generally normal except for weakness of the sternocleidomastoid muscles and ptosis noted in one patient.

Serum enzyme activities are normal. Electromyography reveals an increase in the number of polyphasic potentials and short-duration low-amplitude potentials, usually interpreted as myopathic.

Multicore disease with onset in childhood appears to be nonprogressive. Multicore disease with onset in the adult has been described as a progressive myopathy (Bonnette, Roelofs, and Olson, 1974).

**PATHOLOGY.** Muscle biopsy specimens contain pale, poorly defined areas when stained with hematoxylin and eosin. Under polarized light, these multiple lesions appear as areas of focal loss of cross striations. Cytochemical examination for oxidative enzymes shows a focal decrease in enzymatic activity. Both type I and type II histochemical fiber types are involved, although involvement of type I fibers predominates.

Electron microscopic abnormalities are characterized by a decrease in the number of mitochondria and variable sarcomere disruption, accompanied by Z band streaming.

Multicore disease differs from central core disease in that there are multiple lesions within a single fiber. The lesions are frequently eccentric rather than central and do not extend the length of the muscle fiber. Multicore disease affects both fiber types.

---

**Fig. 7-1. A,** Electron microscopy photomicrograph of muscle biopsy from a patient with central core disease. This cross section stained with NADH-tetrazolium reductase shows dark staining type I fibers and absence of enzyme staining in center of each fiber. Larger and lighter stained type II fibers are less numerous. **B,** Transition between central core area of muscle on left of arrow is delineated from normal muscle on right. Note presence of mitochondria (*M*) in normal area of muscle and absence of mitochondria in central core section. Disruption of Z band (*Z*) with streaming of Z band material is noted at top of photograph at edge of core area. (Courtesy Dr. Stephen A. Smith.)

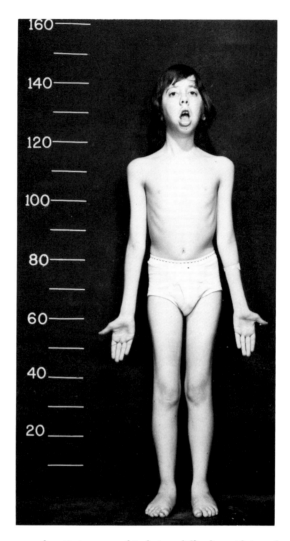

**Fig. 7-2.** Nemaline myopathy. Note myopathic facies, difficulty with jaw closure, and proximal muscle atrophy in upper extremities.

## Nemaline myopathy

CLINICAL FEATURES. Nemaline myopathy was described in 1963 (Shy et al., 1963). The name was derived from the presence of a unique rod- or threadlike structure in the muscle cells. Independently an alternate description of myogranules was given (Conen, Murphy, and Donohue, 1963).

Nemaline myopathy is characterized by hypotonia and weakness at birth. The affected infants have a poor cry, weak suck, dysphagia, and sometimes cyanosis and re-

spiratory difficulty. The disease is generally nonprogressive; however, delayed motor development, including late crawling and walking, is common. In later childhood, a waddling gait is common. Some weakness generally persists into adult life. Intelligence is normal.

On examination the patients appear slender because of reduced muscle bulk. Myopathic facies are common and characterized by lack of facial expression, a long slender face, and some sagging or pursing of the lips

(Fig. 7-2). In addition, dysmorphic features occur, including a high-arched palate, dental malocclusion, kyphoscoliosis, pectus excavatum, and pes cavus. The voice is often high-pitched and nasal. Weakness is usually more prominent in the proximal muscles than in the distal ones, and in some patients the upper extremities appear more involved than the lower extremities. The flexor muscles of the neck are especially weak. In other patients, weakness of the distal muscles of the lower extremities has been manifested by footdrop. Tendon reflexes are generally absent. Sensation is normal.

Although nemaline myopathy is usually nonprogressive, progressive weakness has been described in a 14-year-old girl (Engel, Wanko, and Fenichel, 1964). Rarely, this disease may produce severe weakness and death from pneumonia and respiratory muscle weakness (Kolin, 1967; Neustein, 1973). Serum enzyme activity is generally within normal limits. Electromyography reveals myopathic potentials.

An interesting observation by Afifi, Smith, and Zellweger (1965) is the occurrence of pathologic features of both nemaline myopathy and central core disease in one patient. The combination of these two rare diseases suggests that a genetic defect may be expressed in different ways.

Rod-body myopathy of late onset occurring in adult patients has been described (Engel, 1966b; Heffernan, Rewcastle, and Humphrey, 1968). The clinical manifestations of the infantile nemaline myopathy and the late-onset rod-body myopathy are different, suggesting that they are distinct entities. In the adult, rod-body myopathies have been associated with other diseases of muscle, including dermatomyositis and polymyositis. These diseases may represent a single disease spectrum with an early or late onset (Hopkins, Lindsey, and Ford, 1966).

**PATHOLOGY.** Diagnosis of nemaline myopathy is made from the muscle biopsy specimen, which shows aggregates of rods usually located in the subsarcolemmal area of the muscle fiber (Fig. 7-3). The rods are often overlooked on hematoxylin and eosin stains but can be identified readily with the Gomori's trichrome technique, which stains the rods red and the muscle blue-green.

Electron microscopic studies have suggested that the pathologic rod material of nemaline myopathy represents an abnormality of the Z band material (Price et al., 1965; Gonatas, Shy, and Godfrey, 1966). Histochemical study of muscle biopsy tissue has shown selected involvement of type II fibers (Shy et al., 1963), type I fibers (Gonatas, Shy, and Godfrey, 1966), or no apparent fiber-type selection (Shafiq, Milhorat, and Gorycki, 1967). There is little destruction of muscle tissue, and generally, inflammation, necrosis, or regeneration is not present in muscle fibers. There is no apparent positive correlation between the number of rods in the muscle fiber and the degree of clinical weakness (Nienhuis et al., 1967).

The apparent predominance of type I fibers because of marked decrease or absence of type II fibers suggests the possibility of an innervational defect (Karpati, Carpenter, and Andermann, 1971; Dahl and Klutzow, 1974) but motor innervation studies have not demonstrated denervation (Coërs et al., 1976).

Specificity of the rod body has been questioned because of the occurrence of late-onset progressive myopathy with rod bodies and the presence of rod bodies following experimental tenotomy (Engel, 1966b). However, the congenital form of nemaline myopathy appears to represent a specific clinical disorder.

**BIOCHEMISTRY.** Biochemical abnormalities have been reported in the fragmented sarcoplasmic reticulum and in myosin (Sreter et al., 1976). Sarcoplasmic reticulum ATPase activity and myosin ATPase activity are reduced, and calcium uptake is decreased. Electrophoretic study of normal purified human myosin has revealed three light chains characteristic of fast myosin and two light chains of slow myosin. In one patient with nemaline myopathy, large numbers of light chains of slow myosin and few light chains of fast myosin were present. These studies

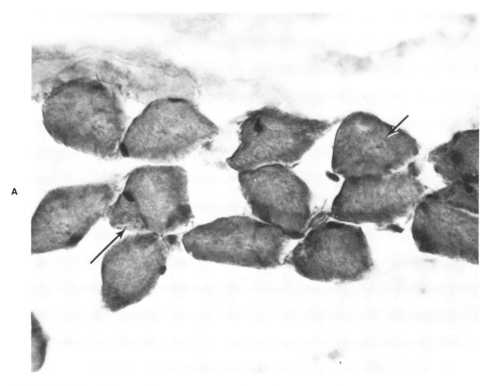

**Fig. 7-3. A,** Muscle biopsy from a patient with nemaline myopathy. Cross sectional examination of H & E stained material shows peripheral clumps and central rods *(arrows)*.

indicate that the abnormal myosin cannot be accounted for simply by an increase in the proportion of type I fibers. The chemical nature of the rod bodies is still unknown, but the rod material may be a breakdown product of the pathologic myosin-type protein. The rod bodies are thought to originate from the Z band and consist of Z band material (Gonatas, Shy, and Godfrey, 1966; Stromer et al., 1976). In the patient studied by Sreter and colleagues (1976), the Z bands were not enlarged, and the electron microscopic appearance of the rods and the Z bands was similar but not identical. Consequently the source of the nemaline bodies remains uncertain.

**GENETICS.** Nemaline myopathy is generally inherited as an autosomal dominant disease (Arts et al., 1978). However, many cases appear to be sporadic or to represent autosomal recessive inheritance. Since nemaline myopathy may be mild or even subclinical,

familial cases may remain undetected without definitive biopsy studies.

**TREATMENT.** Treatment may be needed for dental malocclusion and the orthopedic abnormalities, especially kyphoscoliosis.

### Congenital fiber-type disproportion

Histographic analysis of muscle fiber types in biopsy specimens of children has demonstrated five categories. In normal children, type I and type II muscle fiber diameters vary only slightly in size (Brooke and Engel, 1969).

One category, congenital fiber-type disproportion, is characterized by unusual disparity in size and number of the two major muscle fiber types.

**CLINICAL FEATURES.** The affected infants are weak and hypotonic at birth (floppy infant). The weakness varies in severity but may be so severe as to cause respiratory in-

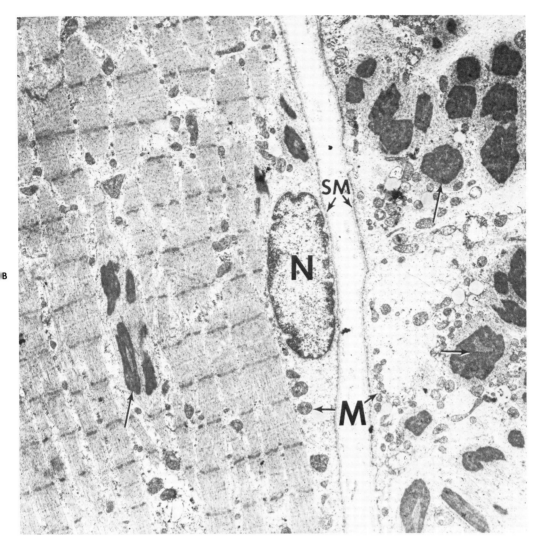

**Fig. 7-3, cont'd. B,** Ultrastructural appearance of a muscle biopsy from a patient with nemaline myopathy demonstrating central and subsarcolemmal clusters of rods *(arrow)*. Mitochondria *(M)*, a muscle nucleus *(N)*, and sarcolemmal membrane *(SM)* are identified. (Courtesy Dr. Stephen A. Smith.)

sufficiency that necessitates assisted ventilation (Lenard and Goebel, 1975). The weakness is generally nonprogressive but seems to be most severe during the first 2 years of life. Acquisition of motor milestones is delayed. The disease generally improves and remains stable, although the patients usually have residual weakness. Intelligence is normal.

Examination reveals muscular weakness in the trunk and extremities. The proximal muscles are somewhat more affected than the distal muscles, and the lower extremities are more involved than the upper extremities. No atrophy, fasciculation, or myotonia is present. The muscles subserved by the cranial nerves are generally normal, although a few patients have had mild facial weakness. Tendon reflexes are decreased or absent. Sensation is reported to be normal.

Over half the patients have contractures,

especially in the hands and feet. Congenital dislocation of the hip, bilateral or unilateral, occurs in one third to one half of the patients. Other associated anomalies are high-arched palate, kyphoscoliosis, and deformities of the feet, including flatfeet or high arches.

Electrodiagnostic studies demonstrate normal conduction velocity and either normal motor unit potentials or low-amplitude short-duration potentials compatible with a myopathic disorder. The serum enzyme activities are usually normal.

**PATHOLOGY.** Routine hematoxylin and eosin stains show little or no abnormality. The fiber-type distribution on routine ATPase reaction shows that type I muscle fibers are smaller and more numerous (predominant) than type II muscle fibers. The largest muscle fibers are type IIB. Oxidative enzyme activity is normal.

The specificity of fiber-type disproportion has been questioned because of its occurrence in Krabbe's disease and Pompe's disease (Martin et al., 1976).

**GENETICS.** Congenital fiber-type disproportion has occurred sporadically and in families, suggesting autosomal dominant inheritance (Brooke, 1973; Curless and Nelson, 1977).

## Myotubular (centronuclear) myopathy

Myotubular myopathy is a unique myopathy thought to represent arrested embryonic development (Spiro, Shy, and Gonatas, 1966). However, other investigators have questioned the embryonic pathogenesis of this disease because the muscle cells are larger than fetal myotubules and the peripheral portions of the muscle cell are similar to normal mature muscle cells (Coleman et al., 1968). The descriptive term "centronuclear myopathy" has been suggested (Sher et al., 1967); however, the historic term "myotubular myopathy" will be retained until the etiology is established.

**CLINICAL FEATURES.** Myotubular myopathy is a progressive disease. Symptoms of weakness may be present at birth or occur in later childhood.

In the infantile form, hypotonia and weakness are present at birth (Campbell, Rebetz, and Walton, 1969; Van Wijngaarden et al., 1969; Kinoshita and Cadman, 1968; Radu et al., 1977). In severe disease, respiratory muscles are involved early, and there is rapid progression to generalized weakness. Motor development is slow. Infants are unable to walk, and death occurs before 3 years of age. If the infant survives the phase of severe respiratory weakness, generalized muscle weakness persists with involvement of extraocular, facial, and neck muscles. Tendon reflexes are absent. Intellectual development is normal. Sensation is normal.

In childhood myotubular myopathy, weakness appears between 2 and 4 years of age. The child has an unsteady, awkward gait and difficulty in climbing stairs. The weakness may progress slowly or rapidly. A number of patients have had motor seizures, focal or generalized. These patients become bedridden in early adult life.

A mild form of myotubular myopathy with mild weakness and disability has been described (Sher et al., 1967). An adult-onset form with mild to moderate weakness and normal longevity has also been described (McLeod et al., 1972).

Myotubular myopathy and type I fiber atrophy have been reported in a single family (Kinoshita, Satoyoshi, and Matsuo, 1975). This observation suggests that myotubular myopathy and type I fiber atrophy are closely related diseases or represent two different phases of the same disease.

Laboratory examination reveals elevated serum creatine phosphokinase (CPK) activity in both the infantile and childhood forms of the disease. Electromyographic findings are variable, with myopathic potentials, fibrillation potentials, and myotonic discharges. Nerve conduction velocity is normal.

**PATHOLOGY.** The pathology of myotubular myopathy generally is similar in both the infantile and later-onset forms (Spiro, Shy, and Gonatas, 1966; Sher et al. 1967). Almost all of the muscle fibers show one or more centrally placed nuclei, with a striking absence of subsarcolemmal nuclei (Fig. 7-4). Surrounding

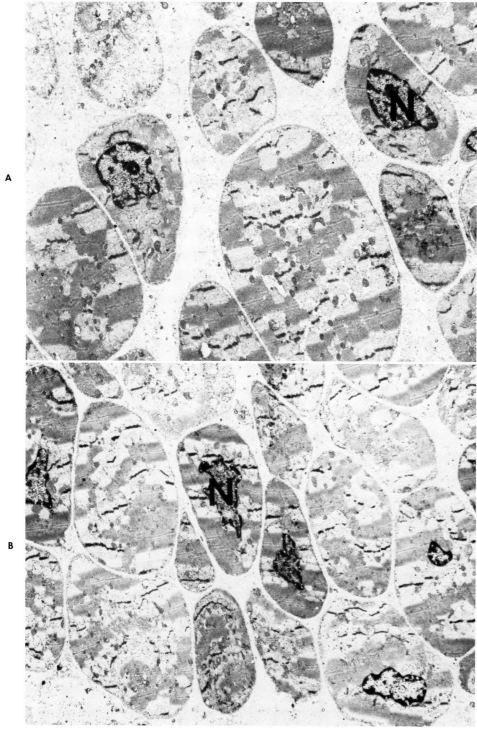

*Continued.*

**Fig. 7-4.** Electron microphotograph of muscle biopsy from an infant with myotubular myopathy. **A** and **B** demonstrate multiple centrally placed nuclei *(N)*, and **C** demonstrates the central myotube *(MT)* area. Scattered central and eccentric disruption of myofibrils is noted in a number of muscle fibers. (Courtesy Dr. Stephen A. Smith.)

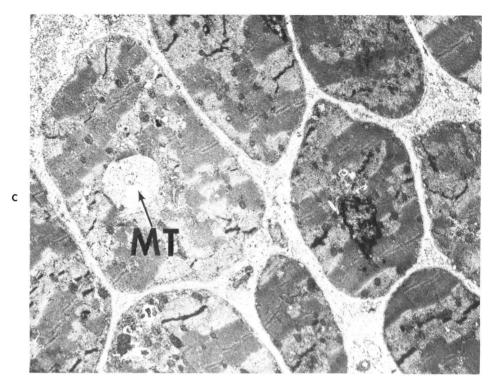

c

MT

**Fig. 7-4, cont'd.** For legend see p. 191.

the central nuclei are clear areas of variable size, which at times occupy almost the entire cell. As a result of these pathologic changes, muscle fibers resemble the normal myotubular stage of embryonic muscle development, which occurs about 10 weeks after conception (see Chapter 2). Cytochemical study reveals two types of abnormal cells. One type lacks oxidative enzyme activity, while the other has increased oxidative enzyme activity in the nuclear, often centrally located, areas of the muscle cell. Myofibrils in the central area are absent, as indicated by negative ATPase reaction. Type I fibers predominate.

Electron microscopic examination shows structural architecture to be well preserved. The central nuclei are associated with aggregates of mitochondria, myelin figures, and dense granules that may represent glycogen. Electron microscopic studies of muscle from the patients with later onset reveal few differences, namely, a lack of myelin figures and, at times, less well-preserved structural architecture.

**GENETICS.** The mode of inheritance may be autosomal dominant (Munsat, Thompson, and Coleman, 1969; McLeod et al., 1972), X-linked recessive (McLeod et al., 1972; Van Wijngaarden et al., 1969), or autosomal recessive (Bradley, Price, and Watanabe, 1970), which suggests that myotubular myopathy is not a single entity.

**TREATMENT.** In the infantile form of the disease, treatment is aimed toward support and maintenance of adequate respiration.

### Type I fiber hypotrophy and central nuclei

Another disease characterized by central nuclei and selective muscle fiber involvement was described as type I fiber hypotrophy and central nuclei (Engel, Gold, and Karpati, 1968). The relationship between

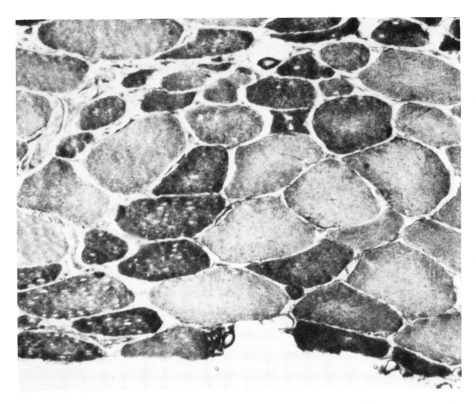

**Fig. 7-5.** Muscle biopsy from a patient with Type I hypotrophy. With NADH-tetrazolium reductase stain, smaller darker type I fibers are identified and compared to larger, lighter type II fibers. (Courtesy Dr. Stephen A. Smith.)

type I fiber hypotrophy with central nuclei and myotubular myopathy is unclear.

**CLINICAL FEATURES.** In the initial report, the infant was apneic and hypotonic at birth and had severe generalized weakness and difficulty sucking and swallowing. Motor abilities were severely delayed. At 11½ months of age, he could raise his arms only over his head, could barely move his legs, and could not roll over.

Examination revealed generalized atrophy and weakness. Cranial nerve examination revealed significant bulbar weakness with difficulty in swallowing and crying, immobile palate, and absent gag reflex. Significantly, the extraocular muscle movements, facial muscles, and tongue were all normal. Tendon reflexes were absent. Sensation was normal. To the extent that mental abilities could be tested, they were normal.

Serum enzyme activities were normal. Electromyographic studies showed increased polyphasic potentials, a few fibrillation potentials, and a mixed interference pattern.

The patient had repeated episodes of pneumonia and died at 18 months of age. A male sibling died of a similar disease at 7 months of age (Meyers et al., 1974).

**PATHOLOGY.** Muscle biopsy and autopsy specimens revealed two populations of muscle fibers: normal muscle fibers (14 to 23 $\mu$) and smaller fibers (5 to 8 $\mu$), many with a central nucleus (Fig. 7-5). All type I muscle fibers were small. Approximately 25% of type II fibers were small and contained central nuclei.

**GENETICS.** Additional reports of cases have emphasized the clinical variability (Inokuchi, Umezaki, and Santa, 1975). Most cases have occurred sporadically, but familial cases and X-linked recessive inheritance have been described (Karpati, Carpenter, and Nelson, 1970). The disease is not necessarily severe or progressive (Bethlem et al., 1969).

### Lysis of myofibrils

Selective involvement of a single histochemical fiber type has been recognized with increasing frequency. Lysis of myofibrils in type I fibers has been described (Cancilla et al., 1971).

**CLINICAL FEATURES.** Two siblings, inactive and weak from birth, demonstrated incoordination, easy fatigability, and delayed motor development.

On neurologic examination, the children were hypotonic and walked with a waddling, slapping gait. The weakness was generalized but more marked proximally. In the older sibling, the muscles were thin but not definitely atrophic. Muscle bulk was normal in the younger boy. The patients had difficulty climbing stairs, and Gowers' sign was present. Tendon reflexes were described as normal. No mention was made of the muscles innervated by the cranial nerves. An electromyogram was normal. The serum lactic dehydrogenase (LDH) and CPK levels were mildly elevated.

**PATHOLOGY.** Muscle biopsy study revealed two populations of muscle fibers. The abnormal muscle fibers were small and irregular with two distinct zones in the sarcoplasm. The central zone contained normal myofibrils, while the peripheral zone lacked myofibrillar striations and appeared homogeneous. At the junction between the central and peripheral areas were chains of vacuoles. Histochemical analysis showed that the small fibers were type I. Electron microscopy of the small fibers revealed a lack of myofibrils in the peripheral portion of the muscle fibers. In many of the myofibrils in the affected fibers, the sarcomeres were normal,

but in other myofibrils the sarcomere pattern was interrupted. Excessive deposition of lipid or glycogen was not evident. The sarcoplasmic reticulum, transverse tubules, sarcolemma, and basement membranes did not appear altered in the affected fibers.

**GENETICS.** No mention was made of consanguinity. This condition may be inherited as an autosomal recessive trait, but additional pedigrees need to be examined.

### Fingerprint-body myopathy

Fingerprint-body myopathy was recognized as a congenital muscle disease in 1972 (Engel, Angelini, and Gomez, 1972). The fingerprint body was regarded as the distinguishing morphologic feature.

**CLINICAL FEATURES.** The original report described a 5-year-old girl with generalized weakness who experienced hypotonia in infancy. Her motor development was slow. She walked unaided at 17 months of age but stumbled frequently and did not run well. No other family members were similarly affected. Neurologic examination showed moderate, diffuse weakness of the trunk and extremities, lordotic posture, and Gowers' sign. The muscles subserved by the cranial nerves were not affected. There was no muscle atrophy. Tendon reflexes were decreased or absent. A static tremor of the upper extremities was noted. Tortuous retinal vessels were present. The patient was reported to have a Stanford-Binet IQ of 80. Serum CPK, glutamic-oxaloacetic transaminase (GOT), and LDH levels were normal. Electrodiagnostic studies documented normal motor and sensory nerve conduction velocities. The motor unit action potentials demonstrated myopathic changes. An electroencephalogram was normal.

**PATHOLOGY.** Muscle biopsy revealed a large number of randomly distributed atrophic fibers. In fresh-frozen sections, type I fibers were atrophic and type II fibers were hypertrophied. Many of the atrophic type I fibers had decreased oxidative enzyme activity in a rimlike peripheral region. Phase microscopy showed numerous abnormal inclusions in normal-sized atrophic fibers. Electron microscopy revealed that they were composed of complex, convoluted lamellae arranged in fingerprint patterns. The fingerprint bodies were not composed of ribosomal protein, glycogen, or known structural proteins. In addition to the fingerprint bodies, the type I fibers displayed focal myofibrillar degeneration and focal decrease in mitochondrial number.

Fingerprint bodies have been described in dermatomyositis (Carpenter et al., 1972) and myotonic dystrophy (Tomé and Fardeau, 1973), raising a question concerning their specificity.

### Sarcotubular myopathy

**CLINICAL FEATURES.** A nonprogressive myopathy, sarcotubular myopathy, was described in two brothers of a Hutterite family whose parents were third cousins (Jerusalem, Engel, and Gomez, 1973). The weakness began in the perinatal period or early infancy. The younger brother had had decreased movement in utero. He walked at 18 months of age with a slow gait and fell frequently. He had difficulty rising from a sitting position, climbing stairs, and running. His mental development was normal. The older brother walked alone at 14 months of age, but his gait was always described as awkward, especially in running, and he had difficulty climbing stairs. His mentation was normal. Neurologic examination of the patients showed moderate symmetric weakness of the proximal muscles of the extremities and neck flexor muscles. The younger child had mild facial muscle weakness. Chest excursions were reduced and the cough was weak. All the affected muscles were reduced in size. The older sibling did not have facial or respiratory muscle weakness but had weakness of the anterior tibialis muscles. Electromyographic examination showed normal motor and sensory nerve conduction velocities. Myopathic motor unit potentials were noted in the older sibling. There was no spontaneous electrical activity. Serum GOT and LDH levels were normal in both boys. The CPK level was elevated in the older child.

**PATHOLOGY.** Segmental vacuolation of type II fibers, resulting from pathologic change in the sarcotubular system, is the distinguishing feature of sarcotubular myopathy. In the two brothers, the myofibrillar markings were separated by multiple small, irregular or polygonal abnormal spaces randomly dispersed throughout the muscle fiber. In longitudinal sections, the abnormal spaces were segmentally distributed. There was a slight to moderate increase in perimysial fibers and fatty connective tissue. Type II fibers were affected more often than type I fibers. Fiber diameter studies revealed moderate hypertrophy of type I fibers and slight hypertrophy of type II fibers. Electron microscopy demonstrated that the small spaces were membrane bound. Ultrastructural and cytochemical studies suggested that the limiting membranes were from the sarcoplasmic reticulum.

### Reducing-body myopathy

Progressive myopathies leading to death in infancy are unusual. Reducing-body myopathy is a severe, progressive myopathy (Brooke and Neville, 1972).

**CLINICAL FEATURES.** Two girls have been described with a severe progressive myopathy. Hypotonia was the major neonatal symptom. There were no feeding problems and the infants appeared to be mentally normal. Motor development was delayed. Neither child could pull to a standing position or support her own weight when standing. One child had mild bilateral ptosis and facial weakness. Both patients had depressed tendon reflexes and weakness that initially was proximal and then became generalized and was accompanied by wasting and atrophy. In one child, bilateral contractures developed in the gastrocnemii and muscles of the forearm and upper arm. Electromyography revealed short-duration polyphasic po-

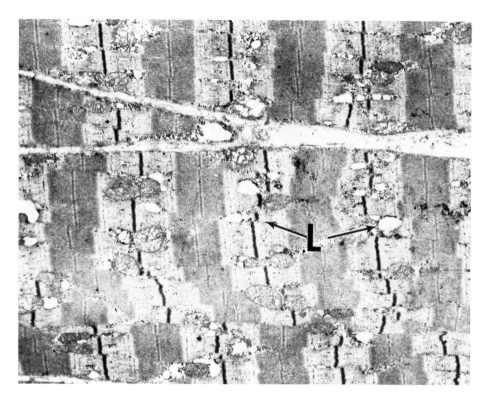

**Fig. 7-6.** Ultrastructural appearance of a muscle biopsy from an infant with excessive lipid storage. Numerous lipid *(L)* droplets can be seen. (Courtesy Dr. Stephen A. Smith.)

tentials. Nerve conduction velocities were normal. Serum CPK activity was elevated in one child. The family history revealed no muscle disease.

Both children had repeated bouts of pneumonia and died from respiratory failure, one at 9 months of age and the other at 30 months.

**PATHOLOGY.** Muscle biopsy specimens showed variability in fiber size, with some mild fibrosis. The most unusual feature was the presence of single round or oval bodies at the periphery of the muscle fiber, termed "reducing bodies." These bodies stained intensely for glycogen, RNA, and sulfhydryl groups. Electron microscopy revealed that the majority of these peripheral bodies occurred near normal nuclei. Some portions of the bodies contained normal mitochondria, triads of transverse tubules, and sarcoplasmic reticulum. The presence of the sulfhydryl

groups in muscles is unusual and remains unexplained, but it was postulated that an abnormality in creatine metabolism may be responsible for their accumulation.

## Lipid myopathy

Lipid myopathy results from a biochemical abnormality in lipid metabolism and may be characterized by excessive storage of lipid material in skeletal muscle (Fig. 7-6). Several lipid abnormalities have been described, including carnitine deficiency (type I lipid storage myopathy), carnitine palmityl transferase deficiency, and pyruvate decarboxylase deficiency (Angelini, 1976).

### Carnitine deficiency

Carnitine is an essential cofactor in the transport of long-chain fatty acids into mitochondria for beta oxidation. Carnitine deficiency results in decreased oxidation of long-chain fatty acids and excessive formation of triglycerides (Engel and Angelini, 1973; Mitchell, 1978). Muscle carnitine concentration is decreased or absent.

**CLINICAL FEATURES.** Carnitine deficiency results in progressive muscular weakness. Onset of symptoms may vary, with mild weakness and clumsiness in early infancy, gait disturbance by 2 years of age (Vandyke et al., 1975), or weakness beginning in the second decade (Isaacs et al., 1976). Achievement of motor milestones is generally not delayed. Mentation is usually normal. Family history usually does not disclose similar disease. However, decreased muscle carnitine levels have been described in the parents of one child (Vandyke et al., 1975).

Examination reveals marked proximal weakness, at times affecting the muscles of respiration. The muscles of the jaw, face, palate, and tongue may be weak. The neck muscles may be severely involved, causing loss of head control. Muscle pain is unusual. Generalized atrophy of the extremities is common. Tendon reflexes are reduced or absent. Sensation is normal.

The serum enzyme activities are usually increased. Serum carnitine concentration is usually normal. Electromyography reveals an increased number of polyphasic potentials and abundant motor unit potentials of decreased duration. In one patient, occasional fibrillation potentials and a decreased interference pattern were noted. Motor and sensory nerve velocities are normal. In general, the electromyographic findings are those of a myopathic process.

A systemic form of carnitine deficiency (Karpati et al., 1975), characterized by acute episodes of cerebral and hepatic dysfunction with hepatomegaly and acidosis, has been described. This condition may be fatal (Engel, Banker, and Eiben, 1977).

Cardiac involvement and fatal cardiomyopathy have also occurred in several patients (Vandyke et al., 1975; Hart et al., 1978).

**PATHOLOGY.** Muscle biopsy reveals many spaces within the muscle fibers adjacent to myofibrils, and some coalesce into irregular globules. Histochemically, type I fibers are most severely affected. The abnormal spaces stain positively with oil red O and Sudan black O, indicating neutral fat and acidic lipids which are presumably fatty acids (Engel and Siekert, 1972). Electron microscopic studies reveal a lack of limiting membrane of the abnormal space. The transverse tubular system and sarcoplasmic reticulum appear normal.

**TREATMENT.** Patients have responded favorably to treatment with prednisone and oral administration of carnitine (Engel and Siekert, 1972; Angelini, 1976).

### Carnitine palmityl transferase deficiency

A familial syndrome of episodic muscle cramps and myoglobinuria without persistent weakness (Bank et al., 1975; Di Mauro and Di Mauro, 1973) occurred in two brothers, with onset at ages 13 and 20 years. They developed normally and could sustain normal physical activity, but muscle cramps occasionally limited strenuous activity. The episodes of myoglobinuria occurred after prolonged exercise associated with fasting. Family history was normal. Neurologic findings were normal.

Laboratory examination revealed persistent elevation of cholesterol, plasma triglycerides, and free fatty acids, with increased beta and prebeta plasma lipoproteins. During fasting, plasma triglyceride and CPK levels increased, and myoglobin was detected in the urine.

Muscle biopsy showed no structural abnormalities or increase in lipids in the muscle fibers. Electron microscopic study of type I fibers revealed some nonmembranous material with low electron density.

Biochemical study of crude muscle extract and mitochondrial fraction revealed absence of carnitine palmityl transferase. Partial deficiency of carnitine palmityl transferase has been associated with recurrent myoglobinuria (Hostetler et al., 1978). Glycogen content and phosphorylase and phosphofructokinase activity were normal. Carnitine content was slightly elevated. The activity of palmityl-coenzyme-A synthetase was normal.

Treatment necessitates adherence to a low-fat diet and avoidance of strenuous exercise.

### Pyruvate decarboxylase deficiency

In the syndrome of intermittent ataxia often associated with choreoathetosis (Blass, Kark, and Engel, 1971), the biochemical abnormality is a defect in synthesis of thiamine-dependent pyruvate decarboxylase. The patient, a 9-year-old boy, developed normally but had episodes of ataxia following febrile illness or nonspecific stress. The patient's father and a paternal uncle had dyspnea and muscle cramps during forced exercise, followed by collapse.

Neurologic examination of the boy during an attack revealed cerebellar ataxia and choreiform movements. Findings related to the cranial nerves were normal, except for slow reaction of the pupils. Tendon reflexes were normal. Sensation was normal, except for decreased sense of vibration. The report did not specifically mention weakness.

Findings at laboratory examination included an elevated venous pyruvate level, a flat glucose tolerance test, normal serum enzyme activity, and retarded bone age. An electromyogram showed conduction velocities and motor unit potentials to be normal. A muscle biopsy specimen prepared with an oxidative enzyme stain showed increased granularity of the muscle fibers; an oil red O stain showed a diffuse, increased amount of droplets in type I fibers. Similar, but less marked, changes were noted in a biopsy specimen from the father.

Treatment with dexamethasone decreased the frequency of attacks, and treatment with thiamine, 600 mg per day orally, reduced the frequency to zero over a 22-month period.

### Other lipid storage myopathies

Another syndrome somewhat similar to carnitine palmityl transferase deficiency was described in identical twin girls (Engel et al., 1970). These children had intermittent muscle cramps following exercise or prolonged immobility. In several severe attacks, myoglobinuria was an associated finding. The symptoms began when the girls were 4 to 5 years old, and each episode lasted from hours to days. Neurologic examination did not disclose any definite weakness. The cranial nerves and respiratory muscles were never involved. No other members of the family were similarly affected.

At laboratory study, serum cholesterol and triglyceride levels were normal. Electromyograms were normal. Muscle biopsy revealed excess lipid droplets in type I fibers. Fasting for 24 to 60 hours induced typical symptoms accompanied by a marked increase in CPK and aldolase levels. Fasting did not produce normal ketosis. A selective defect in the metabolism of long-chain fatty acids was postulated, but the specific enzyme defect was not identified.

Lipid storage myopathy has occurred in the presence of normal carnitine concentration in the muscles (Jerusalem, Spiess, and Baumgartner, 1975); this myopathy is characterized by hypotonia, weakness, and delayed motor development. The nonprogressive, mild weakness did not prevent the child from taking part in normal activity but did limit strenuous exercise and competition in sports. Weakness and easy fatigue continued to occur intermittently. The patient complained of weakness while climbing stairs, rising from a sitting position, and lifting weights over her head. Examination showed mild weakness of the neck and limb and girdle musculature, more evident proximally than distally. Tendon reflexes were decreased and she had valgus deformity of the feet. Electromyography revealed an interference pattern containing an excess of high-frequency potentials and of low-voltage potentials of brief duration. Muscle biopsy showed an excess of lipid droplets in both type I and type II muscle fibers.

## Mitochondrial myopathies

Myopathies have been defined in patients with altered mitochondrial function and structure. Luft and co-workers (1962) gave impetus to the study of the muscle mitochondria and their relation to disease by describing a patient with both structurally and biochemically abnormal mitochondria. Following Luft's description, many isolated case reports have documented structural abnormalities of mitochondria, but there have been relatively few studies of patients with both structural and biochemical abnormalities in relation to the clinical manifestations. In a recent study of consecutive patients with myopathy, about 12% had structurally abnormal mitochondria (Kamieniecka, 1977). The patients were divided into three groups on the basis of symptoms: (1) those with weakness of extraocular muscles, with or without skeletal muscle weakness, (2) those with weakness in the facioscapulohumeral distribution, and (3) a heterogeneous group with central nervous system symptoms, distal myopathy, weakness in a limb-girdle distribution, or polymyositis.

Mitochondria produce energy through activities involving tricarboxylic acid cycle metabolism, fatty acid oxidation, electron transport, and oxidative phosphorylation. Further investigations into the biochemical abnormalities of isolated mitochondria are needed to define and clarify the significance of altered mitochondrial structure. Morphologic changes in mitochondria are not clearly specific for a given disease, for mitochondrial abnormalities have been described in various diseases, including hypothyroid myopathy (Norris and Panner, 1966) and polymyositis (Chou, 1967). Among these morphologic alterations of the mitochondria are variation in number and size, abnormal orientation of cristae, and various inclusions.

## Luft's disease

Two cases of Luft's disease have been described (Luft et al., 1962; Haydar et al., 1971). In Luft's prototype case, the patient had both structural and biochemical abnormalities of mitochondria of unknown etiology.

**CLINICAL FEATURES.** Luft's original patient had symptoms before 7 years of age, while Haydar's patient had onset of symptoms at 14 years of age. The dominant symptomatology indicated a hypermetabolic state and was characterized by profuse perspiration, polydipsia, polyphagia, and extreme heat intolerance. The disease was not progressive, but both patients continued to have symptoms and were capable of only light exercise. Examination revealed tachycardia but no clinical evidence for thyroid disease. Luft's patient had mild to moderate diffuse weakness and absent knee reflexes, while Haydar's patient had normal reflexes. Other neurologic findings were normal. Luft's patient was thin, with atrophy of the subcutaneous tissue. Haydar's patient had unusual discoid erythematous areas, especially over the lower extremities; this finding was thought to reflect an adaptation for heat loss. Electromyography revealed low-amplitude, decreased duration action potentials, increased polyphasic potentials, and a decrease in mean motor unit territory (DeJesus, 1974). Serum enzyme activity was normal.

**PATHOPHYSIOLOGY.** Light microscopic study of muscle from the original patient showed variation in individual fiber diameter and rounded muscle fiber configuration, instead of the normal polygonal configuration. Ultrastructural studies revealed an increase in the number of mitochondria, which collected in zones, varied in size, and contained an increased amount of densely packed cristae in zigzag formation. Some of the mitochondria were altered, with a tubular inner structure and an electron-dense core; small granules surrounded the cylindric mitochondria. Histochemical studies showed subsarcolemmal accumulations of red-blue material (modified trichome stain) and a prominent red intermyofibrillar network. These fibers contained increased oxidative enzyme activity (DiMauro et al., 1976). Both type I and type II fibers appeared to be involved.

Studies with isolated mitochondria revealed an excessive rate of respiration and loosely coupled oxidative phosphorylation. Skeletal muscle mitochondria were characterized by a deficient capability to adjust the cellular respiration to the availability of phosphate or phosphate acceptor, in contrast to an almost normal capacity for coupled oxidative phosphorylation.

An abnormality in divalent calcium ion metabolism has been described (DiMauro et al., 1976). The rate of calcium uptake was normal, but the total amount taken up was reduced and the mitochondria, unable to retain accumulated calcium in normal fashion, spontaneously released it. Divalent calcium ion accumulation requires energy for ion transport. It has been postulated that this alteration in ion transport across the mitochondrial membrane acts as a physiologic uncoupler and continues to stimulate metabolism. The cycling of divalent calcium ions by the skeletal muscle mitochondria may explain the high resting rate of cellular respiration.

Cytochrome content was normal. Glycogen concentration and glycolysis were normal.

**TREATMENT.** Chloramphenicol therapy produces clinical improvement (Haydar et al., 1971), presumably by depressing the synthesis of abnormal mitochondria.

### Oculocraniosomatic neuromuscular disease

A clinical syndrome of progressive external ophthalmoplegia and mitochondrial abnormalities has been described as oculocraniosomatic disease with ragged red fibers (Olson et al., 1972), Kearns-Shy syndrome (Karpati et al., 1973), and ophthalmoplegia plus syndrome (Schneck et al., 1973).

**CLINICAL FEATURES.** Ptosis and external ophthalmoplegia, beginning in childhood or adolescence, are characteristic. Ptosis, initially unilateral, soon becomes bilateral. Some patients have mild proximal weakness in the extremities and muscle fatigue.

Tendon reflexes vary from normal to decreased. Serum CPK activity is often elevated. The electromyogram is generally consistent with that of a myopathy. The basic syndrome involves a variety of nonmyo-

pathic findings, including elevated cerebrospinal fluid protein concentration, sensorineural hearing impairment, ataxia, retinal pigmentary change, small stature, cardiomyopathy, and electrocardiographic conduction defects. Most cases are sporadic; however, two familial cases have been described (Tamura, Santa, and Kuriowa, 1974; Kamieniecka, 1977).

The differential diagnosis includes myasthenia gravis, myotonic dystrophy, myotubular myopathy, type I fiber hypotrophy with central nuclei, and Möbius' syndrome.

**PATHOPHYSIOLOGY.** The muscle biopsy specimen contains abnormally small muscle fibers that have excessive amounts of red-staining subsarcolemmal and intermyofibrillar material. These muscle fibers have been termed "ragged red" fibers. There is an excessive number of cytoplasmic lipid droplets on the oil red O stain. Oxidative enzyme activity is increased in the abnormal fibers, which are generally type I fibers. Ultrastructural studies reveal large mitochondrial clusters with abnormal granular material and paracrystalline structures.

Studies of isolated mitochondria reveal a lack of cellular respiratory control with the presence of alpha-glycerophosphate (DiMauro et al., 1973). Serum lactic acid concentration may be markedly elevated following mild exercise (Scarlato, Pellegrini, and Veicsteinas, 1978).

### Other biochemical defects of mitochondrial function

As biochemical studies of mitochondrial function have become more sophisticated, other defects in mitochondrial energy function have been described.

Schotland and co-workers (1976) described a slowly progressive, congenital mitochondrial myopathy. The patient was weak from early childhood. She walked at a normal age but had difficulty sitting up from a supine position, standing from a squat position, and participating in physical education classes. Family history was normal. Physical examination revealed moderate pes cavus and thoracic scoliosis. Neurologic examination showed moderate proximal weakness in the arms and legs. Remaining neurologic findings, including cranial nerve function, sensation, and gait, were normal. Serum muscle enzyme activity was normal. Electromyography showed an increase in the number of polyphasic potentials and a decrease in the mean duration of action potentials. An electrocardiogram revealed biventricular hypertrophy with strain. A muscle biopsy specimen prepared with modified Gomori's trichrome stain showed increased subsarcolemmal red staining and prominent intermyofibrillar granules. Oxidative enzyme activity in type I fibers was increased. Ultrastructural studies disclosed subsarcolemmal and intermyofibrillar aggregation of mitochondria containing multiple paracrystalline inclusions. The numerous inclusions often completely replaced the inner compartment of the mitochondria. Some mitochondria contained round osmiophilic inclusions and small electron-dense granules.

Biochemical study revealed decreased respiratory rate and respiratory control. However, phosphorylation efficiency was normal. The adenosine triphosphatase (ATPase) activity in the intact mitochondria was decreased. Calcium accumulation by the mitochondria was normal in both rate and extent. The authors postulated that the decrease in respiratory rate resulted from either a defect in the terminal portion of the oxidative chain or reduced phosphorylation at a level common to the three phosphorylative sites. They considered that a defect in ATPase would explain the biochemical alterations. Whether this is a primary or specific defect is not certain. Probably the paracrystalline inclusions replace the functional mitochondrial inner membrane and interfere with mitochondrial metabolism.

An unusual mitochondrial myopathy was described in a patient with excessive desire for salt (Spiro et al., 1970a). The patient was weak from birth and appearance of motor milestones was delayed; he sat at 1 year and walked by 2 years. Intelligence was normal.

Intermittent diarrhea and a gastric ulcer characterized the clinical course. The weakness was nonprogressive. Examination revealed some mild atrophy of the deltoid muscles, slight weakness of the facial and sternocleidomastoid muscles, and proximal weakness in all extremities. Tendon reflexes were absent in the upper extremities and hypoactive in the lower extremities. Sensation was normal. Serum enzyme activities were normal.

Electromyography revealed normal motor nerve conduction velocity and decreased duration of the motor unit potentials consistent with myopathy. The patient had a marked craving for salt, but strength did not appear to be altered during times of salt restriction. Muscle biopsy specimen revealed an increase in red-staining intermyofibrillary network throughout the fiber, especially in the periphery. All fiber types were involved. In addition there was increased staining for lipid material with the Sudan black B stain. Routine histologic studies demonstrated no morphologic abnormalities. Ultrastructural studies showed an overall increase in the number of mitochondria, which were arranged in columns between the myofibrils and beneath the sarcolemma. Lipid droplets were visible in the abnormal accumulations of mitochondria. Mitochondria were larger and more irregular in shape than normal, and many contained an excessive number of cristae. Biochemical study of mitochondrial oxidative phosphorylation indicated a state of loose coupling. Spectrophotometric analysis of the cytochromes was normal.

A dominantly inherited disorder of the central nervous system and muscle was reported by Spiro and colleagues (1970b). This disorder, reported in a man and his 16-year-old son, closely resembled spinocerebellar degenerative disease. The clinical findings consisted of progressive ataxia, proximal muscle weakness, areflexia, bilateral Babinski's signs, and insidious dementia. The son was mentally retarded and had chorioretinitis, intracranial calcification, and bilateral partial external ophthalmoplegia with ptosis and limitation of ocular conversion. A muscle biopsy revealed nonspecific evidence of myopathic and neuropathic processes. There were groups of small fibers, centrally placed nuclei, and increased endomysial connective tissue. An electron microscopic study revealed abnormalities in muscle mitochondria, with increased number and size but normal structure. Biochemical studies indicated loosely coupled oxidative phosphorylation and a marked reduction in cytochrome b.

Morgan-Hughes and colleagues (1977) studied a patient who, at 7 years of age, had progressive symptoms of weakness, excessive fatigability, and leg pain. Examination revealed mild weakness of the facial and neck flexor muscles and muscles of the proximal extremities. Ultrastructural studies showed abnormal mitochondria with extensive branching of cristae, amorphous matrix, and crystalline inclusions. In vitro mitochondrial studies disclosed impaired respiratory rate and control and deficiency of cytochrome b. It was concluded that the patient's excessive fatigability resulted from limitation of adenosine triphosphate synthesis by the oxidative phosphorylation pathway.

### Other structural defects of mitochondria

In other diseases characterized by ultrastructural abnormalities of mitochondria, the biochemical defect remains unknown and further studies are needed.

### Pleoconial myopathy

Pleoconial myopathy is characterized by the presence of many moderately enlarged mitochondria (Shy, Gonatas, and Perez, 1966). Clinically the infant is "floppy" at birth, with pronounced weakness and hypotonia. Motor development is slow. The striking clinical feature is episodic weakness that begins toward evening or in the morning when the patient awakens and develops rapidly, producing severe quadriparesis that lasts from 10 days to 2 weeks. The weakness is more severe proximally, although distal muscle weakness is also noted. Between the episodes of weakness there does not appear

to be any progression. Tendon reflexes are decreased, and sensation is normal. The cranial nerves are normal, and myotonia is absent.

Serum enzyme activity is normal. Electromyography shows the features characteristic of a myopathic process. There is no alteration in gamma globulin concentration, serum electrolyte levels, or basal metabolism rate.

Several attempts to precipitate an attack of weakness have failed. Neither sodium nor potassium administration produces weakness, although these agents do have such an effect on other periodic paralyses. Exercise produces a normal increase in serum lactic acid.

Muscle biopsy tissue, prepared with the routine hematoxylin and eosin and trichrome stains, shows two fiber groups; the first is normal, and the second is characterized by a prominent, purple, intermyofibrillar network. Stains for tricarboxylic acid cycle enzymes (oxidative enzymes) show this purple material to be of mitochondrial origin. Electron microscopic studies confirm the presence of increased numbers of mitochondria of moderately increased size and containing some inclusions (Fig. 7-7).

Pleoconial myopathy is one of several diseases characterized by episodic weakness. Shy (1966) has postulated that pleoconial myopathy and the "normokalemic form of periodic paralysis" (Poskanzer and Kerr, 1961) are both disorders of mitochondria. If further study confirms the mitochondrial abnormality in these disorders, then the situation is analagous to myotubular myopathy, in which there is an early and a late form of the disease with different clinical manifestations.

D'Agostino and associates (1968) have suggested that the alterations seen in pleoconial and megaconial myopathy represent nonspecific biochemical defects found in the mitochondrial myopathies. The patient described in the original report of pleoconial myopathy lacked respiratory control with alpha-glycerophosphate (DiMauro et al., 1973).

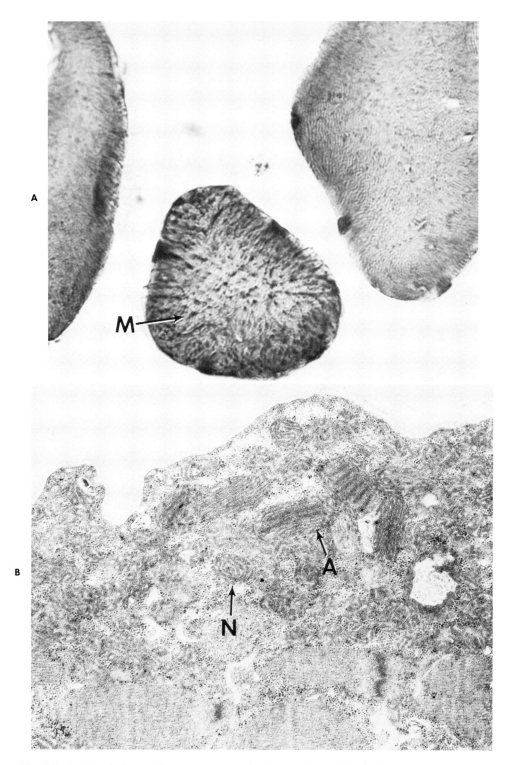

**Fig. 7-7. A,** Muscle biopsy from a patient with pleoconial mitochondrial myopathy. **A** shows prominent mitochondria *(M)* in a type I fiber with a trichrome stain, while **B** shows both normal *(N)* and abnormal *(A)* mitochondria by ultrastructural examination. Paracrystalline inclusions are seen in abnormal mitochondria as compared with normal intercristal pattern. (Courtesy Dr. Stephen A. Smith.)

### Megaconial myopathy

Megaconial myopathy may become manifest in either late infancy (Shy, Gonatas, and Perez, 1966; Hulsmann et al., 1967) or childhood (Coleman et al., 1967). Onset in late infancy is characterized by proximal weakness. Difficulty with physical activities and fatigue are common complaints. The patient has a lordotic posture and a waddling gait and often has difficulty climbing stairs and rising from a supine position. The clinical course is characterized by slow, progressive weakness with loss of motor abilities.

Examination reveals prominent weakness in the muscles of the shoulder and hip girdle, resulting in moderate lordosis and Gowers' sign. Affected muscles may be wasted. The muscles innervated by cranial nerves are unaffected, except for some weakness of the sternocleidomastoid muscles. Tendon reflexes are diminished or absent. Myotonia is not present; sensation is normal.

The serum enzyme activities are normal. The basal metabolism rate and protein-bound iodine (PBI) level are normal. Serum electrophoresis may show hypogammaglobulinemia. In one patient, the electrocardiogram contained depressed ST and T wave segments. Electromyography reveals findings typical of a myopathic process.

In the patient described by Shy and associates (1966), no abnormality was seen in muscle stained with hematoxylin and eosin, while Hulsmann and associates (1967) described abnormal muscle fibers of small diameter and polygonal shape. Numerous vesicular nuclei and granular material were also seen.

Cytochemical examination, using the modified Gomori's stain, reveals large aggregates of red-staining material distributed through the fiber but more prominent in type I muscle fibers than in type II fibers. The mitochondrial origin for these aggregates of red-staining material is indicated by the cytochemical demonstration of increased activity of oxidative enzymes. The lipid content of the cell is also increased. Electron microscopic studies reveal a characteristic cell structure, with giant mitochondria with several inclusions. These inclusions are of three types: round, of low contrast; rectangular; and round, of high contrast. The internal structure of the mitochondria is abnormal because of the lack of cristae (Fig. 7-8).

A second type of megaconial myopathy (Coleman et al., 1967), with different clinical manifestations, has been described. The major clinical difference is the onset at age 7 to 8 years rather than in late infancy. This myopathy is characterized by progressive fatigability and weakness. The patient may occasionally have dysphagia, but otherwise there is no cranial nerve involvement.

### Mitochondrial encephalomyopathy

Several syndromes have been grouped under the term "mitochondrial encephalomyopathies" (Shapira, Harel, and Russell, 1977). These diseases are predominantly degenerative diseases of the central nervous system, but muscle involvement including structural mitochondrial changes have been noted. Several of these syndromes have associated lactic acidemia (Shapira et al., 1975; Hart et al., 1977). Patients have progressive neurologic degeneration, dementia, and seizures, and they may have limitation of extraocular muscle function. In one patient, the muscular weakness and atrophy preceded central nervous system degeneration. No biochemical abnormality has been delineated. Defective oxidation in the cytochrome structure or one of the enzymes in the respiratory chain has been suggested. Definitive biochemical studies are needed to delineate the metabolic disorder.

### Myoadenylate deaminase deficiency

A new muscle disease has been described from the application of a histoenzymatic stain on frozen muscle biopsy specimen. Myoadenylate deaminase deficiency occurred in five male patients representing 1% of a series of muscle biopsies (Fishbein, Armbrustmacher, and Griffin, 1978). Clinically, the patients had symptoms of weakness and muscle cramps following exercise, with

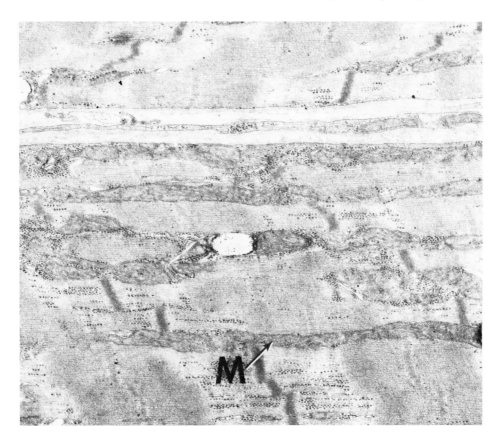

**Fig. 7-8.** Muscle biopsy electron microscopy photograph from a patient with megaconial mitochondrial myopathy showing elongated and numerous mitochondria. One mitochondrion *(M)* extends beyond one sarcomere unit in length. (Courtesy Dr. Stephen A. Smith.)

onset of symptoms in early childhood. Neurologic examination revealed delayed motor development, decreased muscle mass, and weakness in some cases. A few of the patients had frequent childhood infections and allergies.

Serum CPK activity was normal or mildly elevated. Electromyography was normal or showed some polyphasic units and positive waves.

Muscle biopsy specimens were normal in four patients and showed type I muscle fiber atrophy in one patient. All five patients showed no reaction to the adenylate deaminase stain. Adenylate deaminase appears to maintain a high ratio of ATP to ADP during strenuous muscle activity.

Definitive diagnosis requires enzymatic assay on fresh or frozen muscle tissue. A clinical screening test is performed by the simultaneous determination of plasma ammonia and lactate concentration during an ischemic exercise test. Normal controls show a linear response of ammonia to lactate increase during exercise. In the patients, the ratio fell below the normal range. Failure of plasma ammonia concentration to rise can also be used as a screening test.

### Congenital muscular dystrophy

Congenital muscular dystrophy should be considered in the differential diagnosis of the "floppy infant." The majority of patients with this disease have severe hypotonia at birth

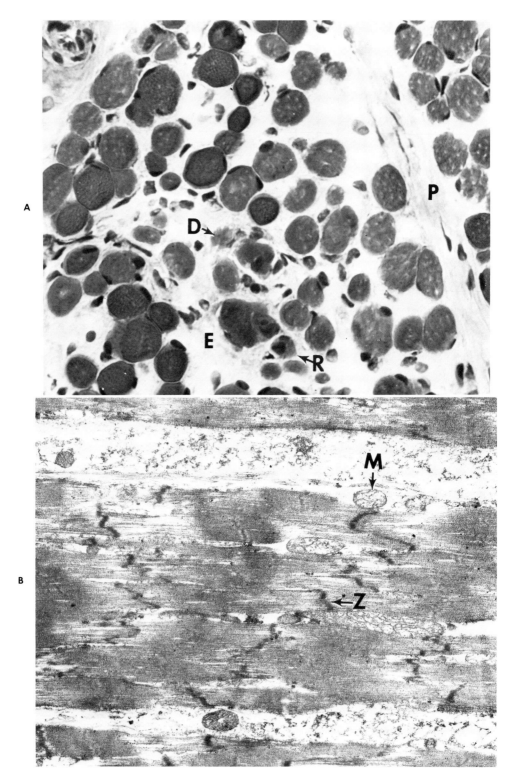

**Fig. 7-9. A,** Muscle biopsy from an infant with congenital muscular dystrophy. Variation in muscle cell size, degenerating *(D),* and regenerating *(R)* muscle fibers are present. An increased amount of endomysial *(E)* and perimysial *(P)* connective tissue is noted. **B,** Ultrastructural appearance of muscle biopsy. Note disruption of sarcomere patterns, myofibrils, and organelles, Mitochondria *(M)* and Z bands *(Z)* can still be recognized. (Courtesy Dr. Stephen A. Smith.)

(Donner, Rapola, and Somer, 1975). However, congenital arthrogryposis with multiple contractures and limitation of joint movement constitutes a separate type of congenital muscular dystrophy (see Chapter 3).

CLINICAL FEATURES. Two forms of congenital muscular dystrophy are seen with hypotonia. A benign form exists with no progression of weakness and gradual improvement in muscular strength (Wharton, 1965). There is also a severe form (Zellweger et al., 1967) characterized either by rapid progression of weakness with death ensuing before the second year of life, or by severe disability with no progression but with marked limitation in activity. Decreased fetal movements have been commonly described.

Examination of the infant at the time of birth reveals marked hypotonia. Sucking and swallowing difficulties are commonly present. The infant may require gavage feeding. The extremities are often thin because of muscular wasting. Contractures are often present at birth. Cranial nerve examination reveals ptosis of the eyelids and absent gag reflex. The diaphragm may be paralyzed, producing intercostal breathing with rapid, labored respirations. The tendon reflexes are diminished or absent. Sensation is normal.

The clinical course in patients with severe muscular dystrophy is characterized by persistent weakness, which is most marked in the extremities and neck flexor muscles. The facial and extraocular muscles may be involved. With time, some of the patients develop contractures about the hips and in the hamstring muscles. Pneumonia is a complication in early infancy because of weak respiratory muscles. The motor milestones are reached very slowly. Sitting is often delayed past the second year, and 40% of the patients are unable to walk without support. In spite of retarded motor development, intelligence is normal. The disease appears to be most active in the first 2 years of life. Congenital muscular dystrophy described in the Japanese literature is characterized by severe mental retardation, seizures, and severe abnormality of the central nervous system (Kamoshita et al., 1976).

LABORATORY FINDINGS. The serum enzyme activity levels are either normal or elevated. The electrocardiogram is generally normal. An electromyographic examination shows low-amplitude, short-duration, polyphasic potentials characteristic of a myopathic process. The motor nerve conduction velocity is normal.

PATHOPHYSIOLOGY. The diagnosis is made by muscle biopsy. Pathologic changes on light microscopy (Greenfield, Corman, and Shy, 1958) show marked variation in fiber size, degeneration of muscle fibers, and increase in connective tissue and fat content. Some of these small muscle fibers have centrally placed nuclei that resemble fetal muscle. Phagocytosis is unusual, and inflammatory cells are uncommon (Fig. 7-9).

GENETICS. Congenital muscular dystrophy appears to be inherited as an autosomal recessive disease.

TREATMENT. Prevention and correction of contractures are major goals of treatment. Muscle-strengthening exercises may benefit those patients in whom the disease process does not progress, but who have residual weakness.

### Myotonia congenita (Thomsen's disease)

Myotonia congenita (Thomsen, 1916) is characterized by delayed relaxation of voluntary muscle contraction (myotonia). Sucking and feeding difficulties are commonly encountered. The infant may show slow motor development, but generally symptoms are not apparent until childhood or adolescence.

Patients with myotonia congenita have difficulty releasing a grasped object quickly or initiating movements such as rising from a chair or climbing stairs. If the movement is performed repeatedly, the abnormal difficulty with relaxation lessens and the patient is able to perform it more rapidly. The myotonia, though often more pronounced in the lower extremities, may be generalized, affecting the muscles innervated by the cranial nerves as well as the extremities. Children often appear awkward and clumsy and may have difficulty in performing physical activities as well as their peers. The myotonia is aggravated by emotional stress and by cold, damp weather. The patient's mentation is normal. The disease is not progressive and tends to lessen in severity as the patient passes through puberty.

These children appear to have generally hypertrophied muscles. This has been referred to as the "Herculean appearance" (Fig. 7-10). Despite the muscular appear-ance, the patient is mildly weak. Several means of detecting myotonia exist. The myotonia is best demonstrated by direct percussion of the thenar eminence, with subsequent prolonged contraction of the muscle, and adduction and opposition of the thumb. Percussion myotonia of the tongue may be demonstrated by placing a tongue blade beneath the patient's tongue and tapping the tongue with a reflex hammer. Contraction of the muscle fibers and a delay in relaxation are seen. The tendon reflexes are normal. Myotonia may also be demonstrated by having the patient grasp the examiner's finger

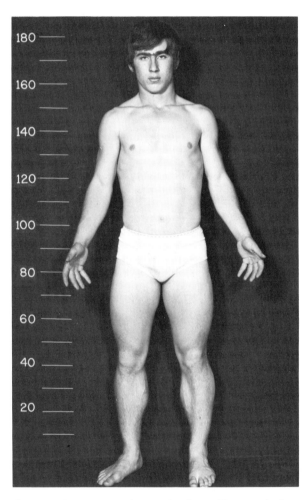

**Fig. 7-10.** Myotonia congenita: autosomal recessive form. Note marked muscle hypertrophy (Herculean appearance). Percussion myotonia could be elicited. Weakness was mild.

and attempt to release the grasp quickly. Myotonia of the eyelids is observed following a forceful voluntary closure of the eyes. The delay in eye opening is obvious.

Myotonia detected clinically and/or electromyographically is encountered in many diseases. These include myotonia congenita, myotonic dystrophy, myotubular myopathy, monomelic myopathy, hyperkalemic periodic paralysis, and glycogen storage disease (acid maltase deficiencies). A pseudomyotonia is observed in patients who have hypothyroidism with delayed muscular relaxation; however, myotonic potentials are absent on electromyography.

Myotonia congenita can be differentiated from myotonic dystrophy by the absence of cataracts, of testicular atrophy, and of evidence for a progressive disease. Myotonia congenita must also be differentiated from hypothyroidism, especially the familial form of cretinism, which is associated with muscular hypertrophy (Debré-Sémélaigne syndrome) and delayed relaxation of tendon reflexes. Hyperkalemic periodic paralysis, which is associated with myotonia, may be differentiated by elevated serum potassium levels during paralysis.

**LABORATORY FINDINGS.** The serum enzyme studies are normal. Electromyography shows myotonic potentials with the characteristic "dive-bomber" sound of myotonic potentials.

**PATHOPHYSIOLOGY.** Pathologic changes in muscle consist mainly of hypertrophied muscle fibers caused by an increased number of myofibrils. Rare, centrally placed nuclei are seen. In contrast to the pathology in myotonic dystrophy, long chains of central nuclei are not seen in myotonia congenita. Histochemical study demonstrates absence of type IIB fibers. The biopsy specimen from the more severely affected patients shows variability of fiber size, atrophic fibers, increased internal nuclei, and fiber hypertrophy (Crews, Kaiser, and Brooke, 1976).

The primary defect in myotonia congenita resides in the muscle cell membrane, which is characterized by a normal resting membrane potential, but with a markedly increased resting resistance related to a decrease in membrane chloride permeability (Lipicky, Bryant, and Salmon, 1971; Barchi, 1975).

**GENETICS.** Two genetic patterns have been identified, one with an autosomal dominant inheritance and the other with an autosomal recessive inheritance (Becker, 1973). The recessive form is more common, and symptoms appear later with more generalized, severe myotonia. Muscle hypertrophy and weakness are more pronounced.

**TREATMENT.** Phenytoin, procainamide, or quinine may be effective in reducing the myotonia (Munsat, 1967).

## Monomelic myopathy

Myopathies in general are characterized by proximal, symmetric muscle weakness, especially in the hip and shoulder girdles. One exception reported observed, however, was in a case of monomelic myopathy (Celesia et al., 1967).

The patient was normal at birth except for an enlarged right lower extremity. The right foot was deformed, with a posterior angulation of the tarsal-metatarsal joints and hallux varus. In early childhood, the condition was characterized by occasional cramps in the right leg, and in later childhood, the patient developed weakness and contractures of the dorsiflexor muscles of the right foot.

On examination, the patient was of normal intelligence. The only abnormality was the enlarged right lower extremity. Muscular hypertrophy was evident in the quadriceps femoris muscle. Palpation of the muscle was normal. A typical myotonic contraction was elicited on percussion of the muscle. In addition, there were spontaneous contractions of a slow, wavelike nature. There was moderate weakness of dorsiflexion of the right foot. The plantar response was normal. Sensation was normal. The tendon reflexes of the right knee and ankle were diminished.

Serum enzyme studies were normal. Electromyography showed characteristic myotonic potentials with bursts of high-frequency discharges. The myotonic discharges accompanied the spontaneous, slow, wavelike contractions of the muscle seen clinically. The motor nerve conduction velocity was normal. Muscle biopsy of the hypertrophic muscle revealed fibers with centrally located chains of nuclei, degeneration of fibers with cellular reaction, and increased fibrosis.

Several conditions must be differentiated from monomelic myopathy. Neurofibromatosis, which may be associated with hypertrophy of one extremity, may be recognized by the characteristic café-au-lait skin lesions and the absence of myotonia. Lymphedema and arteriovenous-shunt malformation are excluded by the clinical examination. Myotonia congenita is a generalized condition often associated with a positive family history. The possibility that monomelic myopathy is a limited form of myotonic dystrophy remains, although the case described has shown no progression or dystrophic features.

### Distal myopathy

An exception to the usual proximal distribution of weakness in myopathies is a form of distal myopathy occurring in early infancy (Magee and DeJong, 1965; van der Does de Willebois et al., 1968). Whether patients with this form of myopathy have symptoms at the time of birth is not conclusively known, but it has been presumed that they do. Distal myopathy, which is inherited as an autosomal dominant trait, has an onset characterized by bilateral footdrop at the time the child begins to walk and is clearly evident by 2 years of age. In the cases described, no obvious progression occurs beyond 18 years of age. Some of these patients have mild extension weakness in the fingers.

The general physical examination reveals no abnormalities. The cranial nerve functions are normal. Sensation and tendon reflexes are normal. No myotonia can be elicited on direct percussion of the muscles. The muscles of the calves are described as somewhat hypertrophic but with no evidence of weakness. The positive findings are most prominent in the anterior tibial and extensor hallucis longus muscles. These muscles show considerable weakness. Weakness in the peroneal muscles is variable (Fig. 7-11).

The serum enzyme activity is within normal limits during childhood. However, the serum aldolase activity may be mildly elevated in adult patients. Electromyography reveals large numbers of polyphasic potentials and short-duration action potentials. These findings are typical of a myopathic process. The conduction velocity is normal. There is no evidence of fibrillation, positive potentials, or myotonic potentials.

Muscle biopsy reveals a marked variation in the diameter size of the muscle fibers, with some increased endomysial connective tissue. The pathologic changes vary in intensity from one muscle bundle to another. The sarcolemmal nuclei show proliferation and

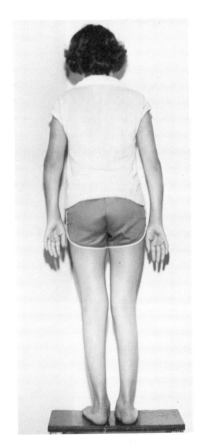

**Fig. 7-11.** Distal myopathy. Note atrophy of forearms and lower legs.

migration to the center of the fiber. The muscle spindles, intramuscular nerves, and blood vessels are normal. The majority of muscle fibers show normal cytochemical activity. The type I fibers have a large diameter compared to the other fibers. The LDH isoenzyme pattern discloses reduction in LDH 5 activity.

Distal myopathy of infancy is a unique disease, because the distribution of weakness differs from that found in the majority of other myopathies. Its inclusion as a congenital disease is somewhat presumptive, because conclusive data are not available to point to onset at the time of birth. Electromyographic findings of typical myopathic potentials and the muscle biopsy confirm this disease as a myopathic process. The normal motor nerve conduction velocity tends to rule out a polyneuropathy. The lack of myotonic potentials makes it unlikely that this is an atypical form of myotonic dystrophy. This form of distal myopathy differs from that seen in adults as described by Welander (1951), in that the adult cases have a mean onset after 40 years of age, and symptoms begin predominantly in the small muscles of the hand. Sporadic cases often manifest symptoms at an earlier age (Markesbery, Griggs, and Herr, 1977).

## GLYCOGEN STORAGE DISEASES

Study of the glycogen storage diseases results in an appreciation of the disparate effects of separate hereditary enzymatic deficiencies along a single metabolic pathway.

Glycogen storage diseases result in the abnormal accumulation in various tissues of glycogen of normal or abnormal configuration (Table 7-2). These diseases are caused by a deficiency or an absence of specific enzyme activity in the metabolic pathway of glycogen. There is general agreement on the numbering system of these conditions up to VI; thereafter viewpoints diverge.

Symptoms and signs of glycogen storage diseases frequently result from free glucose deficiency with ensuing hypoglycemia, occurring separately or in association with increased glycogen storage. Many of these conditions do not involve muscle. The location of the enzymatic block in the pathway determines whether the structure of the glycogen is normal. Both the location in the pathway and the enzyme involved determine whether or not glycogen is accumulated in muscle.

The prime building block in the synthesis of glycogen is the glucose molecule. A number of stepwise reactions are linked in the synthetic process (Fig. 7-12). Glycogen synthesis occurs in many tissues, predominantly in the liver, kidneys, and muscle. Glucose transported in the blood enters the tissue cell, is phosphorylated in a reaction facilitated by the enzyme hexokinase, and becomes glucose-6-phosphate. In the next step, the enzyme phosphoglucomutase mediates the transformation to glucose-1-phosphate. Glucose-1-phosphate, in association with uridine triphosphate (UTP), is transformed to uridine diphosphate (UDP) glucose with the participation of uridine diphosphate glucose pyrophosphorylase. The glucose portion of uridine diphosphate glucose is then affixed by a 1,4 linkage to a terminal glucosyl unit. This reaction is facilitated by the active form of the enzyme glycogen synthetase (UDP-glucose-glycogen glucosyl transferase). After the glucosyl chain reaches 6 to 12 units long, this section is transferred and attached to another glucosyl chain by a 1,6 linkage as a result of the action of the branching enzyme ($\alpha$-1,4-glucan: $\alpha$-1,4 glucan 6-glucosyl transferase). A 1,6 linkage serves as the branch point.

The phosphorylase enzymes split the 1,4 linkages during catabolism, which results in formation of free glucose-1-phosphate molecules from glycogen. There are muscle and hepatic phosphorylase isoenzymes. Activation of phosphorylase takes place through a cascade of reactions ultimately involving phosphorylase b kinase (Fig. 7-13).

As the cleavage of 1,4 bonds moves near the 1,6 branching point, "three-glucose" residues are removed in a block by oligo-1, 4 → 1,4-glucan transferase, and the 1,6 linkage is disrupted by the debranching enzyme (amylo-1,6-glucosidase) with the resultant re-

**Table 7-2.** Glycogen storage diseases

| Name | Clinical manifestations | Glycogen structure | Enzyme defect |
|---|---|---|---|
| Glucose-6-phosphatase deficiency (von Gierke's disease, Cori type I) | Enlarged liver and kidneys<br>Hyperlipidemia<br>Hypoglycemia<br>Ketoacidosis<br>Seizures | Normal | Glucose-6-phosphatase |
| Infantile acid maltase deficiency (Pompe's disease, Cori type II) | Cardiomegaly<br>Death in infancy<br>Progressive hypotonia and weakness<br>Swallowing and respiratory difficulty | Normal | Acid maltase |
| Late infantile acid maltase deficiency, adult acid maltase deficiency | Atonic anal sphincter<br>Calf muscle hypertrophy<br>Hip weakness (Gowers' sign)<br>Slow or regressing motor development, contractures of Achilles tendons | (?) Abnormal: short outer chains | Acid maltase |
| Debrancher deficiency (Forbes' limit dextrinosis, Cori type III) | Hepatomegaly<br>Hypoglycemia<br>Late onset of weakness<br>Mild growth failure<br>Early, severe weakness with myopathy rare | Abnormal: short outer chains, increased branch points | Amylo-1,6-glucosidase |
| Brancher deficiency (Andersen's disease, Cori type IV) | Cirrhosis<br>Growth failure<br>Hepatosplenomegaly<br>Hypotonia<br>Muscle wasting in the lower extremities<br>Slow motor development<br>Weakness | Abnormal: long inner and outer unbranched chains | Amylo-1,4 → 1,6 transglucosidase |
| Myophosphorylase deficiency (McArdle's disease, Cori type V) | Atrophy in older patients<br>Myoglobinuria<br>Poor stamina<br>Severe muscle cramps with exercise | Normal | Muscle phosphorylase |
| Hepatophosphorylase deficiency (Hers' disease, Cori type VI) | Growth retardation<br>Hepatomegaly<br>Hypoglycemia<br>Mild ketosis | Normal | Liver phosphorylase |
| Phosphorylase kinase deficiency (also deficiency of activation sequence including loss of activity of 3′, 5′,-AMP-dependent kinase in muscle and probably liver) | Marked hepatomegaly, with glycogen storage<br>No hypoglycemia<br>No skeletal muscle disease<br>Normal mental development | Normal | Phosphorylase kinase or 3′,5′,-AMP-dependent kinase |
| Phosphoglucomutase deficiency | Calf hypertrophy<br>Mild generalized weakness<br>Regression in motor development<br>Toe walking | Normal | Phosphoglucomutase |
| Phosphohexoisomerase deficiency | Late onset of myopathy<br>Muscle cramps<br>Poor stamina | Normal | Phosphohexoisomerase |

**Table 7-2.** Glycogen storage diseases—cont'd

| Name | Clinical manifestations | Glycogen structure | Enzyme defect |
|---|---|---|---|
| Phosphofructokinase deficiency | Similar to myophosphorylase deficiency | Normal | Phosphofructokinase |
| Glycogen synthetase deficiency | Hypoglycemia<br>Mental retardation<br>Seizures | Normal | Glycogen synthetase |

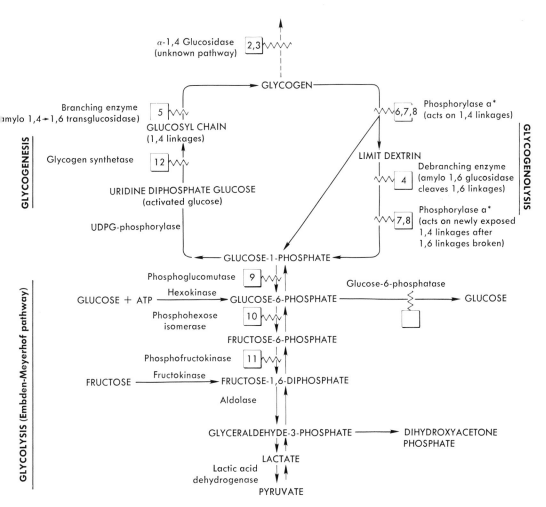

**Fig. 7-12.** Pathways of glycogen metabolism.* See Fig. 7-13 for phosphorylase activation sequence. See Table 7-2 for details of conditions accompanying the enzymatic deficiencies denoted by Arabic numerals. (Modified from Swaiman, K. F.: Glycogen storage diseases. In Swaiman, K. F., and Wright, F. S.: The practice of pediatric neurology, St. Louis, 1975, The C. V. Mosby Co., p. 441.)

lease of a free glucose molecule. Approximately 8% of glucose in glycogen is located at 1,6 branch points and may be released in this free form. This process continues along the branches of the glycogen molecule. Therefore both glucose-1-phosphate and free glucose molecules result from this series of degradation reactions.

The glucose-1-phosphate molecules are subsequently converted to glucose-6-phos-

phate by the action of the enzyme phosphoglucomutase. Subsequently glucose-6-phosphate in the liver and kidney is acted upon by glucose-6-phosphatase, and free glucose results. (Glucose-6-phosphatase activity is absent in skeletal muscle.) The free glucose is transported by the circulation to other organs and utilized. In other organs and in muscle, the glucose-6-phosphate formed upon entry is phosphorylated to fructose-1-6-diphos-

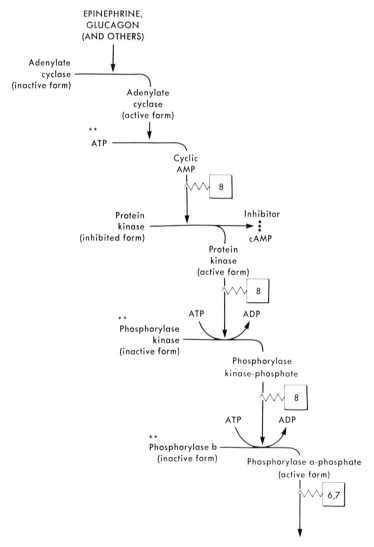

**Fig. 7-13.** Activation sequence of phosphorylase.** Amplification effect of this step. See Table 7-2 for description of the accompanying abnormalities of the enzymatic deficiencies denoted by Arabic numerals. (Modified from Goldberg, N. B.: Hosp. Pract. **9:**127, 1974.)

phate; this, in turn, is transformed by the metabolic steps in the Embden-Meyerhof pathway that lead eventually to the formation of pyruvic and lactic acids.

An increasing number of patients of different ages with glycogen storage disease have been reported to be deficient in the lysosomal enzyme acid maltase ($\alpha$-1,4-glucosidase). The action of this enzyme is unexplained in the "normal" sequence of glycogen degradation.

Among the glycogen storage diseases are a number of conditions that do not involve muscle significantly. Nevertheless, they may be associated with mild symptoms of weakness and hypotonia without explanation. The major glycogen storage diseases, for convenience, are summarized in Table 7-2 and Figs. 7-12 and 7-13. Only those glycogen storage diseases that affect muscle significantly are included in the following detailed discussion.

### Acid maltase deficiency, infantile type (Pompe's disease, idiopathic generalized glycogenosis, Cori type II disease)

**CLINICAL FEATURES.** The infant often develops normally for several weeks to several months, then obvious hypotonia and severe weakness become evident (Fig. 7-14). Little spontaneous movement occurs, and the cry is short-lived and weak. Swallowing is grossly impaired, and secretions accumulate in the posterior oropharynx. Respiratory difficulty caused by weakness is made worse, because the accessory muscles of respiration are compromised. Massive cardiomegaly attributable

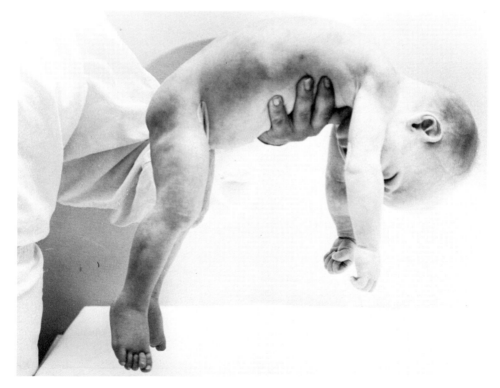

**Fig. 7-14.** Eight-month-old infant with infantile-type acid maltase deficiency (Pompe's disease) manifests marked weakness and hypotonia. Child is virtually motionless and allows himself to hang into space over examiner's hand.

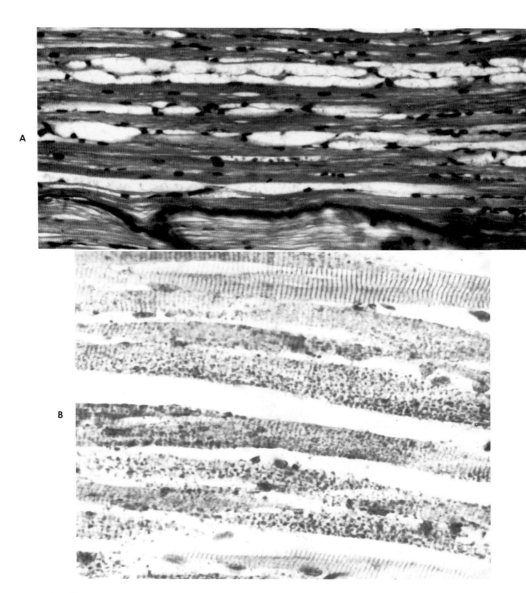

**Fig. 7-15. A,** Gastrocnemius muscle from a patient with infantile acid maltase disease stained with hematoxylin and eosin. Large amounts of stored glycogen are denoted by open spaces remaining after glycogen was dissolved in aqueous dye solution. Only fine connective tissue structure remains. **B,** Skeletal muscle from a patient with infantile acid maltase deficiency. Muscle, stained with Best's carmine stain, demonstrates increased glycogen within muscle fibers. **C,** Electron micrograph of a gastrocnemius muscle from a 20-month-old male with glycogen storage disease. There are an excessive number of dense glycogen granules interspersed throughout muscle fibers ($\times 15,000$). (Courtesy Dr. Stephen A. Smith.)

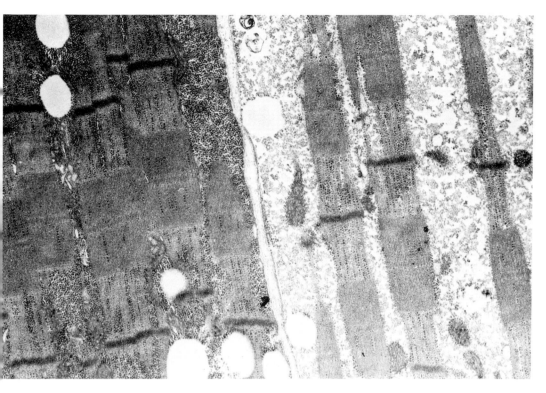

**Fig. 7-15, cont'd.** For legend see opposite page.

to glycogen storage develops, and a soft systolic murmur is usually heard along the left sternal border (Pompe, 1932). Hepatomegaly occurs almost uniformly. The liver has a sharp edge and a very firm consistency. Subcutaneous fat is virtually absent over all areas of the body. The muscles are small and very firm. The tongue is often enlarged and may protrude awkwardly. Intermittent cyanosis ensues because of respiratory and cardiac failure. Deep tendon reflexes are unelicitable by 6 months of age. Affected infants undergo progressive debilitation, and most die by the age of 1 year and almost all by age 2.

### LABORATORY FINDINGS

BIOCHEMISTRY. Hers (1963) first reported the deficiency of activity of the enzyme acid maltase ($\alpha$-1,4-glucosidase). Glycogen structure has usually been normal. Hypoglycemia does not occur.

Activity of the enzyme $\alpha$-1,4-glucosidase at various pH values in infantile, childhood, and adult patients with acid maltase deficiency has been studied. There are only traces of neutral maltase in the heart and significantly decreased neutral maltase activity in the skeletal muscle and liver of an infantile patient. In the late infantile form, neutral acid maltase activity is decreased only in the liver; in the adult form, neutral maltase is not deficient in any tissue. An absolute decrease of leukocyte acid maltase was found in four of five adults with acid maltase deficiency, and a relative decrease was found in one. Decrease in the pH 4:pH 6.5 ratio of leukocyte maltase activity may be of diagnostic importance in adult acid maltase deficiency (Angelini and Engel, 1972).

PATHOLOGY. Infantile and adult cases alike manifest a severe vacuolar myopathy, with accumulation of large amounts of PAS-positive material within muscle fibers (Fig. 7-15). Large amounts of metachromatic material are found within the muscle fibers in the infantile cases. Metachromasia is not seen as often in the adult cases. The metachromasia is probably caused by a glycolipid or glycoprotein and not by storage of mucopolysaccharide. Frequently, scattered, sparse, perivascular lymphocytic infiltrates are seen in the interstitial tissue (Hudgson and Fulthorpe, 1975). Normal amounts of lipids are also seen in the muscle fibers in the infantile cases.

Peripheral lymphocytes may contain morphologic changes consistent with glycogen storage (Coppola, Munoz, and Sher, 1978).

CLINICAL LABORATORY EXAMINATION. Quantity of glycogen and activity of the enzymes involved in glycogen metabolism can be assessed by utilizing skin removed by a vacuum skin blistering technique or by using skin fibroblasts. Among the enzymes in skin are phosphorylase, acid maltase, and the debranching enzyme amylo-1,6-glucosidase (Leathwood and Ryman, 1971). The study of acid maltase activity in skin fibroblasts reveals no acid maltase activity in patients with Pompe's disease, whereas activity is noted in both control cells and cells of heterozygotes (Butterworth and Broadhead, 1977).

Although study of cultured amniotic fluid cells for acid-glucosidase activity must be performed with great care, prenatal detection of Pompe's disease is possible (Fujimoto et al., 1978).

Lymphocytes may be employed for the de-

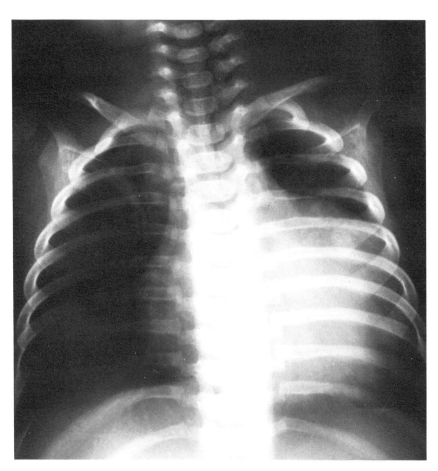

**Fig. 7-16.** Chest x-ray of infant shown in Fig. 7-14. Heart is markedly enlarged. Globular shape is typical of infantile acid maltase deficiency.

tection of decreased acid-glucosidase activity in patients as well as carriers. The use of phytohaemagglutin stimulation enhances the reliability of the studies (Yaniguchi et al., 1978).

Chest x-ray studies reveal massive cardiomegaly (Fig. 7-16) (Ruttenberg at al., 1964). The electrocardiogram is characterized by depressed ST segments, inverted T waves, and a shortened PR interval. These changes may be confused with those of myocarditis.

Electromyography demonstrates myopathic activity; polyphasic potentials and a reduced interference pattern with low voltage are the usual findings. Unusual high-frequency discharges, best described as myotonic-like, are often present (Gutmann, Hogan, and Schmidt, 1967; Hogan et al., 1969). Muscle and liver biopsy specimens contain large amounts of structurally normal glycogen when studied under both light and electron microscopy. Changes in peripheral nerve have also been reported (Araoz et al., 1974).

**GENETICS.** This disease is inherited as an autosomal recessive trait. Prenatal diagnosis has been made (Hug, 1974).

**TREATMENT.** No practical treatment is available. Epinephrine administration has reduced liver glycogen content (Hug, 1974). Administration of specially prepared amyloglucosidase from *A. foetidus* caused decrease in striated muscle glycogen content, lengthened the PR interval, and decreased ventricular electrical forces (Gillette, Nihill, and Singer, 1974).

### Late infantile acid maltase deficiency

**CLINICAL FEATURES.** A number of children have been reported who are deficient in acid maltase activity; however, they do not have clinical symptoms of Pompe's disease (Smith, Amick, and Sidbury, 1966; Smith, Zellweger, and Afifi, 1967; Swaiman, Kennedy, and Sauls, 1968; Tanaka et al., 1979). They are usually asymptomatic during the first year of life and live beyond age 2. Most have slowly progressive weakness but no overt evidence

of accumulation of glycogen in skeletal or heart muscle or in visceral organs.

Clinical manifestations may simulate Duchenne muscular dystrophy. The gastrocnemius and deltoid muscles may be firm and rubbery, and there may be accompanying hypertrophy of the gastrocnemius muscle. Gowers' sign is often present as a result of hip weakness (Fig. 7-17). Waddling gait and increased lumbar lordosis are frequently present. Achilles tendon contractures result in toe walking and further lead to the erroneous diagnosis of Duchenne muscular dystrophy. There is no cardiomegaly, and abnormal heart sounds are occasionally present; there may be an intermittent soft systolic murmur. Two patients have had a patulous anal sphincter.

**LABORATORY FINDINGS**

**BIOCHEMISTRY.** There is accumulation of glycogen that may not be of normal architecture. However, the most distinctive biochemical abnormality is a deficiency of acid maltase activity.

The liver may or may not contain increased glycogen stores (Smith, Amick, and Sidbury, 1966; Smith, Zellweger, and Afifi, 1967). Two patients have been described who had glycogen of abnormal configuration because of shortened outer chains.

**CLINICAL LABORATORY EXAMINATION.** Light and electron microscopic examination of muscle biopsy material displays moderate glycogen storage. When these muscles are stained with hematoxylin and eosin, the glycogen-containing areas appear vacuolated. With electron microscopic examination, monogranular and multigranular deposits of glycogen are found unbound in the sarcoplasm as well as membrane-bound within lysosomes.

Electromyographic study demonstrates polyphasic potentials suggestive of a myopathic process and a reduced, low-voltage interference pattern. The bizarre, myotonic-like potentials described in early infantile acid maltase deficiency are also present in the late infantile form.

**TREATMENT.** One child with late infantile

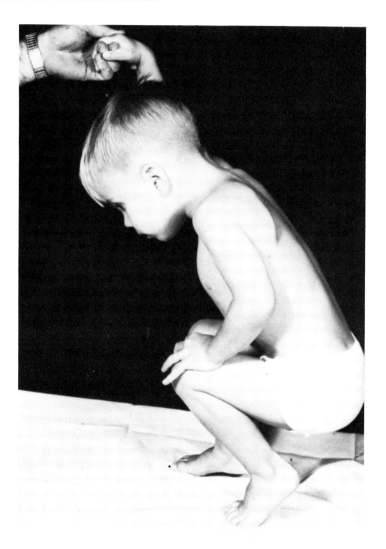

**Fig. 7-17.** A 22-month-old boy with late infantile acid maltase deficiency. He has moderate proximal muscle weakness. He is in the process of manifesting Gowers' sign because of weakness of the hip girdle.

acid maltase deficiency was treated with epinephrine (Swaiman, Kennedy, and Sauls, 1968). After 1 month of injections twice daily, the glycogen content of muscle was decreased. The relative success of this therapeutic method suggests that the conventional pathway for glycogen degradation is intact and can be normally stimulated by epinephrine.

### Adult acid maltase deficiency

Acid maltase deficiency and a slowly progressive myopathy have been described in adult patients. Many have been asymptomatic until adult life. Whether this type of disease is inherited or acquired is unknown (Engel and Dale, 1968).

Adult patients develop weakness associated with acid maltase deficiency during the third through sixth decades of life. Weakness is greater proximally than distally and is more prominent in the pelvic than in the shoulder girdle. Intercostal and diaphragmatic muscles are involved in many patients. Adult patients do not have enlargement of the liver, heart, or tongue.

Each patient has had increased serum enzyme activity of CPK, SGOT, and LDH. Adult cases cannot be delineated from infantile and late infantile cases on the basis of muscle acid maltase activity, but unlike infantile and late infantile cases, neutral acid maltase activity may be normal in adult patients (Askanas et al., 1976). Markedly decreased urinary acid maltase activity has been described (Mehler and DiMauro, 1976).

Glycogen content of muscles in adult patients does not differ from that in infantile and late infantile patients and ranges from 1.8% to 5.8% (Engel et al., 1973).

Epinephrine therapy of adult patients has not usually resulted in any increase in strength, but two adults treated for 3½ and 1½ years, respectively, appeared to gain some strength. Another adult deteriorated during a 2-year treatment period, and four others were unchanged (Engel et al., 1973).

### Amylo-1,6-glucosidase deficiency (debrancher deficiency, Forbes' disease, limit dextrinosis, Cori type III disease)

#### CLINICAL FEATURES

INFANTILE TYPE. This form is usually evident in the first few months of life and is associated with hypoglycemia, failure to thrive, and hepatomegaly (Forbes, 1953). Patients are hypotonic, weak, and have poor head control. Glycogen deposition in cardiac muscle is rarely sufficient to cause clinical disturbances. However, a 3-month-old patient who had gross cardiac involvement with glycogen accumulation and died suddenly has been reported (Miller, Alleyne, and Brooks, 1972).

Association of debranching disease with profound cardiac muscle and skeletal muscle involvement accompanied by thyroid insufficiency has also been reported. The simultaneous presence of these two conditions is unexplained (Goutieres and Aicardi, 1971).

The presence in infancy of hypoglycemia and hepatomegaly in this enzyme deficiency parallels abnormalities found in von Gierke's disease (glucose-6-phosphatase deficiency), but the abnormalities are less pronounced.

ADULT TYPE. Debrancher enzyme deficiency has also been noted in older children and adults (Brunberg, McCormick, and Schochet, 1971). Adult patients with type III glycogenosis and chronic progressive myopathy in middle age have also been reported. Reports of debrancher deficiency have been associated with reports of flaccidity in a 13-year-old patient (Forbes, 1953; Pearson, 1968) and "weak tone" in a 3-year-old patient (van Creveld and Huijing, 1965). There is often a history of a protuberant abdomen during childhood. Patients complain of muscle fatigue without tenderness cramping, or associated hematuria. Persistant diffuse weakness is present, and later, wasting of the hand and forearm muscles with loss of body weight ensues. Sugar-containing foods have no clinical benefit, and no symptoms of hypoglycemia are seen. A history of siblings who have died of similar illness in late childhood may be elicited.

#### LABORATORY FINDINGS

PATHOLOGY. Electron microscopy of biopsied muscle reveals glycogen deposits just inside the sarcolemmal membrane and between the filaments of the I and A bands, as well as between the myofibrils. The abnormalities are not pathognomonic for this glycogenosis (Neustein, 1969).

BIOCHEMISTRY. Debranching enzyme activity may be present in some tissues in patients with clinical symptoms. Approximately 70% of the patients have no activity in all tissues studied. In another 10% of patients, enzyme activity is absent in the liver but present to a small degree in muscle tissue. In yet another group, some activity of the debranching enzyme is present in either or both liver and skeletal muscle. Oligo-1,4 → 1,4-transglucosylase (transferase) activity may be present in muscle and liver tissue of patients with type III glycogenosis but absent in their leukocytes.

Assay of liver tissue of a patient with debrancher enzyme deficiency revealed increased activity of fructose-1,6-diphosphatase. Lack of enzymatic activity limits the breakdown of glycogen, and during fasting, the release of glucose from the liver stems from gluconeogenesis. Probably the increase in fructose-1,6-diphosphatase activity is a reflection of increased gluconeogenesis. Administration of galactose (Hers, 1959), dihydroxyacetone (Brombacher et al., 1964), fructose (Hers, 1959), casein (Fernandes and van de Kamer, 1968), and glycerol (Senior and Loridan, 1968) has resulted in increased blood glucose concentrations, findings that suggest the importance and effectiveness of gluconeogenesis in this condition (Sadeghi-Nejad, Loridan, and Senior, 1970).

In patients with deficient muscle enzyme activity, incorporation of U-$^{14}$C-glucose into red cell glycogen is either very low or absent.

Tissue mosaicism may result from a number of mutational changes in a single enzyme that give rise to a series of abnormal enzymes responsible for both transfer and hydrolytic activity. It is therefore probable that a number of mutant enzymes are present in this condition in different patients (Deckelbaum et al., 1972).

CLINICAL LABORATORY EXAMINATION. Pseudomyotonic discharges are present on electromyographic examination. Serum CPK activity may be increased before and after exercise.

Other laboratory studies demonstrate mild fasting hypoglycemia, fasting ketonuria, and diabetic glucose tolerance curves. Hyperlipemia is frequently present. Blood glucose concentration is not usually responsive to epinephrine or glucagon, but at times a mild response may occur. No abnormalities of galactose, fructose, and glycerol tolerance are found. Abnormally structured glycogen containing short outer chains has been demonstrated in the liver, skeletal muscle, and red and white cells (Brandt and DeLuca, 1966; Van Hoof, 1967; Van Hoof and Hers, 1967).

GENETICS. The infantile type is transmitted as an autosomal recessive trait. Heterozygotes cannot be diagnosed with certainty (Cohn et al., 1975).

### Amylo-1,4 → 1,6 transglucosidase deficiency (brancher enzyme deficiency, Cori type IV disease)

CLINICAL FEATURES. Manifestations of the disease appear in the first 6 months of life and are principally failure to thrive, hepatosplenomegaly, and liver failure with cirrhosis. On occasion, some children have retarded motor development, weakness, hypotonia, and muscle atrophy (Zellweger et al., 1972). Deep tendon reflexes are usually absent or difficult to elicit.

LABORATORY FINDINGS

PATHOLOGY. Glycogen may accumulate disproportionately in the tongue and diaphragm compared to other striated muscles. An electron microscopic study of the deposits reveals branched filaments, osmiophilic granules, and electron-dense amorphous material. The data suggest that the ultrastructural, histochemical, and chemical similarities among the deposits seen in branching enzyme deficiency, in Lafora's bodies and visceral deposits in myoclonus epilepsy, in corpora amylacea, and in basophilic degeneration of the myocardium may represent a commonality of composition and mechanism of synthesis (Schochet, McCormick, and Kovarsky, 1971).

BIOCHEMISTRY. The first patient reported with deficiency of brancher enzyme activity manifested cirrhosis of the liver and glycogen accumulation (Anderson, 1956). In another patient, the muscle glycogen concentration appeared normal (Holleman, van der Haar, and de Vaan, 1966). In yet another patient, muscle glycogen content was decreased (Sidbury et al., 1962).

Brancher enzyme deficiency results in the synthesis of unbranched glycogen composed of elongated chains of glucose molecules joined together by 1,4 linkages. As a result, the glycogen is composed of long outer chains, has few branch points, and resembles the pattern of starch, also known as amylopectin.

The glycogen brancher enzyme has been purified over 3,000-fold from rabbit skeletal muscle. The enzyme appears to have a molecular weight of 92,000 to 103,000, depending upon the choice of reference protein. Amylopectin polysaccharide isolated from the liver of a patient with branching deficiency is branched in the presence of the purified enzyme and $\alpha$-D-glucose-1-phosphate pH 7 (Gibson, Brown, and Brown, 1971).

Study of the fine structure of glycogen from a patient with brancher enzyme deficiency demonstrates that the similarity of abnormal glycogen to amylopectin is in some ways superficial. The abnormal glycogen contains a significant number of short branches. This is consistent with a hypothesis that in these patients there is a normal debranching enzyme system that can participate in a reverse reaction with a resultant small degree of branching activity. The short chains are explained further by the supposition that the glycogen debranching enzyme system would form branch points by the apposition of $1 \rightarrow 6$ bonded $\alpha$-glucose units by amylo-1,6-glucosidase. Further elongation of this chain would occur by transfer of oligosaccharide by the oligo-1,4 $\rightarrow$ 1,4-transferase component of the debranching system. The transferase favors transfer of maltotriosyl residue, which creates a 4-unit branch. Brancher enzyme from muscle or liver tissue ordinarily transfers glucose units of seven glucose molecules. The shorter branches formed by a reversal of the debranching enzyme system are not as readily extended by glycogen synthetase, and indeed, if the units are shorter than four

glucose units, it may be impossible for them to be extended by synthetase (Mercier and Whelan, 1970). The presence of short branches suggests that reversal of the debranching mechanism is operative.

CLINICAL LABORATORY EXAMINATION. Diagnosis of brancher enzyme deficiency by an assay of peripheral white blood activity is feasible.

GENETICS. Studies confirm an autosomal recessive mode of inheritance (Legum and Nitowsky, 1969). Cultured fibroblasts reveal markedly deficient brancher enzyme activity. Dermal enzyme activity was less than control levels in a patient and both parents; this suggests an autosomal recessive mode of inheritance. The correlation between enzyme activity in fibroblasts from normal amniotic fluid cells and activity in normal skin fibroblasts suggests that antenatal diagnosis is possible (Howell, Kaback, and Brown, 1971).

TREATMENT. Treatment with a combination of zinc-glucagon and $\alpha$-glucosidase, attempted in one infant, decreased liver glycogen concentration, but the infant died at 11 months from an infection (Fernandes and Huijing, 1968).

## McArdle's disease (myophosphorylase deficiency, Cori type V disease)

McArdle (1951) reported a condition characterized by weakness, fatigability, and severe muscle cramping with pain following exercise. Later, he reported decreased lactate production in the affected muscles after ischemic work (McArdle, 1951; Pearson, Rimer, and Mommaerts, 1961; Schmid and Mahler, 1959).

CLINICAL FEATURES. Patients manifest decreased stamina and tire easily. Severe cramping pain following minimal exercise is experienced in the involved skeletal muscles and primarily involves distal muscles. Cardiac symptoms have not been reported, but cardiac muscle is compromised (Ratinov, Baker, and Swaiman, 1965). Myoglobinuria follows moderate or strenuous exercise. In adolescence and adulthood, patients may develop persistent weakness and moderate loss of muscle bulk (Schmid and Hammaker, 1961). Prolonged or frequent repetitive episodes of myoglobinuria must be avoided, or chronic renal impairment may ensue. Acute renal failure may not be reversible in these patients (Bank, DiMauro, and Rowland, 1972).

### LABORATORY FINDINGS

PATHOLOGY. Light microscopic studies reveal moderately increased stores of glycogen beneath the sarcolemmal membrane. Electron microscopy shows disorganization of the I band region and distortion of the myofibrils secondary to glycogen deposition (Rowland, Fahn, and Schotland, 1963). Histochemical study of muscle suggests the absence of myophosphorylase activity. Quantitative biochemical studies are necessary to confirm the diagnosis. Critical and definitive diagnosis depends on assay for the enzymatic deficiency in the affected muscle tissue.

BIOCHEMISTRY. Degradation of glycogen to lactate begins with the initial disruption of the 1,4 linkage between glucosyl units. The enzyme myophosphorylase facilitates this reaction in skeletal muscle. Subsequently, glucose-1-phosphate is released and then metabolized to lactate via the Embden-Meyerhof pathway. The myophosphorylase enzyme is itself regenerated in a complex reaction among a number of other enzymes, including phosphorylase kinase (Fig. 7-13).

Deficiency of myophosphorylase activity causes decreased glucose-1-phosphate production; as a result, exercised muscle does not synthesize lactic acid and serum lactic acid concentration is not appropriately elevated (Fig. 7-18). Structure of the accumulated excess glycogen is normal.

Histochemical techniques applied to fresh-frozen sections of skeletal fibers from muscle biopsies of patients demonstrate absence of phosphorylase activity. Studies of immature multinucleated fibers and striated myofibers grown in vitro from these tissues reveal definite evidence of phosphorylase activity. A genetic coding for developing a form of myophosphorylase activity must be present in the

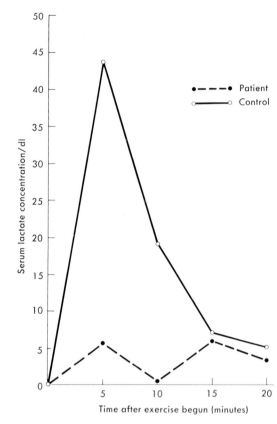

**Fig. 7-18.** Graph depicts relative lack of lactate production in McArdle's disease when compared to a normal individual during an ischemic exercise task.

precursor cells of regenerating skeletal muscle. The observation suggests the presence of the mechanism for loss of activity during maturation of tissues. Feasible explanations include the possibility that muscle maturation results in loss of an enzyme that maintains phosphorylase production, survival, or activity; or that an abnormal specific protease develops with maturity and inactivates myophosphorylase; or that a normally repressed myophosphorylase repressor gene may be "derepressed"; or that a normally present but inactive myophosphorylase-inhibiting or -destroying enzyme is activated and inhibits myophosphorylase enzyme activity or survival (Roelofs, Engel, and Chauvin, 1972).

CLINICAL LABORATORY EXAMINATION. Exercise produces elevated serum CPK activity and an increase in activity of other serum enzymes released from muscle, ostensibly caused by loss of sarcolemmal membrane integrity. The electrocardiogram may show an increased QRS amplitude, a prolonged PR interval, T wave inversion, and bradycardia (Ratinov, Baker, and Swaiman, 1965).

Electromyographic study of contracted muscles after exercise shows a decreased interference pattern; after ischemic exercise, the contracted muscles may show no electrical activity.

Effects of ischemic exercise may be studied by using two blood pressure cuffs, one at the wrist and one just above the elbow. The cuffs are inflated to above systolic pressure and the pressure maintained for 3 minutes. Blood is removed from the antecubital vein at 0, 3, 5, 10, 15, and 20 minutes. After the initial (0 time) blood is drawn, the patient is asked to contract and extend the fingers over a rubber ball or rod while the cuff pressure is maintained. A patient with McArdle's disease, or indeed any of the glycolytic abnormalities that interfere with lactate production, will develop severe contracture and complain bitterly of pain within 30 seconds after the initiation of ischemic exercise. Lactic acid concentration of blood drawn from these patients reveals little or no lactic acid formation during exercise. The basis of the contracture phenomenon may be related to delayed reaccumulation of calcium ions in the sarcoplasmic reticulum (Gruener et al., 1968).

The relaxing factor (accumulation of calcium ions by the sarcoplasmic reticulum) appears to be normal in patients with McArdle's disease (Brody, Gergerg, and Sidbury, 1970).

**GENETICS.** McArdle's disease appears to be transmitted as an autosomal recessive trait.

**THERAPY.** A fat-rich diet was administered to a 21-year-old male patient; he subsequently had a shortened recovery period from the acute physical load and suffered no induration of the deltoid muscle after sustained abduction to 90 degrees. Maximal strength does not appear to be improved by the fat-rich diet, but tolerance of submaximal loads appears to be increased, and recovery from muscle discomfort appears to be accelerated (Viskoper et al., 1975).

### Muscle phosphofructokinase deficiency (Tarui's disease)

**CLINICAL FEATURES.** Motor development is normal during the first decade. Nevertheless, patients do experience decreased exercise tolerance and fatigue easily during childhood. They perform poorly in games requiring physical stamina and complain of muscle stiffness and weakness and occasionally of muscle cramps. Myoglobinuria may follow moderate to strenuous exercise. The physical examination is unremarkable. Usually no evidence of weakness or loss of muscle bulk is seen.

**LABORATORY FINDINGS**

BIOCHEMISTRY. The enzyme phosphofructokinase transforms fructose-6-phosphate to fructose-1,6-diphosphate. Decreased activity of this enzyme results in increased muscle glycogen stores of normal structure and also increased concentration of glucose-6-phosphate and fructose-6-phosphate (Layzer, Rowland, and Ranney, 1967; Tarui et al., 1965; Thomson, MacLaurin, and Prineas, 1963).

CLINICAL LABORATORY EXAMINATION. After exercise, serum CPK activity and activities of other serum enzymes released from muscle may be elevated. Electromyography may be unrevealing. Ischemic exercise testing, as described in the section on McArdle's disease, results in muscle contracture and decreased lactic acid production. The definitive diagnosis is made by an enzymatic assay of muscle tissue.

Phosphofructokinase activity is about 50% of the expected value in the erythrocytes of these patients. A decrease from normal levels of activity is also noted in their parents. Immunologic study suggests that half of the total activity of erythrocyte phosphofructokinase is derived from an enzyme form identical to muscle phosphofructokinase.

**GENETICS.** The condition appears to be transmitted as an autosomal recessive trait.

## *Phosphoglucomutase deficiency (Thomson's disease)*

A patient had numerous episodes of supraventricular tachycardia in early infancy that required digitoxin treatment, then he developed normally until the age of 2½, when he began to walk on his toes (Thomson, MacLaurin, and Prineas, 1963). Examination revealed mild weakness and poor muscle development. His calf muscles were bulky and firm, and the Achilles tendons were shortened. No clinical history of exercise intolerance, muscle pain, or myoglobinuria was elicited.

Serum enzyme activities, including CPK, aldolase, glutamic oxaloacetic, transaminase, and glutamic pyruvic transaminase, were elevated. Examination by electromyography suggested a myopathic process.

In vitro study of biopsy tissue indicated a number of relative enzymatic deficiencies, but phosphoglucomutase deficiency was most pronounced. Glycogen structure appeared normal. There was extensive replacement of muscle tissue by glycogen.

## *Phosphohexoisomerase deficiency (Satoyoshi's disease)*

A family whose members experience muscle pain and stiffness with exercise has been described (Satoyoshi and Kowa, 1967). During childhood, there is exercise tolerance with some muscle pain; the symptoms become more prominent in later life. Muscle contractures do not occur after ischemic exercise.

Routine examination of the patients is normal. Heavy exercise leads to stiffness and tenderness of the muscles, although no weakness is apparent.

The ischemic exercise test does not increase lactic acid concentration. No electromyographic abnormalities have been described. However, serum CPK activity has been increased.

In vitro studies of muscle demonstrate an increase in lactic acid concentration only when fructose-6-phosphate is added to the homogenate. A metabolic defect has been postulated secondary to the deficiency of phosphohexoisomerase activity. Evidence for this hypothesis is weak. It should be noted that activity of this enzyme is normal when the tissue is assayed. Glycogen content is only slightly increased, and its architecture is undetermined.

## EPISODIC WEAKNESS

The diseases characterized by episodic weakness are unique among the myopathies, because the patient is normal between episodes of paralysis. These diseases are characterized by recurrent paralytic attacks, which may progress from mild to profound weakness in all extremities with complete recovery in time. These diseases are most often associated with either low or elevated serum potassium concentration. In addition, there are normokalemic forms of episodic weakness. The classic familial periodic paralyses have an autosomal dominant inheritance, while other diseases associated with low serum potassium are sporadic in occurrence (Table 7-3).

## EPISODIC WEAKNESS WITH ALTERATION IN SERUM POTASSIUM CONCENTRATION
### *Familial hypokalemic periodic paralysis*

CLINICAL FEATURES. This disorder is inherited as an autosomal dominant trait. Males are affected more frequently and have a more severe form than females (McArdle, 1956; Shy et al., 1961). Although the disease may begin in early infancy, the majority of cases develop between 10 and 20 years of age. Typically, the attacks of paralysis occur after a large meal, especially one high in carbohydrates or salt. In addition, the paralysis often develops during a period of rest following strenuous exercise. The attacks commonly occur at night or in the early morning hours, although they may come at any time. Often the patient awakens and finds himself paralyzed, unable to sit up, roll over, or get out of bed. Even with complete paralysis of the limbs, the muscles innervated by the cra-

**Table 7-3.** Diseases characterized by episodic weakness

---

With change in serum potassium concentration
  Classic periodic paralysis
    Familial hypokalemic periodic paralysis
    Familial hyperkalemic periodic paralysis
    ? Paramyotonia congenita
  Aldosteronism
    Pseudoaldosteronism from licorice ingestion
  Thyrotoxicosis with episodic weakness
  Renal disease, diabetic acidosis, diuretics
With no change in serum potassium concentration
  Paramyotonia congenita
  McArdle's disease (myophosphorylase deficiency)
  Mitochondrial myopathy (pleoconial type)
  ? "Familial normokalemic periodic paralysis"

---

nial nerves are usually spared. The frequency of paralytic attacks varies from nightly to several times a week to once in several months.

Examination of the patient during an attack reveals a flaccid paralysis with absent tendon reflexes. The weakness may be asymmetric. It often begins in the lower extremities and extends to the upper extremities, trunk, and neck. The abdominal and cremasteric reflexes are usually unaffected. Sensation is not lost. Mentation and consciousness are preserved. The duration of the paralysis is usually 6 to 12 hours, but it may last up to 36 hours. Examination may reveal myotonia (Resnick, 1965), especially of the eyelids, which produces a pronounced lid lag when the patient looks downward following a period of upward gaze. Myotonia is more commonly detected in hyperkalemic periodic paralysis; it can be demonstrated in the tongue and thenar eminence.

**LABORATORY FINDINGS.** Laboratory studies during an attack usually reveal low serum potassium in the range of 2 to 3 mEq per liter. Electrocardiograms done during the paralysis show bradycardia and sinus arrhythmia, prolongation of Q-T interval, and depression and inversion of T waves. Electromyography (Engel et al., 1965) during an attack discloses many electrically silent areas within the muscle, even during maximal contraction. There are no denervation potentials, and no spontaneous activity is seen. The action potential duration is reduced, and the interference pattern on maximal contraction shows a progressive reduction in the number of motor units that can be activated. The number of polyphasic motor units increases. The motor nerve conduction velocity is normal.

**PATHOPHYSIOLOGY.** Pathologic changes are found in muscle fibers of patients who have had long-standing disease (Pearson, 1964; MacDonald, Rewcastle, and Humphrey, 1968). The predominant changes shown by light microscopy are large vacuoles, loss of cross striations, and hyaline degeneration. Some of the material within the vacuoles is PAS-positive; however, muscle glycogen is not quantitatively increased.

On electron microscopy (Howes et al., 1966; Odor, Patel, and Pearce, 1967), the vacuoles appear to reside in the sarcoplasmic reticulum. During the attack, intracellular water is increased, and the fluid is presumably loculated in the vacuoles seen in both light and electron microscopy.

The basic defect in hypokalemic periodic paralysis is unknown. It has been postulated (Pearson and Kalyaharaman, 1972) that increased mineralocorticoid activity other than aldosterone is a common factor in the pathogenesis of paralysis in patients with hypokalemic periodic paralysis. Treatment of this disease is partially based on the known metabolic alterations present.

**TREATMENT.** The acute attack may be terminated by the oral administration of potassium chloride, beginning with a dose of 2 gm. Careful monitoring of the patient's weakness, electrocardiogram, and serum potassium is necessary. Prophylactically, the patient should avoid large carbohydrate meals and strenuous exercise. The patient also often learns to ward off an impending attack by mild exercise (Campa and Sanders, 1974), which promotes glycogenolysis and glycolysis.

Two other drugs have been used to prevent attacks of paralysis. Their mechanism of

action is unexplained and paradoxical. Spironolactone (Poskanzer and Kerr, 1961), an
aldosterone antagonist, has been effective
despite lack of evidence implicating aldosterone in the pathogenesis of the attacks.
Acetazolamide (Resnick et al., 1968; Vroom,
Jarrell, and Maren, 1975) may reduce the
frequency of attacks.

The prognosis must be somewhat guarded,
for although the attacks are generally more
severe and frequent in the adolescent and
diminish with age, a progressive, persistent
myopathy (see pathophysiology) has been
described in some patients (Buruma and
Bots, 1978).

### Hyperkalemic periodic paralysis (adynamia episodica hereditaria)

CLINICAL FEATURES. Elevated serum potassium concentration during an attack clearly differentiates this form of paralysis from
hypokalemic familial periodic paralysis. Hyperkalemic periodic paralysis is inherited as
an autosomal dominant trait. The disease
may begin early in infancy, and it has been
reported that 90% of the cases have their onset before the age of 10 (Gamstorp, 1956).
The attacks differ from those of hypokalemic
periodic paralysis, because they are usually
milder and of shorter duration, with the paralysis developing rapidly within 30 to 40
minutes. The attack generally lasts only 1 to
2 hours (Fig. 7-19).

In the characteristic onset, the patient reports weakness in the muscles of the back,
thighs, and calves. It then extends to the
arms, hands, and neck. The patient may have
difficulty in swallowing or coughing; however, the muscles of respiration are generally
not affected. One of the earliest signs is the
appearance of a lid lag. This myotonic phenomenon is elicited when the patient looks
downward after first gazing upward, which
produces a marked lag of the superior lid.
Parents often recognize this sign in affected
infants (McArdle, 1962). A point of differentiation from hypokalemic periodic paralysis is
the increased frequency of attacks, which
may occur as often as several times a week or

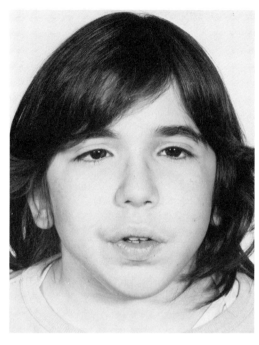

**Fig. 7-19.** Hyperkalemic periodic paralysis. Note
ptosis, flattening of naso-labial folds, and pursing
of lips secondary to myotonic involvement.

even daily in the hyperkalemic form. Although nocturnal attacks are more characteristic of the hypokalemic variety, they have
also been reported in hyperkalemic paralysis. In addition, the patient may initially
complain of paresthesias in an extremity,
which is unusual in the hypokalemic form of
the disease. Attacks typically occur during
rest after a period of physical exertion. There
does not seem to be any relationship between
the attack and ingestion of a carbohydrate
meal, as is true in hypokalemic periodic paralysis. Exposure to cold may increase the
myotonia and weakness.

Physical findings depend upon whether an
attack of paralysis is in progress. In the pre-
attack phase, many adult patients manifest
slight permanent weakness, especially in the
abdominal, hip flexor, and triceps muscles.
The calf muscles may be enlarged. The tendon reflexes are generally normal in the upper extremities, but they may be diminished
at the knee. As mentioned previously, a lid

lag may be present. In addition, percussion myotonia of the tongue and thenar eminence may be elicited (Layzer, Lovelace, and Rowland, 1967). During an attack, there is increased weakness in the muscles previously affected, and the patients often describe a feeling of heaviness or stiffness in the legs or a generally spreading weakness, as described previously. Consciousness is not altered. Respiratory weakness is uncommon. During an attack, the patient often exhibits difficulty rising from a chair or the floor and climbing stairs. The tendon reflexes are diminished or absent but may not bear any consistent relationship to the degree of muscle weakness present.

LABORATORY FINDINGS. Laboratory examination during an attack usually reveals an elevation of serum potassium concentration without any decrease in the excretion of potassium. The rise in serum potassium may be mild and transient. The level of potassium may remain within the normal range, and the rise is apparent only with serial sampling of the patient's serum both before and during an attack. Potassium influx into red blood cells is decreased during attacks (Hoskins et al., 1974). An electrocardiogram taken during the attack reveals typical changes of hyperkalemia with high peaked T waves. Plasma inorganic phosphate and glucose may also be decreased during an induced attack of paralysis. Glucose tolerance tests have been abnormal, and a ketotic odor has been detected during an attack (Hoskins, Vroom, and Jarrell, 1975).

A study of the serum potassium level during an attack of paralysis generally demonstrates an appreciably higher level with a subsequent decrease as the weakness disappears. Although the serum potassium level may still be within the normal range, it appears that patients with hyperkalemic periodic paralysis are sensitive to a rise in the potassium level in the plasma and extracellular fluid. The levels of sodium, calcium, and chloride have been found to be normal during and between attacks.

Electromyography (Buchthal, Engbaek, and Gamstorp, 1958) during an attack shows an increased number of spontaneous potentials, especially fibrillation potentials. There is a reduced number and amplitude of potentials with a maximal contraction, which thus produces a reduction in interference pattern. Excitability to mechanical stimulation is greatly increased during an attack of paralysis. Sensitivity to acetylcholine is also increased. The motor conduction velocity is normal.

PATHOPHYSIOLOGY. Gamstorp (1956) has demonstrated a movement of potassium from the cells to plasma during attacks. An increase in serum potassium without a decrease in urinary potassium excretion suggests that potassium is passing from the intracellular to the extracellular fluid, which should produce a depolarization of the muscle membrane potential and result in weakness. However, the magnitude of decrease in membrane potential during an attack of paralysis has been slight (Creutzfeldt et al., 1963; Brooks, 1969), and it does not appear to be the sole explanation for the changes in excitability seen in this disease. An increase in sodium permeability has been postulated to explain the changes in membrane potential during an attack of paralysis.

Muscle ribosomes show excessive in vitro amino acid incorporation during an induced attack of paralysis (Ionasescu et al., 1973). Whether an abnormal protein interfering with ion movement is synthesized, or abnormality develops in the regulatory proteins of the contractile mechanism, tropomyosin or troponin, is unclear.

Muscle biopsy has revealed pathologic changes similar to those found in hypokalemic periodic paralysis (Pearson, 1964). These changes consist of central myofibrillar and mitochondrial degeneration and vacuole formation.

The differential diagnosis between hyper- and hypokalemic periodic paralysis may be difficult (Layzer, Lovelace, and Rowland, 1967). There is no one single pathognomonic finding (Table 7-4). The most valuable test is the determination of serum potassium dur-

**Table 7-4.** Periodic paralysis

| | Hypokalemic form | Hyperkalemic form | Normokalemic form (? pleoconial myopathy) |
|---|---|---|---|
| Age at onset | First—second decade | Infancy—first decade | First decade |
| Inheritance | Dominant—more common in male | Dominant—more severe in male | Dominant |
| Duration of weakness | Usually 6 to 12 hours | Less than 1 hour | Days to weeks |
| Frequency of attacks | Weekly to monthly | Daily | Every 2 to 3 months |
| Precipitating factors | Rest after exertion, large carbohydrate meal | Rest after exertion | Rest after exertion, sleeping late or long |
| Examination | | | |
|   Cranial nerves | Lid lag | Lid lag | Weakness of mastication and cough |
|   Tendon reflexes | Absent | Diminished to absent | Absent |
|   Sensory symptoms | None | Paresthesias | Rare hyperthesia |
|   Myotonia | None (except lid lag) | Tongue and thenar eminence hyperesthesia | None |
| Laboratory | | | |
|   Serum potassium | Low | High | Normal |
|   EKG | Depression and inversion of T waves | High peaked T waves | Normal |
|   EMG | Myopathic potentials, silent areas | Increased spontaneous and insertion potentials with fibrillation and myotonic discharges | Myopathic potentials |
| Diagnostic provocation | Glucose and insulin, NaCl | KCl | KCl |
| Treatment of attack | KCl | Calcium gluconate, salbutamol | NaCl |
| Prophylaxis against attack | Avoid large carbohydrate meals and strenuous exercise, acetazolamide, low sodium diet | Acetazolamide, mild exercise after exertion | Acetazolamide, NaCl, mild exercise after exertion |

ing an attack. If the degree of paralysis is mild, however, serum potassium may be normal in either condition. The best provocative test is the potassium loading test, which, if weakness is produced with elevated serum potassium levels, is diagnostic of hyperkalemic periodic paralysis. This test must be carried out under carefully controlled conditions with electrocardiographic monitoring. In addition, it is important that only small oral doses of potassium chloride (2 to 3 gm) be administered at the beginning of the test.

The electromyogram may be useful in detecting myotonia even if it is not clinically apparent. Evidence of myotonia favors the diagnosis of hyperkalemic periodic paralysis.

**TREATMENT.** Most attacks end spontaneously. In a severe attack, however, resolution of the paralysis may be brought about with the intravenous infusion of 10 to 20 ml of 10% calcium gluconate (Gamstorp, 1956). Prophylaxis for the prevention of the paralytic attacks has been brought about through the use of acetazolamide, a carbonic anhydrase inhibitor. The effectiveness of the carbonic anhydrase inhibitor (McArdle, 1962) varies from patient to patient. Paradoxically, acetazolamide is also useful in preventing attacks in the hypokalemic form of periodic paralysis. The paralytic episode may be treated by inhalation of salbutamol (Wang and Clausen, 1976).

### Paramyotonia congenita

Paramyotonia congenita is characterized by myotonia aggravated by cold, episodic weakness, and an autosomal dominant inheritance (Thrush, Morris, and Salmon, 1972). The symptoms of myotonia and weakness begin in early childhood; they are not progressive and are not accompanied by muscle wasting. Magee (1963) has emphasized the occurrence of paradoxical myotonia, that is, myotonia aggravated rather than improved with exercise. The myotonia occurs at any temperature but more rapidly and with less exertion when the patient is exposed to cold. Paramyotonia congenita is also characterized by episodic flaccid weakness of the muscles of the hip and shoulder girdles. The weakness occurs as the myotonia lessens and may even occur in absence of myotonia.

Several authors (Drager, Hammill, and Shy, 1958; Layzer, Lovelace, and Rowland, 1967) have suggested that paramyotonia congenita and familial hyperkalemic periodic paralysis are the same disease. The episodic weakness is similar in both conditions. However, precipitation of muscular weakness by a potassium chloride loading test has not been constant. The paradoxical myotonia seems to be a unique feature of paramyotonia congenita. The absence of a common metabolic abnormality linking paramyotonia congenita and familial hyperkalemic periodic paralysis prevents confirmation of the identical nature of these diseases.

Neurologic examination of the patient with paramyotonia congenita is generally normal, except for the presence of percussion myotonia in the muscles of the thenar eminence and tongue. Exposure to cold aggravates the myotonia, which then may develop in the facial muscles and the flexor muscles of the hands. If the patient is examined during an attack of weakness, flaccid paralysis will be present with decreased tendon reflexes in the affected regions. The weakness may persist for hours but can often be relieved by warming the patient.

Serum enzyme activity is normal. The serum potassium concentration is generally within the normal range. Electromyography shows typical myotonic potentials. A significant reduction (80%) in the amplitude of the evoked response occurs with repetitive stimulation at 25 to 50 Hz (Burke, Skuse, and Lethlean, 1974). Histologically, the muscle may be normal or contains sarcoplasmic masses and ringbinden formation.

Avoidance of exposure to cold appears to be the most effective form of therapy. The prognosis is good, since there appears to be no progression of the myotonia or weakness.

### Primary aldosteronism

CLINICAL FEATURES. In patients with primary aldosteronism, there is an inappropriate, excessive secretion of aldosterone. This disease is usually caused by an adrenal adenoma, but it may also be seen in patients with adrenal hyperplasia or adrenal carcinoma. The original report (Conn, 1955) emphasized the clinical picture of intermittent and episodic weakness, with paralysis of the lower extremities. Primary aldosteronism is largely a disease of adults but has been described in children (Kretchmer et al., 1959). The clinical picture is one of episodic muscle weakness that may progress to paralysis. The lower extremities are predominantly affected, although the weakness may become generalized. Muscles innervated by the cranial nerves are rarely affected. The patient exhibits polyuria and polydipsia and often complains of headache.

Examination reveals hypertension, a cardinal feature of this disease. The diastolic pressure is frequently elevated. The patient's headache is probably related to hypertension. Between attacks of weakness, the patient's neurologic status is normal. During an attack, there are decreased tendon reflexes and muscle weakness, the latter resulting from potassium depletion.

**LABORATORY FINDINGS.** Primary aldosteronism may be suspected by the constellation of clinical and laboratory findings. The characteristic laboratory findings are hypokalemia, hypernatremia, and alkalosis. The specific diagnosis of primary aldosteronism depends upon the demonstration of elevated secretion of aldosterone. Subsequent treatment consists of adrenal exploration, with removal of the tumor or adrenalectomy in the cases of adrenocortical hyperplasia.

A myopathy mimicking primary aldosteronism occurs following the ingestion of large quantities of licorice (Conn, Rovner, and Cohen, 1968). The active ingredient in licorice producing the sodium retention and potassium loss is glycyrrhizinic acid. Licorice myopathy is therefore characterized by hypokalemia, hypernatremia, alkalosis, and hypertension, although aldosterone secretion is not increased. Myoglobinuria has occurred in a patient with licorice myopathy.

### Thyrotoxic periodic paralysis

Engel (1961) has reviewed 228 cases of thyrotoxic periodic paralysis. Over 90% of these are reported from Japan. This disease usually has its onset during adult life, with only 8% of the cases reported developing paralytic attacks before age 19. There is a dominant male distribution, with the male-female ratio higher than six to one. Thyrotoxic periodic paralysis occurs as a sporadic disease in contrast to familial periodic paralysis. The thyrotoxic form also differs from the familial form in its later age of onset and marked predominance in males. The attacks of weakness generally appear after the onset of the thyrotoxicosis. However, some patients have experienced attacks of weakness before the symptoms of thyroid disease were evident. In other patients, both disorders began simultaneously. Thyrotoxic episodic weakness is similar to familial periodic paralysis, in that it is precipitated by a large carbohydrate intake and occurs in the evening or night or when the patient is at rest following strenuous exercise. The episodes of paralysis last from hours to days, and they may occur as frequently as several times a week.

Examination reveals the symptoms and signs of hyperthyroidism. Generally, the patients are not weak between the attacks, and the tendon reflexes are normal. During an attack of paralysis, the weakness may predominate in the lower extremities or become generalized. Tendon reflexes are depressed in the areas of weakness.

Serum CPK activity is elevated between attacks and increases with the onset of weakness. During the paralysis, the serum potassium concentration is low, while the sodium concentration is normal. Typical myopathic potentials are seen with electromyography (Ramsay, 1965).

The weakness produced in thyrotoxic paralysis appears to be related to the hypokalemia. In an extensive study by Shizume and associates (1966), a constant positive arterial-venous difference of serum potassium was present during the development of the paralysis. These data support the hypothesis that there is a cellular uptake of potassium, resulting in hypokalemia and weakness. The mechanism for initiating these changes is not known.

Muscle biopsy obtained in the nonparalytic state is generally normal by light microscopy. There are occasional degenerating muscle fibers. With electron microscopy (Engel, 1966a; Norris, Panner, and Stormont, 1968; Norris, Clark, and Biglieri, 1971), the muscle fibers are found to contain numerous membrane-limited vesicles. These vesicles generally occur adjacent to the I bands and occasionally about the Z bands. These abnormalities seem to lie in the tubular system, and these vesicles contain a low-density granular material. There may be some vacuolization and disruption of myofibrils. A few muscle fibers contain subsarcolemmal collections of glycogen. Generally the remaining organelles are normal.

The attacks of paralysis are relieved by treatment of hyperthyroidism.

### Renal disease

Chronic renal diseases with loss of potassium may be associated with episodic paralysis (Evans and Milne, 1954). Periodic attacks of weakness have been described with renal tubular acidosis, Fanconi's syndrome, and pyelonephritis. Although the patient may have no weakness between the attacks of paralysis, excessive fatigue is common.

Episodic paralysis secondary to renal disease is differentiated from familial periodic paralysis by the lack of family history, later age of onset, persistence of hypokalemia, and mild persistent weakness between more severe attacks. The episodes of weakness are generally more severe in patients with chronic renal disease. Diagnosis of chronic renal disease is based on the careful documentation of impairment of renal function. There is a decrease in serum potassium concentration.

### Episodic weakness with no change in serum potassium concentration

Paramyotonia congenita and McArdle's disease have been previously discussed.

Poskanzer and Kerr (1961) described episodic paralysis with normal or slightly low serum potassium concentration. Relief of the attack was obtained by infusion with sodium chloride. Shy (1966) considered this form of episodic paralysis to be a mitochondrial disease (see pleoconial myopathy). The patients originally described were normal at birth and had onset of paralysis within the first decade of life. Gradual onset over 2 to 3 days and prolonged duration of days to weeks characterize this form of episodic paralysis. Chemically, the serum potassium concentration is normal during an attack. No myotonic potentials were seen. The attacks of paralysis have been shortened and improved by

oral sodium chloride or intravenous normal saline. Since no electron microscopic studies were undertaken in these patients, the presence of a mitochondrial abnormality remains speculative.

## ENDOCRINE MYOPATHIES

Hormonal factors exert profound control over glycogen and protein metabolism, as well as over intracellular and extracellular ionic concentration. Endocrine disorders consequently produce both metabolic and structural changes within the muscle cell.

Clinically, administration of adrenal steroids and parathyroid and thyroid disorders commonly produce muscle disease.

### Steroid myopathy

A myopathy occurs in Cushing's syndrome (Cushing, 1932; Müller and Kugelberg, 1959), in animals following experimental administration of adrenal steroids (Awad, Swaiman, and Kottke, 1965; Ritter, 1967), and in patients who have been on prolonged steroid therapy for rheumatic fever (Byers, Bergman, and Joseph, 1962), blood dyscrasias, and other collagen diseases (Perkoff et al., 1959).

In the steroid myopathy produced in patients, the disease has resulted from use of cortisone, prednisone, and triamcinolone. The halogenated steroids are more likely to produce a myopathy. Common therapeutic doses, as well as excessive dosage of steroids, have produced myopathy (Dubowitz, 1976). The exact mechanism of steroid myopathy is unknown, although corticosteroids affect the metabolic processes involving glucose and the metabolism of protein.

The onset of weakness is usually noted several weeks after starting the steroid. Patients have difficulty walking and especially climbing stairs. If the patient remains on steroid treatment, the weakness progressively worsens and may become so generalized that the patient is bedridden.

On examination, the cranial nerves are normal. The most pronounced weakness occurs in the hip and thigh muscles, although the dorsiflexor muscles of the feet may be involved. The tendon reflexes are depressed or absent. Sensation is normal. There is no bladder or bowel involvement.

Electromyography may reveal normal potentials or myopathic potentials. Muscle biopsy may be relatively normal or show myopathic changes of rounding of muscle fibers, increased sarcolemmal nuclei, and some scattered fiber necrosis. Type II fibers are selectively involved (Stern et al., 1972). Electron microscopy shows more profound changes even in those muscle fibers that appear normal under light microscopy. Engel (1966a) has described sarcolemmal projections containing aggregates of mitochondria surrounded by glycogen. Vacuolated mitochondria and myelin figures were also seen.

Steroid myopathy is treated by reducing the dosage or discontinuing the steroid. The patients generally recover over a period of weeks to months.

### Hyperparathyroidism

Subjective complaints of fatigue and weakness commonly occur in patients with hyperparathyroidism (Bischoff and Esslen, 1965; Frame et al., 1968). Less commonly, objective weakness, atrophy, and muscle pain may occur as an early manifestation of this disease. The muscle weakness often is manifested by difficulty in walking and climbing stairs (Bjernulf et al., 1970; Patten et al., 1974). These symptoms, which suggest a myopathy, may precede the classic symptoms of hyperparathyroidism, namely, irritability, constipation, vomiting, headache, and polydipsia. Anorexia and weight loss are also common findings.

Neurologic examination reveals normal cranial nerves. The tendon reflexes are generally normal but may be increased. There is no evidence of spasticity, clonus, or Babinski's sign. Muscle tenderness is variable. There are no visible fasciculations. The muscle weakness is largely proximal, involving the shoulders, hips, and thighs. Patients often have striking difficulty in abduction of the arms. They commonly manifest a positive Gowers' sign. Sensation is normal.

The diagnosis is suggested by increased serum calcium and decreased serum phosphorus concentrations. The alkaline phosphatase activity is also elevated. Electromyography reveals increased polyphasic potentials and a reduced interference pattern. Motor nerve conduction velocity is normal.

Muscle biopsy shows diffuse, scattered areas of muscle fiber degeneration with increased sarcolemmal nuclei of both type I and type II muscle fibers. Increased polymorphonuclear cells have been reported.

The muscular symptoms appear to be prominently related to the aberration in calcium metabolism. These symptoms are relieved following surgical removal of the parathyroid adenoma. The mechanism by which calcium dysfunction results in the myopathy is unknown. Calcium, which has been implicated in the electromechanical coupling in muscle fibers (Henson, 1966), appears to play a major role in the coupling reaction between adenosine triphosphate attached to myosin and the reactive sites on the actin filaments. The hypercalcemia undoubtedly alters this normal function. A neuropathic origin for the neuromuscular symptoms encountered in primary hyperparathyroidism has also been suggested (Patten et al., 1974).

### Thyroid disease

Disorders of thyroid metabolism may have profound effects on the neuromuscular apparatus. Periodic paralysis and a myasthenic syndrome are associated with hyperthyroidism as well as with hypothyroidism. However, the most common muscular abnormality associated with thyroid disease is a chronic thyrotoxic myopathy (Rosman, 1976).

#### Chronic thyrotoxic myopathy

Hyperthyroidism in children is rare, constituting approximately 5% of the total incidence of this disease (McClintock, Frawley, and Holden, 1956; Saxena, Crawford, and Talbot, 1964). Early adolescence is the time of peak onset. The etiology of hyperthyroidism is unknown. The presence of abnormal thyroid-stimulating substances and their relation with the hypothalamus has led to speculation that these substances play a role in the production of hyperthyroidism. Clinically, hyperthyroidism occurs most commonly in females in a ratio of four to one. There is a high familial predisposition to thyroid disease. In addition, hyperthyroidism often follows severe physical or psychic stress.

Hyperthyroidism begins insidiously with a predominance of central nervous system symptoms. These symptoms include nervousness, irritability, emotional lability, fatigability, and deterioration of school performance. The earliest signs include an enlarged thyroid gland, tachycardia, and prominence of the eyes resulting in a staring appearance.

Thyrotoxic myopathy may merely increase fatigability or loss of stamina, or the patient may show severe weakness, with difficulty climbing stairs and rising from a chair. The severity of the weakness depends on the duration of the hyperthyroidism.

Examination reveals proximal weakness, involving especially the muscles of the shoulders and hips. In long-standing disease, there may be weakness of distal muscles. The proximal distribution of weakness generally remains confined to muscles of the trunk and extremities but may occasionally involve the bulbar muscles. The patient exhibits a fine tremor of the outstretched hands and tongue, so severe at times as to resemble chorea. There may be striking wasting and atrophy of muscles, especially about the shoulder girdle. The tendon reflexes are brisk. The active tendon reflexes constitute an unusual feature of this type of myopathy in contrast with most other myopathies, which are associated with either decreased or absent reflexes.

Serum CPK activity may be elevated. Electromyography (Ramsay, 1968) reveals myopathic potentials characterized by decreased duration of the action potential and an increase in polyphasic potentials. Muscle biopsy has often shown normal histologic appearance. When changes occur in the muscle fibers, they consist merely of an increase in sarcolemmal nuclei, muscle fiber degeneration, and an increase in fat between muscle fibers. Electron microscopic studies by Engel (1966a) have shown abnormal mitochondria. focal dilatation of the transverse tubular system, and slender projections on the surface of the muscle fiber.

The basic mechanism responsible for thyrotoxic myopathy is unknown. The thyroid hormone has a prominent effect on the mitochondrial membrane. These organelles are important in the production of high-energy bonds, and alteration in the mitochondria could reasonably be expected to lead to the clinical symptom of weakness. Thyroid hormone also affects phosphocreatine and cellular potassium. Electron microscopic studies have shown the alteration of transverse tubular systems, which may interfere with the contraction mechanism of the muscle fiber. The observation that the weakness disappears with the treatment of the hyperthyroidism suggests that the myopathy is predominantly metabolic in nature, and that the structural alterations seen, at least at some stage of the disease, are reversible.

### Hypothyroid myopathy

Weakness, slowness of muscular contraction and relaxation, and generalized hypotonia occur in the infant with cretinism and in the older child with myxedema (Wilkins, 1957). These symptoms and signs of muscular involvement from hypothyroidism are generally reversible by treatment with thyroid hormone.

The infant with congenital hypothyroidism or cretinism is generally normal at birth, unless there is evidence of maternal thyroid deficiency. However, in the ensuing weeks and months, a characteristic clinical picture emerges. The infant has poor feeding, poor weight gain, and slow growth and development. The infant is apathetic, lethargic, has a hoarse cry, and often has marked constipation.

In the hypothyroid infant, the diagnosis is generally suspected from the examination.

The skin is pale, dry, and mottled. The hair is sparse over the scalp and eyebrows. The forehead is often wrinkled. The tongue is thick and protruding. The supraclavicular and axillary fat pads are prominent. The bridge of the nose is flat and widened. The abdomen is protuberant, and an umbilical hernia is often present. The infant exhibits hypotonia with normal or depressed tendon reflexes. The relaxation phase of the tendon reflex is prolonged.

A rare combination of muscular hypertrophy with the signs of hypothyroidism has been described in infants (Debré-Sémélaigne syndrome) (Debré and Sémélaigne, 1935; Spiro et al., 1970a; Najjar, 1974). The muscles of the extremities appear large, creating a false impression of increased strength in contrast to the obvious clinical weakness. The muscles are firm to palpation, but muscular movements are slow, both in contraction and relaxation. The facial muscles may be enlarged. There is often increased stiffness on passive movement of the extremities. Percussion myotonia is not seen. The serum CPK, LDH, and SGOT activity are elevated. Bone age is retarded.

Electromyography reveals normal action potentials with no myotonic discharges (Norris and Panner, 1966). Muscle biopsy studies show only rare muscle fiber degeneration with light microscopy. Electron microscopic studies in an adult patient reveal scattered areas of increased sarcolemmal nuclei, central nuclei, and mitochondrial alterations.

The diagnosis may be suspected from the clinical manifestations and confirmed by a low serum thyroxin ($T_4$) and $T_3$ resin uptake with a resultant low thyroid index. The thyroid stimulating hormone (TSH) concentration is usually elevated.

The weakness, hypotonia, altered tendon reflexes, and muscular hypertrophy when present disappear with treatment of the hypothyroidism.

The differential diagnosis of muscular hypertrophy must include myotonia congenita, late infantile acid maltase deficiency, Duchenne muscular dystrophy, and adreno-cortical hyperplasia. Hypothyroidism is generally excluded in these diseases by the lack of the characteristic findings of thyroid deficiency.

## MYOPATHIES ASSOCIATED WITH MYOGLOBINURIA

Myoglobinuria signals a condition of diverse etiology that is characterized by sudden onset of muscle pain and weakness, followed by passage of dark brown urine, a result of the excretion of the muscle protein myoglobin (Rowland and Penn, 1972; Robotham and Haddow, 1976). Myoglobin is an iron-containing protein that can release oxygen during muscle contraction.

The presence of myoglobinuria indicates only an alteration in muscle membrane permeability. Although the basic mechanism for the appearance of myoglobinuria is unknown, it is assumed that an acute, extensive injury or disease to skeletal muscle disrupts the sarcolemmal membrane and leads to the entry of myoglobin and muscle enzymes into the blood and to the subsequent urinary excretion of these substances.

Although there is no satisfactory classification of the etiologies of myoglobinuria, Table 7-5 presents some known causes. It should be emphasized that before the diagnosis of idiopathic myoglobinuria is made, the known causes should be sought. In general, a traumatic, vascular, or toxic-metabolic etiology will be readily apparent from the history. In cases where the etiology is obscure, a metabolic defect should be excluded.

A common denominator among the ischemic, anoxic, and metabolic causes of myoglobinuria has been suggested (Rowland et al., 1964). Patients have been described in whom the attack occurred under circumstances that might interfere with oxidative or glycolytic metabolism; such circumstances included the presence of diabetic acidosis (Rainey et al., 1963), barbiturate intoxication (Fahlgren, Hed, and Lundmark, 1957; Penn, Rowland, and Fraser, 1972), carbon monoxide poisoning (Jackson et al., 1959), hypokalemia secondary to regional enteritis,

**Table 7-5.** Myoglobinuria

Idiopathic
Metabolic
   Glycolytic enzyme deficiency
      Myophosphorylase deficiency (McArdle's disease)
      Phosphofructokinase deficiency
   Carnitine palmityl transferase absence
   Drug—barbiturate, narcotic
   Carbon monoxide poisoning
   Diabetic acidosis
   Hypokalemia—enteritis, licorice ingestion, familial periodic paralysis
   Haff disease—eel ingestion
   Sea snake bite poison
Traumatic
   Crush injury—weights, coma
   Burns
   Convulsions—electric shock, status epilepticus
   Severe exertion
   Malignant hyperthermia
Infection—systemic
Vascular
   Arterial occlusion

cortisone therapy (Heitzman, Patterson, and Stanley, 1962), and carnitine palmityl transferase absence (Bank et al., 1975).

There is often a striking relationship between exercise and the occurrence of myoglobinuria, and previous classifications have stressed the occurrence of exertional and nonexertional types of myoglobinuria. The patients studied by Korein and associates (1959) were equally divided into exertional and nonexertional groups. In the exertional group, there was a preponderance of males, of multiple attacks, and of onset in adolescence and young adulthood. In the nonexertional group, onset occurred at all ages but was clustered in the first decade of life; in addition, there was a preponderance of females in this group, and the myoglobinuria was more often associated with an antecedent infection. Although multiple attacks occurred less frequently in the nonexertional group, the muscle damage seen by biopsy was more severe, and the mortality rate was higher. As mentioned above, it is necessary to elim-

inate a biochemical abnormality in the patients in whom no obvious cause for the myoglobinuria is found.

There may be familial tendency in idiopathic myoglobinuria. Favara and associates (1967) have described a familial form of paroxysmal myoglobinuria in children. Although no specific metabolic disorder was uncovered, excessive phosphorylase activity was present in the skeletal muscle of one child and his mother, which suggests a genetically determined disease. There was no increase in glycogen within the muscle in this family. (For a discussion of myophosphorylase deficiency, see the section on glycogen storage disease.)

**CLINICAL FEATURES.** The clinical manifestations of myoglobinuria present a characteristic picture. The onset of an attack is abrupt and characterized by pain, tenderness, and weakness most often in the calf and thigh muscles. However, any muscles of the trunk or extremities may be involved. The patient often has difficulty walking, rising from a sitting position, or climbing stairs. The patient may pass dark brown urine several hours after the onset of pain and weakness.

Examination shortly after an attack reveals swollen, firm, tender muscles. There is mild to moderate weakness in the affected muscles. The tendon reflexes may be depressed. There is often limitation of motion as a result of pain and swelling. In addition to these clinical manifestations, systemic signs of fever, malaise, lethargy, chills, and abdominal pain are often present.

**PATHOPHYSIOLOGY.** Study of muscle removed during an acute attack shows extreme necrosis of muscle fibers without evidence of interstitial inflammatory reaction. The presence of inflammatory cells depends upon the time of the biopsy. Biopsies have been reported normal during an attack. Evidence of regeneration of muscle may be seen.

**LABORATORY FINDINGS.** The identification of the pigment excreted in the urine is of the utmost importance. Three pigments need to be considered, namely, hemoglobin, porphyrin, and myoglobin. The diagnosis can be made on the basis of simple laboratory examinations. The presence of a guaiac- or benzadine-positive pigment excludes porphyrin. If the serum is clear and the urine contains only a few red blood cells, the diagnosis of myoglobinuria is supported. A positive diagnosis of myoglobin can be made by spectrophotometric examination. Urine to be examined should be freshly collected, neutralized, and preferably examined immediately or refrigerated until the time of examination. Another laboratory test that differentiates hemoglobinuria is the measurement of the serum haptoglobin. The haptoglobin is generally normal in myoglobinuria, whereas after an episode of hemolysis, the bound haptoglobin must be regenerated, resulting in a low serum haptoglobin level. The erythrocyte sedimentation rate is often elevated.

Several other laboratory tests may show adnormalities, namely, the levels of the muscle enzymes LDH, CPK, and GOT, all of which are generally elevated during the course of an attack. Serum myoglobin levels may be predicted from the serum enzyme activity level (Olerud, Homer, and Carroll, 1975).

TREATMENT. The myoglobinuria generally lasts only a few days and usually patients recover normal function over a period of several weeks. Although myoglobinuria is a self-limiting process, serious complications may result. Renal tubular necrosis may lead to renal failure and death (Schaar, 1955). Another serious complication is respiratory failure from involvement of respiratory muscles. The renal failure has been treated by dietary restriction of fluids and potassium; at times, peritoneal dialysis has been necessary. Respiratory failure may require a tracheotomy and artificial respiration.

Cardiac arrhythmias may lead to cardiac arrest. These cardiovascular changes may result from the extensive release of potassium and phosphorus during muscle cell destruction. Serum calcium concentration may decrease because of deposition of calcium into the damaged muscle cell (Savage, Forbes, and Pearce, 1971). Serum electrolyte concentrations and electrocardiographic activity need to be monitored during the acute stage, especially if there is renal failure.

## CONGENITAL DEFECTS OF MUSCLE
### Congenital absence of muscle

Congenital absence of muscle is usually limited to one muscle or muscle group (Adams, 1975). Absence of certain muscles, particularly the palmaris longus, pyramidalis abdominis, and the plantaris muscles, does not cause any clinical difficulty. The defect is rarely bilateral. Of the muscles that are associated with clinical symptoms, the pectoralis muscle is the most frequently absent (Bing, 1902). The sternal portion of the pectoralis muscle is most commonly involved. The absence of pectoral muscles has been noted in association with certain cases of Duchenne muscular dystrophy and facioscapulohumeral dystrophy. After the pectoralis, the muscles that are most frequently absent and that cause clinical difficulties are the trapezius, serratus anterior, and quadratus femoris muscles (Horan et al., 1977; Carnevale et al., 1976; Haller, 1977).

Absence of the pectoral muscle may be associated with absence of the mammary glands and with presence of microdactyly and syndactyly.

Absence of the muscles of the abdomen has been reported on a number of occasions. Respiration and urination are greatly impaired. There may also be associated anatomic abnormalities of the urinary tract. Shortened life expectancy is frequently noted in these children.

### Congenital muscular torticollis

Congenital muscular torticollis (wryneck) is caused by unilateral shortening or contracture of the sternocleidomastoid muscle (Ling and Low, 1972). Experimental studies by Brooks (1922), in which he ligated the vein draining the sternocleidomastoid muscle but did not disturb the artery, resulted in changes that, over a period of time, produced fibrosis of the sternocleidomastoid muscle.

Forceps and breech presentations are relatively common in children with this deformity. The abnormal muscle may contain a palpable mass shortly after birth, which later shrinks and ostensibly leads to fibrosis. Pathologic studies reveal only that fibrous tissue has replaced the normal muscle architecture (Lidge, Bechtol, and Lambert, 1957).

Torticollis occurs more frequently in girls than boys. The shortening of the muscle results in a tilt of the head toward the same side and causes the chin to be turned to the opposite side.

If the condition is untreated, pronounced asymmetry of the head and face occurs with growth. Stretching the muscle with exercise often proves efficacious. If exercise is not successful or the patient is seen after he is a year or 2 old, the muscle is sectioned, usually at its distal insertion. Following surgery, stretching exercises are instituted after a short period and special head appliances are utilized to hold the head with the chin pointing toward the affected side (Tachdjian, 1967).

Torticollis, or more commonly unusual positions of the head in relation to the shoulders, may be caused by abnormalities of the atlas and occiput or by deformities of the cervical vertebrae. Torticollis may be acquired after infection or trauma to these bony parts, anterior horn cell involvement of the upper cervical area (such as that occurring in poliomyelitis), posterior fossa tumors, and strabismus. These conditions should be considered before the disease is characterized as congenital muscular torticollis.

### Congenital ptosis and defects in other muscles innervated by cranial nerves

Although congenital ptosis, or ptosis that becomes apparent in the first few months of life, may be associated with a number of different conditions (including Horner's syndrome, myasthenia gravis, myotonic dys-trophy, congenital paresis of cranial nerve III, congenital muscular dystrophy, and myotubular myopathy), there may be no apparent reason for the ptosis. On occasion, the levator may retract when the patient opens the jaw and relaxes when the jaw is closed. In some patients, the lid may open briefly as the jaw is closed, and in other patients, the lid may retract upon lateral movement of the jaw. These combinations of events are known as the "Marcus-Gunn" or "jaw-winking" phenomena. They are probably associated with a mixture of fibers of cranial nerves III and V, which causes a pattern of aberrant innervation of the levator.

Surgical treatment of ptosis is available to enable the patient to use the affected eye or eyes. Often epicanthal folds that restrict upward elevation of the eyelid are present. These contractures and restrictive abnormalities must be corrected before the ptosis is repaired. At times, exercise alone will strengthen the levators significantly after these folds are surgically corrected.

Shortening of the levators is best carried out between 2 and 3 years of age. The removed portion of the muscle should be scrutinized carefully for histologic abnormalities. If no levator strength is present, operations utilizing fascia lata to form a frontalis sling are sometimes beneficial.

Of special interest is congenital absence of the pterygoid and masseter muscles. Ford (1966) reports that in this condition the mandible is narrow. When the patient closes the mouth so that his molars touch, a wide gap between his upper and lower incisors still exists. Mild paresis of the bulbar muscles may also be present.

Another congenital condition involving muscles innervated by cranial nerves is congenital facial diplegia. The infant usually has bilateral involvement of muscles innervated by cranial nerve VII, which leads to inability to close the eyes during sleep and immobile facies during crying. Loss of subcutaneous tissue often occurs in the involved areas, and the skin cannot be moved freely. There is little wrinkling as compared to acquired cranial nerve VII paresis. The degree of weakness may not be complete, and infrequently it may involve only one side of the face or only the upper or lower portions of the face. Associated deformities of the ears, feet, and hands or absence of the pectoral muscles may be seen. Facial diplegia may be found associated with paralysis of one or both lateral rectus muscles (Möbius' syndrome, see Chapter 3).

The etiology of this difficulty is unknown, and indeed it is not known whether it is primarily neural or myopathic in origin. Familial incidence has been reported. Failure of the development of the involved cranial nerve nuclei has been supported by some pathologic evidence (Richter, 1960). This syndrome may be a part of progressive ocular dystrophy.

### Sprengel's deformity (congenital high scapula)

Sprengel's deformity is a congenital abnormality in which the scapula is abnormally high and rotated as a result of a developmental error.

In the third fetal month, the scapula usually descends from the cervical area to its normal position. Failure of this migration leads to the abnormality. The abnormal scapula is usually small and malformed to match the contour of the upper thorax. It is reduced in height, and its transverse dimension is increased beyond normal. It is usually attached to the vertebrae by means of bone, cartilage, or a fibrous band. The connection is usually from the superior angle of the scapula to the transverse process or spinous process of one of the lower cervical vertebrae. The inferior angle of the scapula is rotated to bring it toward the vertebral column.

Clinically, there is obvious asymmetry with elevation and lack of abduction of the shoulder. Other associated congenital abnormalities are often present, including scoliosis, cervical ribs, fusion of ribs, fusion of vertebrae, hemivertebrae, and Klippel-Feil syndrome. The inferior portion of the trapezius muscle is frequently absent. There is occasional fibrosis of the rhomboid muscles and hypoplasia and weakness of the serratus anterior muscles.

Early therapy consisting of passive and active motion is helpful. Surgical therapy in which the scapula is freed, placed in normal position, and held there by wire traction is recommended. The muscles that are sectioned to permit this maneuver are then reattached to the scapula to help fix it in position. Surgery is usually carried out between 4 and 7 years of age (Ross and Cruess, 1977).

### Congenital clubfoot

Clubfoot appears in the form of a number of abnormal positions of the feet. The word "talipes" is a generic term for congenital deformities of the foot. The most common deformity is that of talipes equinovarus, in which there is plantar flexion of the foot along with adduction and inversion. The combination of dorsiflexion of the foot accompanied by adduction and inversion is known as "talipes calcaneovarus." If the foot is in a position of abduction and eversion, the condition is known as talipes valgus.

Talipes equinovarus is more common in boys than girls by a two to one ratio. The deformity may be very mild, or it may be so severe that the toes almost touch the medial portion of the leg. The condition may be unilateral or bilateral. The congenital deformity does not relent when manual attempts to place the foot into normal positions are made. The abnormal position becomes more pronounced with growth. The gastrocnemius, soleus, and posterior tibial muscles are shortened.

The etiology of clubfoot is unknown (Lichtblau, 1972). A few cases have been convincingly explained on the basis of cord lesions. However, the vast majority of cases are unexplained. Vander Eecken and associates (1962) noted a marked decrease in the average diameter of fibers of the peroneal and anterior tibial muscles in two 25- to 30-week-old fetuses. Muscles that favor the maintenance of the abnormal position had normal fiber diameter, while the fibers of the peroneal and anterior tibial muscles were statistically smaller in diameter. Whether this discrepancy is primary or secondary to other factors is not known.

Irani and Sherman (1963, 1972) studied eleven fetal equinovarus foot deformities. Their studies led them to believe that congenital medial deviation of the anterior portion of the talus is the fundamental defect.

Most cases are nonfamilial. Palmer (1964) concluded from a study of 108 unrelated families that a positive family history will produce a chance of one in ten that subsequent children will have talipes equinovarus.

Early therapy is important to success and should begin in the first days of life. The foot should be manipulated into position regularly, and after a few days, a cast should be applied from the toes to the upper leg. The casts are changed frequently to accommodate growth. If conservative therapy of this type is unsuccessful, surgical intervention is necessary (Shaw, 1977; Bleck, 1977).

## REFERENCES

Adams, R. D.: Congenital neuromuscular disease. In Adams, R. D., editor: Diseases of muscle: a study in pathology, Hagerstown, Md., 1975, Harper & Row, Publishers, p. 230.

Afifi, A. K., Smith, J. W., and Zellweger, H.: Congenital non-progressive myopathy: central core disease and nemaline myopathy in one family, Neurology **15:** 371, 1965.

Anderson, D. H.: Familial cirrhosis of the liver with storage of abnormal glycogen, Lab. Invest. **5:**11, 1956.

Angelini, C.: Lipid storage myopathies—review of metabolic defect and of treatment, J. Neurol. **214:**1, 1976.

Angelini, C., and Engel, A.: Comparative study of acid maltase deficiency, Arch. Neurol. **26:**344, 1972.

Araoz, C., et al.: Glycogenosis type II (Pompe's disease): ultrastructure of peripheral nerves, Neurology **24:**739, 1974.

Arts, W. F., et al.: Investigations on the inheritance of nemaline myopathy, Arch. Neurol. **35:**72, 1978.

Askanas, V., et al.: Adult-onset maltase deficiency: morphologic and biochemical abnormalities reproduced in cultured muscle, N. Engl. J. Med. **294:**573, 1976.

Awad, E. A., Swaiman, K. F., and Kottke, F. J.: Changes in the structure, innervation, electromyographic patterns and enzymes of skeletal muscle resulting from experimental treatment with triamcinolone, Arch. Phys. Med. Rehabil. **46:**297, 1965.

Bank, W., DiMauro, S., and Rowland, L.: Renal failure in McArdle's disease, N. Engl. J. Med. **287:**1102, 1972.

Bank, W. J., et al.: A disorder of muscle lipid metabolism and myoglobinuria: absence of carnitine palmityl transferase, N. Engl. J. Med. **292:**443, 1975.

Barchi, R.: Myotonia: an evaluation of the chloride hypothesis, Arch. Neurol. **32:**175, 1975.

Becker, P. E.: Generalized non-dystrophic myotonia. In Desmedt, J. E., editor: New developments in electromyography and clinical neurophysiology, Basel, 1973, S. Karger, p. 407, vol. 1.

Bethlem, J., et al.: Neuromuscular disease with type I fiber atrophy, central nuclei and myotube-like structures, Neurology **19:**705, 1969.

Bing, R.: Ueber angeborene muskeldefecte, Virchows Arch. Pathol. Anat. **170:**175, 1902.

Bischoff, A., and Esslen, E.: Myopathy with primary hyperparathyroidism, Neurology **15:**64, 1965.

Bjernulf, A., et al.: Primary hyperparathyroidism in children: brief review of the literature and a case report, Acta Paediatr. Scand. **59:**249, 1970.

Blass, J. P., Kark, R. A. P., and Engel, W. K.: Clinical studies of a patient with pyruvate decarboxylase deficiency, Arch. Neurol. **25:**449, 1971.

Bleck, E. E.: Congenital clubfoot: pathomechanics. Radiographic analysis and results of surgical treatment, Clin. Orthop. **125:**119, 1977.

Bonnette, H., Roelofs, R., and Olson, W. H.: Multicore disease: report of a case with onset in middle age, Neurology (Minneap.) **24:**1039, 1974.

Bradley, W. G., Price, D. L., and Watanabe, C. K.: Familial centronuclear myopathy, J. Neurol. Neurosurg. Psychiatry **33:**687, 1970.

Brandt, I. K., and DeLuca, V. A., Jr.: Type III glycogenosis: a family with an unusual tissue distribution of the enzyme lesion, Am. J. Med. **40**(5):779, 1966.

Brody, I., Gerberg, C., and Sidbury, J., Jr.: Relaxing factor in McArdle's disease, Neurology **20:**555, 1970.

Brombacher, P. J., et al.: A report on two adult patients with glycogen storage disease, Acta Med. Scand. **176:** 269, 1964.

Brooke, M. H.: Congenital fiber-type disproportion. In Kakulas, B. A., editor: Clinical studies in myology, Amsterdam, 1973, Excerpta Medica.

Brooke, M. H., and Engel, W. K.: The histolographic analysis of human muscle biopsies with regard to fiber type, Neurology **19:**221, 1969.

Brooke, M. H., and Neville, H. E.: Reducing body myopathy, Neurology **22:**829, 1972.

Brooks, B.: Pathological changes in muscle as a result of disturbance of circulation, Arch. Surg. **5:**188, 1922.

Brooks, J. E.: Hyperkalemic periodic paralysis: intracellular electromyographic studies, Arch. Neurol. **20:** 13, 1969.

Brunberg, J. A., McCormick, W. F., and Schochet, S. S., Jr.: Type III glycogenosis: an adult with diffuse weakness and muscle wasting, Arch. Neurol. **25:** 171, 1971.

Buchthal, F., Engbaek, L., and Gamstorp, I.: Paresis and hyperexcitability in adynamia episodica hereditaria, Neurology **8:**347, 1958.

Burke, D., Skuse, N. F., and Lethlean, A. H.: Contractile properties of the abductor digiti minimi muscle in paramyotonia congenita, J. Neurol. Neurosurg. Psychiatry **37:**894, 1974.

Buruma, O., and Bots, G.: Myopathy in familial hypokalemic periodic paralysis independent of paralytic attacks, Acta Neurol. Scand. **57:**171, 1978.

Butterworth, J., and Broadhead, D.: Diagnosis of Pompe's disease in cultured skin fibroblasts and primary amniotic fluid cells using 4-methylumbelliferyl-alpha-D-glucopyranoside as substrate, Clin. Chim. Acta **78:**335, 1977.

Byers, R. K., Bergman, A. B., and Joseph, M. C.: Steroid myopathy, Pediatrics **29:**26, 1962.

Campa, J. F., and Sanders, D. B.: Familial hypokalemic periodic paralysis: local recovery after nerve stimulation, Arch. Neurol. **31:**110, 1974.

Campbell, M. J., Rebetz, J. J., and Walton, J. N.: Myotubular, centronuclear or peri-centronuclear myopathy? J. Neurol. Sci. **8:**425, 1969.

Cancilla, P. A., et al.: Familial myopathy with probable lysis of myofibrils in type I fibers, Neurology **21:**579, 1971.

Carnevale, A., et al.: Congenital absence of gluteal muscles: report of 2 sibs, Clin. Genet. **10:**135, 1976.

Carpenter, S., et al.: Childhood dermatomyositis and familial collagen disease, Neurology **22:**425, 1972.

Celesia, G. G., et al.: Monomelic myopathy: congenital hypertrophic myotonic myopathy limited to one extremity, Arch. Neurol. **17:**69, 1967.

Chou, S. M.: Myxovirus-like structures in a case of human chronic polymyositis, Science **158:**1453, 1967.

Coërs, C., et al.: Changes in motor innervation and histochemical pattern of muscle fibers in some congenital myopathies, Neurology **26:**1046, 1976.

Cohn, J., et al.: Amylo-1,6-glucosidase deficiency (glycogenosis type III) in the Faroe Islands, Hum. Hered. **25:**115, 1975.

Coleman, R. F., et al.: New myopathy with mitochondrial enzyme hyperactivity, J.A.M.A. **199:**624, 1967.

Coleman, R. F., et al.: Histochemical investigation of "myotubular" myopathy, Arch. Pathol. **86:**365, 1968.

Conen, P. E., Murphy, E. G., and Donohue, W. L.: Light and electron microscopic studies of "myogranules" in a child with hypotonia and muscle weakness, Can. Med. Assoc. J. **89:**983, 1963.

Conn, J. W.: Primary aldosteronism, a new clinical syndrome, J. Lab. Clin. Med. **45:**6, 1955.

Conn, J. W., Rovner, D. R., and Cohen, E. L.: Lico-rice-induced pseudoaldosteronism, J.A.M.A. **205:** 492, 1968.

Coppola, A., Munoz, A., and Sher, J.: Morphologic changes of lymphocytes in Pompe disease, J. Pediatr. **93:**824, 1978.

Creutzfeldt, O. D., et al.: Muscle membrane potentials in episodic adynamia, Electroencephalogr. Clin. Neurophysiol. **15:**508, 1963.

Crews, J., Kaiser, K., and Brooke, M. H.: Muscle pathology of myotonia congenita, J. Neurol. Sci. **28:**449, 1976.

Curless, R. G., and Nelson, M. B.: Congenital fiber type disproportion in identical twins, Ann. Neurol. **2:**455, 1977.

Cushing, H.: Basophilic adenomas of the pituitary body and their clinical manifestations, Bull. Johns Hopkins Hosp. **50:**137, 1932.

D'Agostino, A. N., et al.: Familial myopathy with abnormal muscle mitochondria, Arch. Neurol. **18:**388, 1968.

Dahl, D. S., and Klutzow, F. W.: Congenital rod disease: further evidence of innervational abnormalities as the basis for the clinicopathologic features, J. Neurol. Sci. **23:**371, 1974.

Debré, R., and Sémélaigne, G.: Syndrome of diffuse muscular hypertrophy in infants causing athletic appearance, Am. J. Dis. Child. **50:**1351, 1935.

Deckelbaum, R., et al.: Type III glycogenosis: atypical enzyme activities in blood cells in two siblings, J. Pediatr. **81:**955, 1972.

DeJesus, P. V.: Neuromuscular physiology in Luft's syndrome, Electromyogr. Clin. Neurophysiol. **14:**17, 1974.

Denborough, M. A., Dennett, X., and Anderson, R. M. D.: Central core disease and malignant hyperpyrexia, Br. Med. J. **1:**272, 1973.

DiDonato, S., et al.: Mitochondria-lipid-glycogen myopathy, hyperlactacidemia, and carnitine deficiency, Neurology **28:**1110, 1978.

DiMauro, S., and DiMauro, P. M. M.: Muscle carnitine palmityltransferase deficiency and myoglobinuria, Science **182:**929, 1973.

DiMauro, S., et al.: Progressive ophthalmoplegia, glycogen storage and abnormal mitochondria, Arch. Neurol. **29:**170, 1973.

DiMauro, S., et al.: Luft's disease: further biochemical and ultrastructural studies in the second case, J. Neurol. Sci. **27:**217, 1976.

Donner, M., Rapola, J., and Somer, H.: Congenital muscular dystrophy: a clinico-pathological and follow-up study of 15 patients, Neuropädiatrie **6:**239, 1975.

Drager, G. A., Hammill, J. F., and Shy, G. M.: Paramyotonia congenita, Arch. Neurol. Psychiatry **80:**1, 1958.

Dubowitz, V.: Treatment of dermatomyositis in childhood, Arch. Dis. Child. **51:**494, 1976.

Dubowitz, V., and Brooke, M. H.: Muscle biopsy: a modern approach, Philadelphia, 1973, W. B. Saunders Co., p. 78.

Dubowitz, V., and Pearse, A. G. E.: Oxidative enzymes and phosphorylase in central core disease of muscle, Lancet **2:**23, 1960.

Ellis, F. R., et al.: Screening for malignant hyperpyrexia, Br. Med. J. **3:**559, 1972.

Engel, A. G.: Thyroid function and periodic paralysis, Am. J. Med. **30:**327, 1961.

Engel, A. G.: Electron microscopic observations in thyrotoxic and corticosteroid-induced myopathies, Mayo Clin. Proc. **41:**785, 1966a.

Engel, A. G.: Late onset rod myopathy, Mayo Clin. Proc. **41:**713, 1966b.

Engel, A. G., and Angelini, C.: Carnitine deficiency of human skeletal muscle with associated lipid storage myopathy: a new syndrome, Science **173:**899, 1973.

Engel, A. G., and Dale, A. J.: Glycogenosis of late onset with mitochondrial abnormalities, Proc. Staff Mayo Clin. **43:**233, 1968.

Engel, A. G., and Gomez, M. R.: Congenital myopathy associated with multifocal degeneration of muscle fibers, Trans. Assoc. **91:**222, 1966.

Engel, A. G., and Siekert, R. G.: Lipid storage myopathy responsive to prednisone, Arch. Neurol. **27:**174, 1972.

Engel, A. G., Angelini, C., and Gomez, M. R.: Fingerprint body myopathy: a newly recognized congenital muscle disease, Mayo Clin. Proc. **47:**377, 1972.

Engel, A. G., Banker, B. Q., and Eiben, R. M.: Carnitine deficiency: clinical, morphological, and biochemical observations in a fatal case. J. Neurol. Neurosurg. Psychiatry **40:**313, 1977.

Engel, A. G., Gomez, M. R., and Groover, R. V.: Multicore disease: a recently recognized congenital myopathy associated with multifocal degeneration of muscle fibers, Mayo Clin. Proc. **46:**666, 1971.

Engel, A. G., et al.: Clinical and electromyographic studies in a patient with primary hypokalemic periodic paralysis, Am. J. Med. **38:**626, 1965.

Engel, A. G. et al.: The spectrum and diagnosis of acid maltase deficiency, Neurology **23:**95, 1973.

Engel, G. D., et al.: Malignant hyperthermia and central core disease in a child with congenital dislocating hips—case presentation and review, Arch. Neurol. **35:**189, 1978.

Engel, W. K., Gold, G. N., and Karpati, G.: Type I fiber hypotrophy and central nuclei: a rare congenital muscle abnormality with a possible experimental model, Arch. Neurol. **18:**435, 1968.

Engel, W. K., Wanko, T., and Fenichel, G. M.: Nemaline myopathy: a second case, Arch. Neurol. **11:**22, 1964.

Engel, W. K., et al.: Central core disease—an investigation of a rare muscle cell abnormality, Brain **84:**167, 1961.

Engel, W. K., et al.: A skeletal-muscle disorder associated with intermittent symptoms and a possible defect of lipid metabolism, N. Engl. J. Med. **282:**697, 1970.

Evans, B. M., and Milne, M. D.: Potassium-losing nephritis presenting as a case of periodic paralysis, Br. Med. J. **2:**1067, 1954.

Fahlgren, H., Hed, R., and Lundmark, C.: Myonecrosis and myoglobinuria in alcohol and barbiturate intoxication, Acta Med. Scand. **158:**405, 1957.

Favara, B. E., et al.: Familial paroxysmal rhabdomyolysis in children, Am. J. Med. **42:**196, 1967.

Fernandes, J., and Huijing, F.: Branching enzyme-deficiency glycogenosis: studies in therapy, Arch. Dis. Child. **43:**347, 1968.

Fernandes, J., and van de Kamer, J. H.: Hexose and protein tolerance tests in children with liver glycogenosis caused by a deficiency of the debranching enzyme system, Pediatrics **41:**935, 1968.

Fishbein, W. N., Armbrustmacher, V. W., and Griffin, J. L.: Myoadenylate deaminase deficiency: a new disease of muscle, Science **200:**545, 1978.

Forbes, G. B.: Glycogen storage disease: report of a case with abnormal glycogen structure in liver and skeletal muscle, J. Pediatr. **42:**645, 1953.

Ford, F. R.: Diseases of the nervous system: in infancy, childhood and adolescence, ed. 5, Springfield, 1966, Charles C Thomas, Publisher, p. 54.

Frame, B., et al.: Myopathy in primary hyperparathyroidism, Ann. Intern. Med. **68:**1022, 1968.

Fujimoto, A., et al.: The change of the pH 4 and pH 6 forms of alpha-glucosidase in cultured amniotic fluid cells and its implication in prenatal diagnosis of Pompe's disease. Clin. Chim. Acta **90:**157, 1978.

Gamstorp, I.: Adynamia episodica hereditaria, Acta Paediatr. [Suppl.] (Uppsala) **108:**1, 1956.

Gibson, W., Brown, B., and Brown, D.: Studies of glycogen branching enzyme: preparation and properties of $\alpha$-1,4-glucan-$\alpha$-1,4-glucan 6-glycosyltransferase and its action on the characteristic polysaccharide of the liver of children with type IV glycogen storage disease, Biochemistry **10:**4253, 1971.

Gillette, P. C., Nihill, M. R., and Singer, D. B.: Electrophysiological mechanism of the short PR interval in Pompe disease, Am. J. Dis. Child. **128:**622, 1974.

Gonatas, N. K., Shy, G. M., and Godfrey, E. H.: Nemaline myopathy: the origin of nemaline structures, N. Engl. J. Med. **274:**535, 1966.

Gonatas, N. K., et al.: Central "core" disease of skeletal muscle: ultrastructural and cytochemical observations in two cases, Am. J. Pathol. **47:**503, 1965.

Goutieres, F., and Aicardi, J.: Glycogénose par deficit en amylo-1,6-glucosidase associée à un trouble de l'hormonosynthèse thyroidienne, Arch. Fr. Pediatr. **28:**699, 1971.

Greenfield, J. G., Corman, T., and Shy, G. M.: The prognostic value of the muscle biopsy in the "floppy infant," Brain **81:**461, 1958.

Gruener, R., et al.: Contracture of phosphorylase deficient muscle, J. Neurol. Neurosurg. Psychiatry **31:**268, 1968.

Gutmann, L., Hogan, G., and Schmidt, R.: Electromyography and histology of Pompe's disease, Bull. Am. Assoc. EMG Electrodiag. **14:**13, 1967.

Haller, P.: Hereditary abductor-opponens agenesis: report of a family with congenital muscle defects of the thenar eminence, J. Neurol. **214:**235, 1977.

Hart, Z. H., et al.: Familial poliodystrophy, mitochondrial myopathy, and lactate acidemia, Arch. Neurol. **34:**180, 1977.

Hart, Z. H., et al.: Muscle carnitine deficiency and fatal cardiomyopathy, Neurology **28:**147, 1978.

Haydar, N. A., et al.: Severe hypermetabolism with primary abnormality of skeletal muscle mitochondria: functional and therapeutic effects of chloramphenicol treatment, Ann. Intern. Med. **74:**548, 1971.

Heffernan, L. P., Rewcastle, M. B., and Humphrey, J. G.: The spectrum of rod myopathies, Arch. Neurol. **18:**529, 1968.

Heffner, R., et al.: Multicore disease in twins, J. Neurol. Neurosurg. Psychiatry **39:**602, 1976.

Heitzman, E. J., Patterson, J. F., and Stanley, M. M.: Myoglobinuria and hypokalemia in regional enteritis, Arch. Intern. Med. **110:**117, 1962.

Henson, R. A.: The neurologic aspects of hypercalcemia: with special reference to primary hyperparathyroidism, J. Roy. Coll. Physicians Lond. **1:**41, 1966.

Hers, H. G.: Études enzymatique sur fragments hepatiques: application á la classification des glycogénoses, Rev. Int. Hepatol. **9:**35, 1959.

Hers, H. G.: α-Glucosidase deficiency in generalized glycogen storage disease (Pompe's disease), Biochem. J. **86:**11, 1963.

Hogan, G. R., et al.: Pompe's disease, Neurology **19:**894, 1969.

Holleman, L. W. J., van der Haar, J. A., and de Vaan, G. A. M.: Type IV glycogenosis, Lab. Invest. **15:**357, 1966.

Hopkins, I. J., Lindsey, J. R., and Ford, F. R.: Nemaline myopathy—a long term clinicopathologic study of affected mother and daughter, Brain **89:**299, 1966.

Horan, F. T., et al.: Bilateral absence of the trapezius and sternal head of the pectoralis major muscle: a case report, J. Bone Joint Surg. **59A:**133, 1977.

Hoskins, B., Vroom, F., and Jarrell, M. A.: Hyperkalemic periodic paralysis, Arch. Neurol. **32:**519, 1975.

Hoskins, B., et al.: Acetazolamide and potassium flux in red blood cells, Arch. Neurol. **31:**187, 1974.

Hostetler, K. Y., et al.: Partial deficiency of muscle carnitine palmitoyltransferase with normal ketone production, N. Engl. J. Med. **298:**553, 1978.

Howell, R., Kaback, M., and Brown, B.: Type IV glycogen storage disease: branching enzyme deficiency in skin fibroblasts and possible heterozygote detection, J. Pediatr. **78:**638, 1971.

Howes, E. L., et al.: Hypokalemic periodic paralysis, electromicroscopic changes in the sarcoplasm, Neurology **16:**242, 1966.

Hudgson, P., and Fulthorpe, J. J.: The pathology of type II skeletal muscle glycogenosis: a light and electronmicroscopic study, J. Pathol. **116:**39, 1975.

Hug, G.: Enzyme therapy and prenatal diagnosis in glycogenosis type II, Am. J. Dis. Child. **128:**614, 1974.

Hulsmann, W. C., et al.: Myopathy with abnormal structure and function of muscle mitochondria, J. Neurol. Neurosurg. Psychiatry **30:**519, 1967.

Inokuchi, T., Umezaki, H., and Santa, T.: A case of type I muscle fibre hypotrophy and internal nuclei, J. Neurol. Neurosurg. Psychiatry **38:**475, 1975.

Ionasescu, V., et al.: Biochemical abnormalities of muscle ribosomes during attacks of hyperkalemic periodic paralysis, J. Neurol. Sci. **19:**389, 1973.

Irani, R. N., and Sherman, M. S.: The pathologic anatomy of clubfoot, J. Bone Joint Surg. **45A:**45, 1963.

Irani, R. N., and Sherman, M. S.: The pathological anatomy of idiopathic clubfoot, Clin. Orthop. **84:**14, 1972.

Isaacs, H., and Barlow, M. B.: Central core disease associated with elevated creatine phosphokinase levels: two members of a family known to be susceptible to malignant hyperpyrexia, S. Afr. Med. J. **48:**640, 1974.

Isaacs, H., Heffron, J. J. A., and Badenhorst, M.: Central core disease: a correlated genetic histochemical, ultramicroscopic, and biochemical study, J. Neurol. Neurosurg. Psychiatry **38:**1177, 1975.

Isaacs, H., et al.: Weakness associated with the pathological presence of lipid in skeletal muscle: a detailed study of a patient with carnitine deficiency, J. Neurol. Neurosurg. Psychiatry **39:**1114, 1976.

Jackson, R. C., et al.: Case of carbon monoxide poisoning with complications: successful treatment with artificial kidney, Br. Med. J. **2:**1130, 1959.

Jerusalem, F., Engel, A. G., and Gomez, M. R.: Sarcotubular myopathy: a newly recognized, benign, congenital, familial muscle disease, Neurology **23:**897, 1973.

Jerusalem, F., Spiess, H., and Baumgartner, G.: Lipid storage myopathy with normal carnitine levels, J. Neurol. Sci. **24:**273, 1975.

Kamieniecka, Z.: Myopathies with abnormal mitochondria, Acta Neurol. Scand. **55:**57, 1977.

Kamoshita, S., et al.: Congenital muscular dystrophy as a disease of the nervous system, Arch. Neurol. **33:**513, 1976.

Karpati, G., Carpenter, S., and Andermann, F.: A new concept of childhood nemaline myopathy, Arch. Neurol. **24:**291, 1971.

Karpati, G., Carpenter, S., and Nelson, R. F.: Type I muscle fibre atrophy and central nuclei, J. Neurol. Sci. **10:**489, 1970.

Karpati, G., et al.: Infantile myotonic dystrophy: histochemical and electron microscopic features in skeletal muscle, Neurology **23:**1066, 1973.

Karpati, G., et al.: The syndrome of systemic carnitine deficiency, Neurology **24:**16, 1975.

King, J. O., Denborough, M. A., and Zapf, P. W.: Inheritance of malignant hyperpyrexia, Lancet **1:**365, 1972.

Kinoshita, M., and Cadman, T. E.: Myotubular myopathy, Arch. Neurol. **18:**265, 1968.

Kinoshita, M., Satoyoshi, E., and Matsuo, N.: "Myotubular myopathy" and "type I fiber atrophy" in a family, J. Neurol. Sci. **26**:575, 1975.

Kolin, I.: Nemaline myopathy: a fatal case, Am. J. Dis. Child. **114**:95, 1967.

Korein, J., Coddon, D. R., and Mowrey, F. H.: Clinical syndrome of paroxysmal paralytic myoglobinuria, report of two cases and analytical review of literature, Neurology **9**:767, 1959.

Kretchmer, N., et al.: Primary aldosteronism in a nine year old child, Pediatrics **23**:1115, 1959.

Layzer, R. B., Lovelace, R. E., and Rowland, L. P.: Hyperkalemic periodic paralysis, Arch. Neurol. **16**:455, 1967.

Layzer, R. B., Rowland, L. P., and Ranney, H. M.: Muscle phosphofructokinase deficiency, Arch. Neurol. **17**:512, 1967.

Leathwood, P., and Ryman, B.: Enzymes of glycogen metabolism in human skin with particular reference to differential diagnosis of the glycogen storage disease, Clin. Sci. **40**:261, 1971.

Legum, C. P., and Nitowsky, H. M.: Studies on leukocyte brancher enzyme activity in a family with type IV glycogenosis, J. Pediatr. **74**:84, 1969.

Lenard, H. G., and Goebel, H. H.: Congenital fiber-type disproportion, Neuropaediatrie **6**:220, 1975.

Lichtblau, S.: Etiology of clubfoot, Clin. Orthop. **84**:21, 1972.

Lidge, R. T., Bechtol, R. C., and Lambert, C. N.: Congenital muscular torticollis: etiology and pathology, J. Bone Joint Surg. **39A**:1165, 1957.

Ling, C. M., and Low, Y. S.: Sternomastoid tumor and muscular torticollis, Clin. Orthop. **86**:144, 1972.

Lipicky, R., Bryant, S., and Salmon, J.: Cable parameters, sodium, potassium, chloride and water content, and potassium efflux in isolated external intercostal muscle of normal volunteers and patients with myotonia congenita, J. Clin. Invest. **50**:2091, 1971.

Luft, R., et al.: A case of severe hypermetabolism of non-thyroid origin with a defect in the maintenance of mitochondrial respiratory control: a correlated clinical, biochemical and morphological study, J. Clin. Invest. **41**:1776, 1962.

MacDonald, R. N., Rewcastle, N. B., and Humphrey, J. G.: The myopathy of hyperkalemic periodic paralysis, Arch. Neurol. **19**:274, 1968.

Magee, K. R.: A study of paramyotonia congenita, Arch. Neurol. **8**:461, 1963.

Magee, K. R., and DeJong, R. N.: Hereditary distal myopathy with onset in infancy, Arch. Neurol. **13**:387, 1965.

Markesbery, W. R., Griggs, R. C., and Herr, B.: Distal myopathy: electron microscopic and histochemical studies, Neurology **27**:727, 1977.

Martin, J. J., et al.: Is congenital fibre type disproportion a true myopathy? Acta Neurol. Belg. **76**:335, 1976.

McArdle, B.: Myopathy due to a defect in muscle glycogen breakdown, Clin. Sci. **10**:13, 1951.

McArdle, B.: Familial periodic paralysis, Br. Med. Bull. **12**:226, 1956.

McArdle, B.: Adynamia episodica hereditaria and its treatment, Brain **85**:121, 1962.

McClintock, J. C., Frawley, T. E., and Holden, J. H.: Hyperthyroidism in children: observations in 50 treated cases, including an evaluation of endocrine factors, J. Clin. Endocrinol. **16**:62, 1956.

McLeod, J. G., et al.: Centronuclear myopathy with autosomal dominant inheritance, J. Neurol. Sci. **15**:375, 1972.

Mehler, M., and DiMauro, S.: Late-onset acid maltase deficiency, Arch. Neurol. **33**:692, 1976.

Mercier, C., and Whelan, W.: The fine structure of glycogen from type IV glycogen-storage disease, Eur. J. Biochem. **16**:579, 1970.

Meyers, K. R., et al.: Familial neuromuscular disease with myotubes, Clin. Genet. **5**:327, 1974.

Miller, C., Alleyne, G., and Brooks, S.: Gross cardiac involvement in glycogen storage disease type III, Br. Heart J. **34**:862, 1972.

Mitchell, M. E.: Carnitine metabolism in human subjects. I. Normal metabolism, Am. J. Clin. Nutr. **31**:293, 1978.

Morgan-Hughes, J. A., et al.: A mitochondrial myopathy characterized by a deficiency in reducible cytochrome b, Brain **100**:617, 1977.

Müller, R., and Kugelberg, E.: Myopathy in Cushing's syndrome, J. Neurol. Neurosurg. Psychiatry **22**:314, 1959.

Munsat, T. L.: Therapy of myotonia, Neurology **17**:359, 1967.

Munsat, T. L., Thompson, L. R., and Coleman, R. F.: Centronuclear ("myotubular") myopathy, Arch. Neurol. **20**:120, 1969.

Najjar, S. S.: Muscular hypertrophy in hypothyroid children: the Kocher-Debré-Sémélaigne syndrome: a review of 23 cases, J. Pediatr. **85**(2):236, 1974.

Neustein, H. B.: Fine structure of skeletal muscle in tyep III glycogenesis, Arch. Pathol. **88**:130, 1969.

Neustein, H. B.: Nemaline myopathy: a family study with three autopsied cases, Arch. Pathol. **96**:192, 1973.

Neville, H. E., and Brooke, M. H.: Central core fibers; structured and unstructured. In Kakulas, B. A., editor: Basic research in myology, Amsterdam, 1973, Excerpta Medica.

Nienhuis, A. W., et al.: Nemaline myopathy: a histopathologic and histochemical study, Am. J. Clin. Pathol. **48**:1, 1967.

Norris, F. H., Jr., and Panner, B. J.: Hypothyroid myopathy, Arch. Neurol. **14**:574, 1966.

Norris, F. H., Jr., Clark, E. C., and Biglieri, E. G.: Studies in thyrotoxic periodic paralysis, J. Neurol. Sci. **13**:431, 1971.

Norris, F. H., Jr., Panner, B. J., and Stormont, J. M.: Thyrotoxic periodic paralysis, Arch. Neurol. **19**:88, 1968.

Odor, D. L., Patel, A. N., and Pearce, L. A.: Familial

hypokalemic periodic paralysis with permanent myopathy. J. Neuropathol. Exp. Neurol. **26**:98, 1967.

Olerud, J. E., Homer, L. D., and Carroll, H. W.: Serum myoglobin levels predicted from serum enzyme values, N. Engl. J. Med. **293**::483, 1975.

Olson, W., et al.: Oculocraniosomatic neuromuscular disease with "ragged-red" fibers, Arch. Neurol. **26**:193, 1972.

Palmer, R. M.: The genetics of talipes equinovarus, J. Bone Joint Surg. **46A**:542, 1964.

Patten, B. M., et al.: Neuromuscular disease in primary hyperparathyroidism, Ann. Intern. Med. **80**:182, 1974.

Pearson, C. M.: The periodic paralyses: differential features and pathological observations in permanent myopathic weakness, Brain **87**:341, 1964.

Pearson, C. M.: Glycogen metabolism and storage diseases of type III, IV and V, Am. J. Clin. Pathol. **50**:29, 1968.

Pearson, C. M., and Kalyaharaman, K.: The periodic paralyses. In Stanbury, J. B., Wyngaarden, J. B., and Fredrickson, D. S., editors: The metabolic basis of inherited disease, ed. 3, New York, 1972, The McGraw-Hill Book Co., p. 905.

Pearson, C. M., Rimer, D. G., and Mommaerts, W. F. H. M.: A metabolic myopathy due to absence of muscle phosphorylase, Am. J. Med. **30**:502, 1961.

Penn, A. S., Rowland, L. P., and Fraser, D. W.: Drugs, coma, and myoglobinuria, Arch. Neurol. **26**:336, 1972.

Perkoff, G. T., et al.: Studies in disorders of muscle: XII. Myopathy due to the administration of therapeutic amounts of 17-hydroxycorticosteroids, Am. J. Med. **26**:891, 1959.

Pompe, J. C.: Over idiopatische hypertrophy van het hart, Ned. Tijdschr. Geneeskd. **76**:304, 1932.

Poskanzer, D. C., and Kerr, D. N.: Periodic paralysis with response to spironolactone, Lancet **2**:511, 1961.

Price, H. M., et al.: New evidence for excessive accumulation of Z-band material in nemaline myopathy, Proc. Natl. Acad. Sci. U.S.A. **54**:1398, 1965.

Radu, H., et al.: Myotubular (centronuclear) (neuro-) myopathy. I. Clinical, genetical and morphological studies, Eur. Neurol. **15**:285, 1977.

Rainey, R. L., et al.: Myoglobinuria following diabetic acidosis, Arch. Intern. Med. **111**:564, 1963.

Ramsay, I.: Thyrotoxic muscle disease, Postgrad. Med. J. **44**:385, 1968.

Ramsay, I. D.: Electromyography in thyrotoxicosis, Q. J. Med. **34**:255, 1965.

Ratinov, G., Baker, W. P., and Swaiman, K. F.: McArdle's syndrome with previously unreported electrocardiographic and serum enzyme abnormalities, Ann. Intern. Med. **62**:328, 1965.

Resnick, J. S.: Episodic muscle weakness, Clin. Orthop. **39**:63, 1965.

Resnick, J. S., et al.: Acetazolamide prophylaxis in hypokalemic periodic paralysis, N. Engl. J. Med. **278**:582, 1968.

Richter, R. B.: Unilateral congenital hypoplasia of the facial nucleus, J. Neuropathol. Exp. Neurol. **19**:33, 1960.

Ritter, R. A., Jr.: Effect of cortisone on the structure and strength of skeletal muscle, Arch. Neurol. **17**:403, 1967.

Robotham, J. L., and Haddow, J. E.: Rhabdomyolysis and myoglobinuria in childhood, Pediatr. Clin. North Am. **23**:279, 1976.

Roelofs, R., Engel, W., and Chauvin, P.: Histochemical phosphorylase activity in regenerating muscle fibers from myophosphorylase-deficient patients, Science **177**:795, 1972.

Rosman, N. P.: Neurological and muscular aspects of thyroid dysfunction in childhood, Pediatr. Clin. North Am. **23**:575, 1976.

Ross, D. M., and Cruess, R. L.: The surgical correction of congenital elevation of the scapula: a review of seventy-seven cases, Clin. Orthop. **125**:17, 1977.

Rowland, L. P., and Penn, A. S.: Myoglobinuria, Med. Clin. North Am. **56**:1233, 1972.

Rowland, L. P., Fahn, S., and Schotland, D. L.: McArdle's disease, Arch. Neurol. **9**:325, 1963.

Rowland, L. P., et al.: Myoglobinuria, Arch. Neurol. **10**:537, 1964.

Ruttenberg, H. D., et al.: Glycogen-storage disease of the heart: hemodynamic and angiocardiographic features in 2 cases, Am. Heart J. **67**:469, 1964.

Sadeghi-Nejad, A., Loridan, L., and Senior, B.: Studies of factors affecting gluconeogenesis and glycolysis in glycogenoses of the liver, Pediatrics **76**:561, 1970.

Satoyoshi, E., and Kowa, H.: A myopathy due to glycolytic abnormality, Arch. Neurol. **17**:248, 1967.

Savage, D. C., Forbes, M., and Pearce, G. W.: Idiopathic rhabdomyolysis, Arch. Dis. Child. **46**:594, 1971.

Saxena, K. M., Crawford, J. D., and Talbot, N. B.: Childhood thyrotoxicosis: a long term perspective, Br. Med. J. **2**:1153, 1964.

Scarlato, G., Pellegrini, G., and Veicsteinas, A.: Morphologic and metabolic studies in a case of oculo-cranio-somatic neuromuscular disease, J. Neuropathol. Exp. Neurol. **37**:1, 1978.

Schaar, F. E.: Paroxysmal myoglobinuria, Am. J. Dis. Child. **89**:23, 1955.

Schmid, R., and Hammaker, L.: Hereditary absence of muscle phosphorylase (McArdle's syndrome), N. Engl. J. Med. **264**:223, 1961.

Schmid, R., and Mahler, R.: Chronic progressive myopathy with myoglobinuria: demonstration of a glycogenolytic defect in the muscle, J. Clin. Invest. **38**:2044, 1959.

Schneck, L., et al.: Ophthalmoplegia plus with morphological and chemical studies of cerebellar and muscle tissue, J. Neurol. Sci. **19**:37, 1973.

Schochet, S., Jr., McCormick, W., and Kovarsky, J.: Light and electron microscopy of skeletal muscle in type IV glycogenosis, Acta Neuropathol. (Berl.) **19**:13, 1971.

Schotland, D. L., et al.: Neuromuscular disorder associated with a defect in mitochondrial energy supply, Arch. Neurol. **33**:475, 1976.

Senior, B., and Loridan, L.: Functional differentiation of glycogenosis of the liver with respect to the use of glycerol, N. Engl. J. Med. **279**:965, 1968.

Shafiq, S. A., Milhorat, A. T., and Gorycki, M. A.: Fine structure of human muscle in neurogenic atrophy, Neurology **17**:934, 1967.

Shapira, Y., Harel, S., and Russell, A.: Mitochondrial encephalomyopathies: a group of neuromuscular disorders with defects in oxidative metabolism, Isr. J. Med. Sci. **13**:161, 1977.

Shapira, Y., et al.: Familial poliodystrophy, mitochondrial myopathy, and lactate acidemia, Neurology **25**:614, 1975.

Shaw, N. E.: Treatment and prognosis in clubfoot, Br. Med. J. **1**:219, 1977.

Sher, J. H., et al.: Familial centronuclear myopathy, Neurology **17**:727, 1967.

Shizume, K., et al.: Studies on electrolyte metabolism in idiopathic and thyrotoxic periodic paralysis. I. Arteriovenous differences of electrolytes during induced paralysis, Metabolism **15**:138, 1966.

Shy, G. M.: Chemical and morphological abnormalities in muscle disease, Ann. N.Y. Acad. Sci. **138**:232, 1966.

Shy, G. M., and Magee, K. R.: A new congenital nonprogressive myopathy, Brain **79**:610, 1956.

Shy, G. M., Gonatas, N. K., and Perez, M.: Two childhood myopathies with abnormal mitochondria 1. megaconial myopathy 2. pleoconial myopathy, Brain **89**:133, 1966.

Shy, G. M., et al.: Studies in familial periodic paralysis, Exp. Neurol. **3**:53, 1961.

Shy, G. M., et al.: Nemaline myopathy, a new congenital myopathy, Brain **89**:793, 1963.

Sidbury, J. B., Jr., et al.: Type IV glycogenosis: report of a case proven by characterization of glycogen and studied at necropsy, Johns Hopkins Med. J. **111**:157, 1962.

Smith, H., Amick, L. D., and Sidbury, J.: Type II glycogenosis, Am. J. Dis. Child. **11**:475, 1966.

Smith, J., Zellweger, H., and Afifi, A. K.: Muscular form of glycogenosis type II (Pompe): report of a case with unusual features, Neurology **17**:537, 1967.

Spiro, A. J., Shy, G. M., and Gonatas, N. K.: Myotubular myopathy: persistence of fetal muscle in an adolescent boy, Arch. Neurol. **14**:1, 1966.

Spiro, A. J., et al.: Cretinism with muscular hypertrophy (Kocher-Debré-Sémélaigne syndrome), Arch. Neurol. **23**:340, 1970a.

Spiro, A. J., et al.: A cytochrome-related inherited disorder of the nervous system and muscle, Arch. Neurol. **22**:259, 1970b.

Sreter, F. A., et al.: Characteristics of myosin in nemaline myopathy, J. Neurol. Sci. **27**:99, 1976.

Stern, L. F., et al. The fine structure of cortisone-induced myopathy, Exp. Neurol. **36**:530, 1972.

Stromer, M. H., et al.: Nemaline myopathy, an integrated study: selective extraction, Exp. Neurol. **50**:402, 1976.

Swaiman, K. F., Kennedy, W. R., and Sauls, H. S.: Late infantile acid maltase deficiency, Arch. Neurol. **18**:642, 1968.

Tachdjian, M. O.: Diagnosis and treatment of congenital deformities of the musculoskeletal system in the newborn and the infant, Pediatr. Clin. North Am. **14**:307, 1967.

Tamura, K., Santa, T., and Kuriowa, Y.: Familial oculocranioskeletal neuromuscular disease with abnormal mitochondria, Brain **97**:665, 1974.

Tanaka, N., et al.: Muscular form of glycogenosis type-II (Pompe's disease), Pediatrics **63**:124, 1979.

Taniguchi, N., et al.: Alpha-glucosidase activity in human leucocytes: choice of lymphocytes for the diagnosis of Pompe's disease and the carrier state, Clin. Chim. Acta, **89**:293, 1978.

Tarui, S., et al.: Phosphofructokinase deficiency in skeletal muscle: a new type of glycogenosis. Biochem. Biophys. Res. Comm. **19**:517, 1965.

Telerman-Toppet, N., Gerard, S. M., and Coërs, C.: Central core disease: a study of clinically unaffected muscle, J. Neurol. Sci. **19**:207, 1973.

Thomsen, J.: Myotonia congenita, Edinburgh Med. J. **16**:216, 1916.

Thomson, W. H. S., MacLaurin, J. C., and Prineas, J. W.: Skeletal muscle glucogenosis: an investigation of two dissimilar cases, J. Neurol. Neurosurg. Psychiatry **26**:60, 1963.

Thrush, D. C., Morris, C. J., and Salmon, M. V.: Paramyotonia congenita: a clinical, histochemical and pathological study, Brain **95**:537, 1972.

Tomé, F. H., and Fardeau, M.: Fingerprint inclusions in muscle fibers in dystrophia myotonica, Acta Neuropathol. **24**:62, 1973.

van Creveld, S., and Huijing, F.: Glycogen storage disease, Am. J. Med. **38**:554, 1965.

van der Does de Willebois, A. E., et al.: Distal myopathy with onset in early infancy, Neurology **18**:383, 1968.

Vander Eecken, H., Pearson, C. M., and Adams, R. D.: Congenital defects of skeletal muscle. In Adams, R. D., Denny-Brown, D., and Pearson, C.M., editors: Diseases of muscle, ed. 2, New York, 1962, Paul B. Hoeber, Inc., p. 306.

Vandyke, D. H., et al.: Hereditary carnitine deficiency of muscle, Neurology **25**:154, 1975.

Van Hoof, F.: Amylo-1,6-glucosidase activity and glycogen content of the erythrocytes of normal subjects, patients with glycogen storage disease and heterozygotes, Eur. J. Biochem. **2**:271, 1967.

Van Hoof, F., and Hers, H. G.: The subgroups of type III glycogenosis, Eur. J. Biochem. **2**:265, 1967.

Van Wijngaarden, G. K., et al.: Familial myotubular myopathy, Neurology **19**:901, 1969.

Viskoper, R., et al.: McArdle's syndrome: the reaction to a fat-rich diet, Am. J. Med. Sci. **269**:217, 1975.

Vroom, F. Q., Jarrell, M. A., and Maren, T. H.: Acetazolamide treatment of hypokalemic periodic paralysis. Arch. Neurol. **32:**385, 1975.

Wang, P., and Clausen, T.: Treatment of attacks in hyperkalaemic familial periodic paralysis by inhalation of salbutamol, Lancet **1:**221, 1976.

Welander, L.: Myopathia distalis tarda hereditaris: 249 examined cases in 72 pedigrees, Acta Med. Scand. (suppl.) **265:**1, 1951.

Wharton, B. A.: An unusual variety of muscular dystrophy, Lancet **1:**248, 1965.

Wilkins, L.: The diagnosis and treatment of endocrine disorders in childhood and adolescence, ed. 2, Springfield, Ill., 1957, Charles C Thomas, Publisher, p. 91.

Zellweger, H., et al.: Severe congenital muscular dystrophy, Am. J. Dis. Child. **114:**591, 1967.

Zellweger, H., et al.: Glycogenosis IV: a new cause of infantile hypotonia, J. Pediatr. **80:**842, 1972.

# CHAPTER 8

# Myositis

"Myositis" refers to a group of conditions in which there is inflammation of muscles. These conditions can be divided into two broad categories: (1) inflammation of unknown causes, thought to be related to processes similar to those that lead to the collagen diseases and (2) inflammation secondary to infection with known microbial agents.

Myositis is relatively rare in childhood, but the idiopathic diseases are more common than those secondary to known microbial agents (Pearson, 1962). Table 8-1 outlines the classification of myositis.

## Myositis of unknown etiology
### Dermatomyositis

Childhood dermatomyositis is a relatively rare nonsuppurative inflammatory condition characterized by an underlying angiitis that is multisystemic but affects predominantly the muscles and skin. Unverricht (1887) was among the first to describe the clinical manifestations.

By convention, the term "dermatomyositis" is employed when there are skin manifestations and "polymyositis" when no skin lesions are present.

The childhood form differs from the adult form because of the prominent angiitis and the increasingly severe clinical course that often occurs. The angiitis and accompanying thrombosis and infarction (Banker and Victor, 1966) have been treated with corticosteroids and more recently with immunosuppressive agents. The efficacy of corticosteroid therapy appears to be established, and the value of immunosuppressive therapy in selected children is becoming evident. Prior to current drug therapy programs, one third of patients recovered fully within a year (Bitnum et al., 1964).

**CLINICAL FEATURES.** The child complains initially of fatigue, malaise, and anorexia and lacks interest in the environment. The symptoms may appear abruptly, and the patient may become weakened over a period of days;

**Table 8-1.** Myositis in childhood

Myositis of unknown etiology
    Dermatomyositis
    Polymyositis
Myositis associated with systemic disease
    Myositis associated with lupus erythematosus
    Myositis associated with scleroderma
    Myositis associated with rheumatoid arthritis
    Myositis associated with rheumatic fever
    Myositis associated with polyarteritis nodosa
    Myositis associated with mixed connective tissue disease
    Myositis associated with other conditions
Infectious myositis
    Bacterial
        Staphylococcus, streptococcus, gas gangrene, tuberculosis
    Viral
        Coxsackie, rubella, influenza
    Parasitic
        Trichinosis, cysticercosis, echinococcosis, toxoplasmosis, trypanosomiasis
    Spirochetal
        Syphilis, leptospirosis
    Fungous
        Actinomycosis, nocardiosis

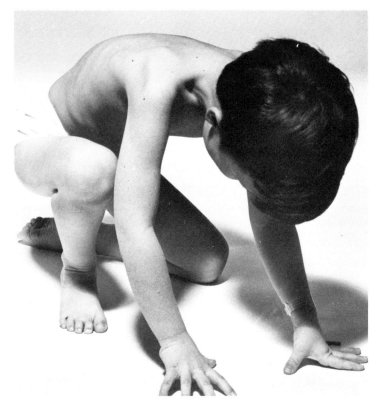

**Fig. 8-1.** This 6-year-old boy with dermatomyositis has diffuse weakness, which is predominantly proximal in distribution. He is attempting to arise and is engaged in the Gowers' maneuver.

more often the disorder is chronic and insidious over a period of weeks, sometimes with periods of relative remission.

Muscle involvement is usually heralded by proximal weakness of the hip girdle (Fig. 8-1) and occasionally of the shoulder girdle (Fig. 8-2). The patient has difficulty climbing steps and rising from the floor. This pattern of weakness may lead to the erroneous diagnosis of Duchenne muscular dystrophy. Moderate to profound weakness of the neck flexor muscles often occurs (Fig. 8-3).

Pain in the limbs that is poorly localized in skin, subcutaneous tissue, or muscle is common although pain is absent in at least a third of these patients (Banker and Victor, 1966). Arthralgia is occasionally present; true arthritis is uncommon.

Low-grade fever is frequently present and is usually the symptom that leads to medical attention (Sullivan et al., 1972). The skin lesions described in the following paragraph may precede or succeed the signs and symptoms of muscle disease; they often occur simultaneously. Weakness of the pharyngeal muscles may develop, documented by difficulties with swallowing and speaking. Respiratory muscle function is impaired in a small number of children.

Skin lesions pathognomonic of dermatomyositis include erythematous or violaceous (heliotrope) patches on the eyelids, which may spread to the periorbital areas and over the cheeks and may circumscribe a butterfly distribution about the nose. There may be mild to moderate periorbital edema. Subungual telangiectasia may occur. Reddened or violaceous patches in the periungual areas

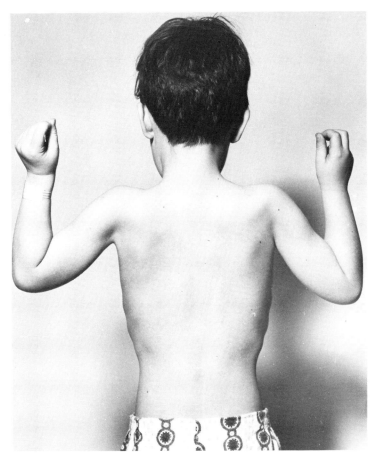

**Fig. 8-2.** Same patient as in Fig. 8-1. He is attempting to raise his arms above his head. Note marked muscle wasting in shoulder and scapular areas and relative sparing of deltoid muscles.

or over the interphalangeal joints of the hands are common (Fig. 8-4), and they may also occur over the extensor surfaces of the elbows and knees. Brawny edema that appears to be subcutaneous has been described (Wedgwood, Cook, and Cohen, 1953). These areas may be extremely tender or pain free; absence of pain is usually associated with the chronic forms. In late stages, the skin may manifest atrophic changes, abnormal pigmentation, and telangiectasia.

The progressive weakness may culminate in death secondary to pharyngeal dysfunction and resultant inability to swallow or respiratory muscle failure. The usual duration of progression is about a month, but the disease

may run its course in less than a week or may remain active for several years. Rarely, myocardial insufficiency or cardiac dysrhythmia is present.

The patient may be left with profound atrophy and weakness. Severe contractures about the hips, knees, and elbows are common. Extensive atrophy and tightness of the skin following dermatomyositis may prove highly incapacitating. Most patients who die of the disease do so in the first 2 years; death from dermatomyositis has become unusual (DeVere and Bradley, 1975).

Calcification of muscles, much more prevalent in children than in adults, is thought to represent a favorable prognostic sign (Fig.

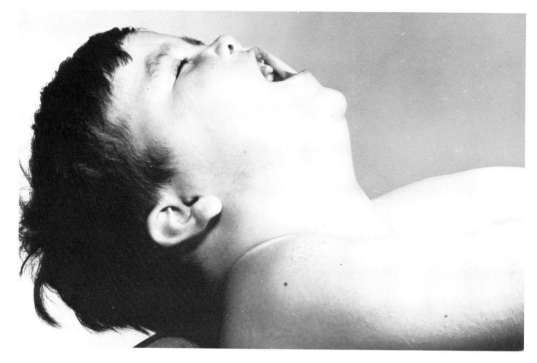

Fig. 8-3. Same patient as in Figs. 8-1 and 8-2. Patient is being pulled forward by arms while sitting in a chair with his head resting on backrest. He is unable to flex his neck to bring his head upright. Weakness of neck flexor muscles commonly occurs in dermatomyositis.

8-5). Cook and associates (1963) reported that calcification developed in 60% of children who lived more than 2 years. The calcification may become widespread; this condition is called "calcinosis universalis." Superficial nodules may appear and ulcerate with subsequent extrusion of calcium deposits.

Perforation of the gastrointestinal tract was the most frequent cause of death in cases reported by Banker and Victor (1966). Hemorrhagic and ulcerative lesions occurred along the entire gastrointestinal tract. Everett and Curtis (1957), on the other hand, reported that during the first year, their patients more often died of bulbar paralysis or cardiac failure. In their series, the children who died, but lived beyond 1 year, usually died of infection.

Recent reports indicate that even after 5 years, acute inflammatory changes, with or without associated muscle weakness, may continue. This prolonged period of inflammation necessitates frequent observation and sometimes continuous therapy.

Of a group of 118 patients with dermatomyositis-polymyositis, 21 were 20 years of age or less when first seen. The ratio of females to males in this young group was 2.5:1. Those in whom the disease developed during the first decade had less residual disability than those in whom it developed during the second decade. However, the average patient had little or no functional impairment at reexamination. Only one young patient in this series died (DeVere and Bradley, 1975). Long-term functional impairment or death are also uncommon in other reports (Sullivan et al., 1972).

LABORATORY DIAGNOSIS

MORPHOLOGY. Childhood dermatomyositis is a diffuse angiopathic process involving

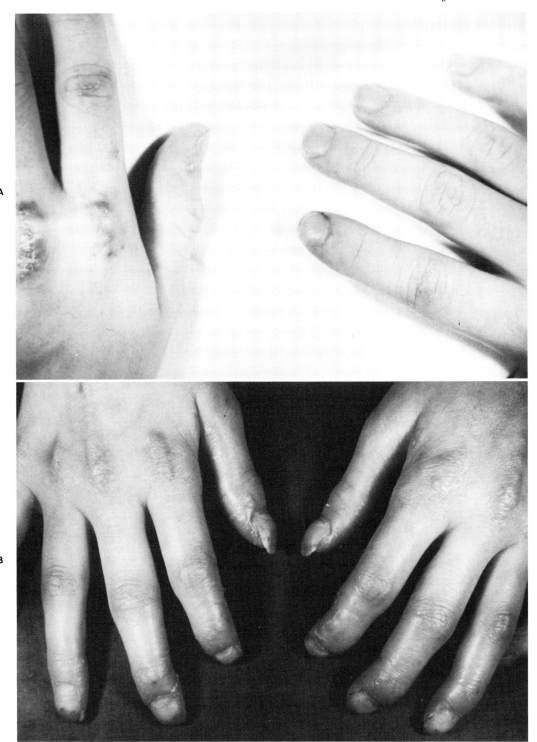

**Fig. 8-4. A,** Roughened, violaceous patches over periungual areas and interpharyngeal joints are seen frequently in dermatomyositis. **B,** Progression of skin lesions often leads to shiny, atrophic discolored skin over knuckles, interphalangeal joints, and distal fingers.

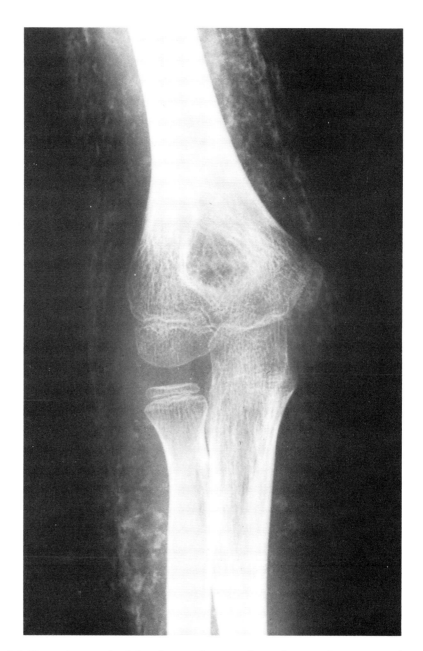

**Fig. 8-5.** X-ray photograph of the elbow and surrounding soft tissue demonstrates the subcutaneous calcification that often develops in dermatomyositis.

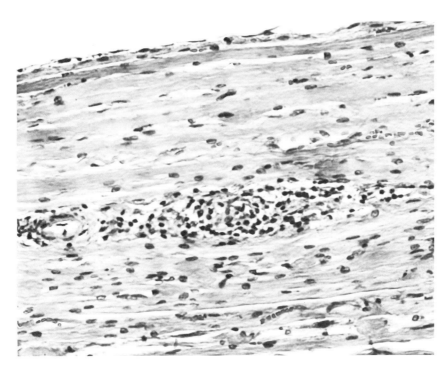

**Fig. 8-6.** Muscle from a patient with dermatomyositis demonstrates moderate numbers of mononuclear cells, primarily lymphocytes, that surround small blood vessels. Cellular infiltration is limited to vessel wall and perivascular spaces. Nearby muscle fibers are unaffected. Hematoxylin and eosin stain.

muscle, skin, gastrointestinal tract, and the smaller nerves. Early changes are predominantly those of perivascular inflammation (Fig. 8-6). Initially, the inflammatory cells are polymorphonuclear, but later, chronic lymphocytic infiltrate and some plasma cells are noted. Hyperplasia of the intima of many of the arteries and veins progresses until the lumen is occluded and fibrin thrombi are evident. Changes occur in vessels of all sizes but are more prevalent in the perimysial vessels. Recanalization of thrombi is a frequent finding. Infarction is visible in almost all sections of muscle, but little inflammatory reaction occurs about the destroyed tissue. The areas of infarction are discrete, and each section displaying infarction also contains normal muscle fibers (Banker and Victor, 1966). Some childhood patients do not manifest the morphologic changes of angiitis (Pearson and Bohan, 1977).

Denervation atrophy is evidenced by fascicles of small, rounded muscle fibers typical of the grouped lesion of neurogenic atrophy (Chapter 2). In the acute stages, inflammatory cells infiltrate the muscle spindles. These changes may account for the loss of tendon reflexes in these patients.

Electron microscopy reveals unusual masses of undulating tubules within the smooth endoplasmic reticulum of endothelial cells as well as in lymphocytes, pericytes, and pseudosatellite cells. Before the atrophic process is evident, muscle cells show mitochondrial elongation, Z band streaming, focal myofibrillary loss, and scattered loss of thick filaments (Carpenter et al., 1976).

SERUM STUDIES. The studies of serum enzyme activity regularly employed in diagnosing muscle disease (see Chapter 2), including measurements of creatine phosphokinase (CPK) and glutamic oxaloacetic transaminase

(GOT), are among the most helpful in the diagnosis of dermatomyositis (Sullivan et al., 1972). Although the elevations in serum enzyme activities are usually moderate in comparison to those observed in children with Duchenne muscular dystrophy, they are sufficient to be helpful in diagnosing the disease in patients who are mildly affected or do not have discomfort or tenderness.

A positive reaction to the serum antinuclear antibody test was reported in one patient with fulminating dermatomyositis. This finding is highly unusual (Hanson and Kornreich, 1967). Dermatomyositis has been associated with lymphocytic leukemia in a 4-year-old boy (Singsen et al., 1976).

ELECTROMYOGRAPHY. Electromyographic examination does not yield results pathognomonic of dermatomyositis, but certain characteristics are routinely present (Chapter 2). Polyphasic potentials of short duration and low amplitude occur with spontaneous potentials of short duration. Other bursts of potentials similar to those in myotonia, but more prolonged, frequently are present.

**PATHOPHYSIOLOGY.** Childhood dermatomyositis probably results from deposition of immunoglobulin and complement in blood vessels (Whitaker and Engel, 1972, 1973). Other studies suggest that the pathogenesis of dermatomyositis includes a lymphocyte-mediated immunologic reaction directed at skeletal muscle (Dawkins and Mastaglia, 1973). Additionally, there have been reports of particles of myxovirus (Chou, 1967; Sato et al., 1971), picornavirus (Chou and Gutmann, 1970), and paramyxovirus (Fidziańska, 1973) in muscle tissues of polymyositis patients.

Interviews with parents of 42 children with polymyositis-dermatomyositis and with parents of controls matched for sex and age revealed no significant differences in medical history, residential and family history, animal exposure history, and immunization history between the two groups. A suggestive difference was exposure to bacteriologically confirmed streptococcal disease in 20 affected children as compared with 13 controls (Koch, Brody, and Gillespie, 1976).

TREATMENT. No consensus exists concerning the value of drug treatment in childhood dermatomyositis, but high-dosage steroid therapy has achieved wide acceptance despite lack of definitive evidence from studies. Early investigators found ACTH and corticosteroids to be of questionable value (Cook, Rosen, and Banker, 1963; Everett and Curtis, 1957). Steroid therapy always carries with it the possibility of complications, such as hypokalemia, hypertension, gastrointestinal bleeding, infection including tuberculosis, growth retardation, and vertebral compression fractures secondary to osteoporosis. The cushingoid appearance is typical, but changes in the body habitus and facial features usually return to normal when therapy is discontinued. Behavioral changes ranging from mild mood swings to depression and acute psychosis may occur. Gastric and duodenal ulcers often develop in children treated with steroids (Carlisle and Good, 1959); such treatment therefore increases the risk of perforation attendant to the natural course of the disease.

High-dosage prednisone therapy, 1.5 to 2 mg/kg/day for as long as 2 months, has often been successful (Dubowitz, 1976). Reduction of clinical symptoms and decrease in serum enzyme activity are the criteria of improvement. Dosage is then reduced by 2.5 mg every 4 to 6 days. After initial therapy, a maintenance dosage of 0.25 mg/kg/day is often necessary to prevent relapse. Every-other-day therapy may suffice and may forestall side effects of steroid therapy. Therapy usually must be continued for 1 to 3 years (Rose, 1974).

Immunosuppressive drugs have been used with variable success (Goel and Shanks, 1976; Currie and Walton, 1971). The drugs employed include azathioprine, methotrexate, cyclophosphamide, and 6-mercaptopurine. These drugs are often administered in combination with steroids. They should not be prescribed until there is evidence that the symptoms do not respond to steroid therapy.

If corticosteroid therapy is unsatisfactory or there are still significant symptoms, azathioprine, 2.5 to 3 mg/kg/day in divided doses, may be given. The lymphocyte count should not be allowed to go below 1,000 cu mm. Most patients respond rapidly, but high dosages of both drugs may be necessary for up to 6 months. If this therapy is successful, after 2 years, the drugs should be gradually discontinued. If recurrence is evident, the drugs should be administered at the previous control level; after an additional year, withdrawal should be attempted again (Bradley and Walton, 1976).

Methotrexate has also been used with some success, and it is probably less toxic than azathioprine, although possibly less effective. Some advocate its use before azathioprine (Fischer, 1979). The drug is given orally or intravenously. One regimen consists of biweekly injections of methotrexate (2 to 3 mg/kg/dose or 7 mg/kg/dose with citrovorum factor rescue) (Jacobs, 1977). There are varying reports concerning the prevalence of untoward reactions that consist of pleuritis, pneumonitis, hepatitis, and buccal ulcers. The maximum response in one series occurred after 13 weeks of therapy (Sokoloff, Goldberg, and Pearson, 1971).

Calcium deposition appears to be related primarily to duration of the disease. There are inconclusive reports of benefit derived from the use of chelating agents such as ethanehydroxydiphosphate (10 mg/kg/day).

If in the acute phase palatal insufficiency or respiratory dysfunction dominate the clinical picture, meticulous pulmonary care, including postural drainage and suction, is necessary. In fulminating cases, tracheostomy and mechanical ventilation may be necessary to maintain an adequate airway.

After the inflammatory process has dissipated, physical therapy is often of benefit for those patients with contracture formation and weakness.

### Polymyositis

In many reviews, dermatomyositis and polymyositis are grouped together, and indeed it is not clear that childhood polymyositis should be accorded a special, separate division from childhood dermatomyositis. Furthermore, often no differentiation is made between childhood polymyositis and adult polymyositis, although childhood polymyositis is almost never associated with malignancy.

If a distinction is made between childhood dermatomyositis and childhood polymyositis, it is based on the presence or absence of skin lesions. For purposes of this discussion, polymyositis includes only patients who lack the typical skin lesions of dermatomyositis. The problem of classification will be clarified only when a better understanding of the underlying causes of these conditions is available.

**CLINICAL FEATURES.** Relatively few cases of childhood polymyositis without skin involvement have been reported (Walton and Adams, 1958; Rose and Walton, 1966; Dowben et al., 1965; Thompson, 1968). Despite the lack of documentation in the literature, however, experienced clinicians can cite experience with a handful of childhood polymyositis patients without skin manifestations who have not had a collagen disease or an evident systemic disease. In general, these patients have proximal weakness of the limbs without the gross systemic manifestations that accompany dermatomyositis. Gowers' sign is often present. Pseudohypertrophy has been reported. The clinical course is one of prolonged, relatively static or slowly progressive weakness, which, coupled with lack of systemic manifestations, often leads to an erroneous diagnosis of muscular dystrophy (Dowben et al., 1965).

Cardiac conduction defects may occur in childhood polymyositis. The abnormalities include arrhythmias and atrioventricular block (Singsen et al., 1976).

Polymyositis with a facioscapulohumeral distribution has been described with onset between the ages of 9 and 13 years (Munsat et al., 1972; Rothstein, Carlson, and Sumi, 1971). The children experienced progressive weakness of the face and shoulder muscles, modest increase in serum muscle enzyme activity, and the microscopic changes of inflammatory myopathy. Decrease in serum CPK activity during prednisone therapy of facioscapulohumeral polymyositis initially may be associated with clinical improvement, but the decrease does not necessarily parallel therapeutic improvement (Munsat and Bradley, 1977).

Inflammatory myopathy associated with cardiomyopathy and scapulo-ilio-peroneal distribution of atrophy has been reported in two families. Onset of the disease occurred in the third decade (Jennekens et al., 1975).

Polymyositis in conjunction with multisystemic disease including renal failure, all caused by phenytoin hypersensitivity, has been described in an adult (Michael and Mitch, 1976).

**LABORATORY FINDINGS.** Electromyography reveals a myopathic pattern with decrease in amplitude of action potentials (Chapter 2). Elevation of serum enzyme activities of CPK, aldolase, and lactate dehydrogenase (LDH) is common. Nemaline structures have been associated with chronic polymyositis in childhood (Cape, Johnson, and Pitner, 1970).

### Myositis associated with systemic diseases

Myositis has been reported in association with all of the conventionally designated collagen diseases, which include lupus erythematosus, scleroderma, rheumatoid arthritis, rheumatic fever, and polyarteritis nodosa.

**MORPHOLOGY.** Except for polyarteritis nodosa, the polymyositis associated with these conditions has been referred to as interstitial or focal polymyositis (Adams, 1975). The morphologic pattern of the myositis in each of these conditions is uniform. The most common lesions are minute inflammatory nodules in skeletal muscles. The lesions are composed of inflammatory cells that aggregate in perimysial and endomysial locations, usually perivascular areas predominantly near small veins; however, small arteries, arterioles, and capillaries may also be at the nidus. Most of the cells are lymphocytes; plasma cells, mast cells, histiocytes, epithelioid cells, and rare multinucleated giant cells are also evident. Polymorphonuclear leukocytes appear in varying numbers.

The muscle fibers that are adjacent to the area of cellular aggregation are seen in various stages of degeneration with associated vacuolation and hyalinization. If necrosis ensues, macrophages become evident. Focal fiber loss frequently gives way to fibrosis.

**MYOSITIS ASSOCIATED WITH LUPUS ERYTHEMATOSUS.** Although as many as 25% of adults with lupus erythematosus have symptoms of overt myositis, muscle weakness is not as common in children. The muscle weakness is almost always proximal. CPK activity is usually elevated in the presence of clinical symptomatology.

The focal muscle lesions described earlier are prominently seen in muscle biopsy material. The possibility of vacuolar myopathy secondary to corticosteroid therapy must be kept in mind when considering both the clinical course and the morphologic features of the disease.

**MYOSITIS ASSOCIATED WITH SCLERODERMA.** Skeletal muscles develop profound atrophy if joint movement is grossly impaired by swelling and pain. In this situation, atrophic changes are superimposed upon the already described pathology of focal myositis.

Although CPK activity is increased in one third of children with scleroderma, many of these children do not have clinical manifestations of muscle pain or weakness (Dabich, Sullivan, and Cassidy, 1974).

**MYOSITIS ASSOCIATED WITH RHEUMATOID ARTHRITIS.** Rheumatoid arthritis may occur with profound weakness associated with myositis and may be enhanced by disuse atrophy and poor nutrition (Brooke and Kaplan, 1972; Sokoloff, Wilens, and McEwen, 1950; Magyar et al., 1977).

Felty's syndrome, which consists of rheumatoid arthritis, splenomegaly, and leukopenia, is frequently associated with myositis.

Sjögren's syndrome, which consists of rheumatoid arthritis, keratoconjunctivitis, sicca, and xerostomia, has also been reported to be associated with myositis (Bunim, 1961).

The features of focal myositis may be augmented further with severe changes consistent with atrophy.

**MYOSITIS ASSOCIATED WITH RHEUMATIC FEVER.** The focal myositis associated with collagen diseases has been reported in many cases (Clawson, Nobel, and Lufkin, 1947; Sokoloff, Wilens, and Bunim, 1951). All in all, little is written about the clinical and pathologic changes in muscle that accompany rheumatic fever; nevertheless, changes are undoubtedly present.

**MYOSITIS ASSOCIATED WITH POLYARTERITIS NODOSA.** Polyarteritis nodosa in childhood has been associated with skeletal muscle changes. The changes are unlike those in the other collagen diseases. The diffuse arteritis involves not only muscle but also many other organs, including peripheral nerves (Chapter 5) and the central nervous system. The arteritis can result in perivascular inflammation in the surrounding muscle, muscle atrophy caused by peripheral nerve involvement, or necrosis from interruption of blood flow because of thrombosis or hemorrhage secondary to the arteritis.

Laboratory studies of patients with calf pain virtually always demonstrate increased serum aldolase, GOT, and CPK activities along with accompanying myopathic potentials revealed during electromyographic study. There may be sterile subcutaneous nodules associated with the muscle pain. Both pain and nodules are usually responsive to corticosteroid therapy. Immunosuppressive agents have been of value in some patients who have not responded to corticosteroids.

**MYOSITIS ASSOCIATED WITH OTHER CONDITIONS.** Both children and adults have been described with a new syndrome—mixed connective tissue disease. These patients have a combination of features usually found in scleroderma, dermatomyositis, rheumatoid arthritis, and systemic lupus erythematosus (Singsen et al., 1977; Fraga et al., 1978). The condition is associated with laboratory findings of high titers of speckled, fluorescent antinuclear antibody and a specific hemagglutinating antibody for ribonucleoprotein (Sharp, 1976).

An inflammatory myopathy involving proximal limb and facial muscles has been reported in association with intestinal malabsorption and IgA deficiency. Both myopathy and malabsorption improve with corticosteroid treatment. Serum LDH and CPK concentrations, which had increased during the course of disease, decreased after therapy (Silverman et al., 1976).

Penicillamine therapy may cause myositis. The use of penicillamine in the therapy of rheumatoid diseases may prove confounding when myositis appears during the course of therapy (Machtey et al., 1977).

### Infectious myositis

Inflammatory disease of muscle secondary to microbial agents is a relatively rare condition.

#### Bacterial myositis

Suppurative myositis secondary to bacterial infection may result as an extension of an infection from a neighboring organ, such as bone or skin. Rarely, it is primary, becoming established on a hematogenous basis.

Bacterial infection with pus formation is usually associated with staphylococcal or streptococcal (Barrett and Gresham, 1958; Grose, 1978) infection. Focal pain and swelling occur in the affected area. Some systemic manifestations are associated with abscess formation no matter what the anatomic location; these include anorexia, fever, chills, and lethargy. An abscess often forms if the infection is contained, and surgical removal of purulent material is necessary. Further therapy is based on sensitivity of the organism to antibiotics.

Another form of bacterial infection of muscle is that of the gas gangrene organism (*Clostridium perfringens*). The bacteria are introduced through a wound, and the damaged muscle proves to be a suitable medium for bacterial growth. Carbon dioxide forms during the rapid destruction of muscle tissue. The local area is swollen and painful; crepitus is easily found. The surrounding skin is suffused and may later become brownish yellow. The disease is associated with fever and extreme toxicity.

The rapid destruction of muscle tissue is due to enzymatic activity. Gram-positive bacilli are easily visible microscopically. Clostridial myositis can follow parenteral administration of medication and is accompanied by high mortality (Berggren et al., 1964; Nahir et al., 1978).

Therapy of gas gangrene infection consists of surgical removal of the affected muscle tissue. Polyvalent antiserum has not proved helpful (Howard and Inui, 1954), but hyperbaric oxygen therapy (Brummelkamp, 1965) appears to have merit.

Tuberculous myositis, a rare form, is usually the result of extension of infection in other involved tissues, frequently bone (Plummer, Sanes, and Smith, 1934). It is rarely associated with miliary tuberculosis.

Clinical evidence of myositis is unusual in sarcoidosis, but histologic evidence is relatively common (Harvey, 1959).

### Viral myositis

Coxsackieviruses can be divided into types A and B on the basis of lesions developed in susceptible animals. Injection of type A coxsackievirus into mice leads to diffuse, severe degeneration of striated muscle. Tongue and heart are not usually affected, and there are few lesions elsewhere. When type B viruses are injected into mice, the central nervous system is grossly involved, but lesions in muscle are characteristically focal and limited (Horsfall and Tamm, 1965).

Laboratory studies with chick embryos into which coxsackievirus A2 was injected intravenously in the seventh day of incubation produced severe myositis and paralysis within 48 hours. Electron microscopic and immunofluorescence techniques confirmed the presence of the virus in muscle cells. After 3 or 4 days, the muscle was profoundly atrophied, and ankylosis of joints occurred similar to human arthrogryposis (Drachman et al., 1976).

Both types A and B coxsackieviruses can cause aseptic meningitis, although type B is much more commonly the offender. Type B viruses also cause myocarditis and pericarditis in the neonatal period.

Acute transient myositis in humans has been associated with both types A and B influenza viruses (Barton and Chalhub, 1975; Schwartz, Swash, and Gross, 1978). In one series of 17 children with influenza B myositis, the gastrocnemius and soleus muscles were almost exclusively involved (Dietzman et al., 1976). Postinfectious polymyositis has also been described (Schwartz, Swash, and Gross, 1978).

Rubella infection in the prenatal period is commonly associated with mental deficiency, microcephaly, spasticity, deafness, cataracts, hepatomegaly, generalized heart disease, abnormal dermatoglyphics, and growth retardation (Korones et al., 1965). Spiro and Rorke (1966) reported the presence of skeletal muscle lesions in the congenital rubella syndrome. Muscle architecture was normal in many areas but many muscle bundles consisted of empty connective tissue tubes in which only a few small fibers with darkly staining nuclei were present. The capsules of the spindles in the abnormal areas contained excessive connective tissue. There were no signs of regeneration, and no inflammatory cells were seen. Changes in the intramuscular nerves or blood vessels were not apparent. Myositis with inclusion bodies has been reported in adults (Carpenter et al., 1978).

### Myositis secondary to parasitic infection

Parasitic infection is an uncommon cause of myositis. Various types of tapeworm are among the parasites that cause myositis. Trichinosis is caused by a worm that enters its human host through ingestion of undercooked pork (Kagan, 1960). Encysted *Trichinella spiralis* are released in the human digestive tract and develop there. Following fertilization, the female penetrates the mucosa of the upper small intestine and deposits young. These embryos are transported by the lymphatics, enter the circulation, and are then found in all tissues, including striated muscle, the tissue best suited to their further development. The severity of human disease is proportional to the number of organisms present.

The course of the disease usually runs several months and is characterized by fever, muscle pain, maculopapular rash, subungual splinter hemorrhages, periorbital edema, and weakness. Biopsy of the muscle demonstrates the encysted parasites in the muscle fibers. Cardiac muscle is also involved. The muscle fibers are swollen and fragmented. Eosinophilic and polymorphonuclear cells are present in the neighboring connective tissue. Eosinophilic leukocytosis is also present in the peripheral blood.

A skin test with antigen prepared from larvae is useful. Therapy is supportive in mild cases. In severe cases, ACTH and corticosteroid usually ameliorate gross discomfort and myocarditis. Ingestion of the pork tapeworm *Taenia solium* leads to the liberation of the larvae *Cysticercus cellulosae* in the bloodstream and their subsequent deposition in various body tissues (Obrador, 1948). Areas of tenderness may be noted in muscles. Central nervous system symptoms of a multifocal nature are present, and later, calcification of the parasites within the muscle, brain, and other tissues can be documented by x-ray studies.

Other diseases such as echinococcosis (Hutchinson and Bryan, 1960), toxoplasmosis (Siim, 1960; Samuels and Rietschel, 1976; Henrickx et al., 1979), and American trypanosomiasis (Laranja et al., 1956), are known to involve skeletal muscle.

### Spirochetal myositis

Luetic myositis occurs only in tertiary syphilis. The most common lesion, the gumma, is usually solitary and may be accompanied by an area of palpable swelling. The sternocleidomastoid and biceps muscles are most frequently involved, but other muscle involvement has been reported. The pathologic picture is one of replacement of normal tissue with dense, fibrous connective tissue.

A less common form of luetic myositis is diffuse myositis, which involves one or more muscles, sometimes in a consecutive pattern. The sternocleidomastoid and upper arm muscles are among those reported to be affected. The pathologic lesion consists of loss of muscle fibers in large areas and their replacement by connective tissue.

Leptospirosis is caused by a number of serotypes, but most commonly *Leptospira icterohemorrhagiae*, *L. canicola*, and *L. pomona* cause disease in man (Galton et al., 1962). The clinical picture consists of headache, nausea, vomiting, prostration, fever, and injection of the conjunctivae with myalgia. The disease is dominated by symptoms other than myositis. Penicillin therapy may prove beneficial.

### Fungous myositis

Infection of the jaw with *Actinomyces bovis* may occur after trauma or tooth extraction. Actinomycosis results in painful swelling of all tissues in the area. Suppuration appears on areas of skin, denoting the presence of multiple abscesses and fistulas. The fluid that drains from the fistulas is filled with yellow granules consisting of mycelial filaments. Penicillin or tetracycline therapy usually is effective (Lane, Kutscher, and Chaves, 1953).

Nocardiosis, infection with *Nocardia asteroides*, is another uncommon cause of myositis. Myositis may result from metastatic abscesses in the muscle secondary to pulmonary involvement (Weed et al., 1955). Nocardial infection of the foot is one of the causes of Madura foot, along with infection by a number of other genera of fungi. Madura foot is treated with drainage and surgical exposure of the numerous fistulas. Treatment with sulfadiazine appears to be the best form of antimicrobial therapy in nocardiosis (Weed et al., 1955).

### REFERENCES

Adams, R. D.: Diseases of muscle: a study in pathology, ed. 3, Hagerstown, Md., 1975, Harper & Row, Publishers, p. 357.

Banker, B. Q., and Victor, M.: Dermatomyositis (systemic angiopathy) of childhood, Medicine **45**:261, 1966.

Barrett, A. M., and Gresham, G. A.: Acute streptococcal myositis, Lancet **1**:347, 1958.

Barton, L., and Chalhub, E.: Myositis associated with influenza A infection, J. Pediatr. **87**:1003, 1975.

Berggren, R. B., et al.: Clostridial myositis after parenteral injections, J.A.M.A. **188**:1044, 1964.

Bitnum, S., et al.: Dermatomyositis, J. Pediatr. **64:**101, 1964.

Bradley, W., and Walton, J.: Treatment of dermatomyositis, Br. Med. J. **2:**43, 1976.

Brooke, M., and Kaplan, H.: Muscle pathology in rheumatoid arthritis, polymyalgia rheumatica and polymyositis, Arch. Pathol. **94:**101, 1972.

Brummelkamp, W. H.: Considerations on hyperbaric oxygen therapy at three atmospheres absolute for Clostridial infections type welchii, Ann. N.Y. Acad. Sci. **117:**688, 1965.

Bunim, J. J.: A broader spectrum of Sjøgren's syndrome and its pathogenetic implications, Ann. Rheum. Dis. **20:**1, 1961.

Cape, C. A., Johnson, W. W., and Pitner, S. E.: Nemaline structures in polymyositis: a nonspecific pathological reaction of skeletal muscles, Neurology **20:**494, 1970.

Carlisle, J. W., and Good, R. A.: Dermatomyositis in childhood: report of studies on 7 cases and a review of literature, Lancet **79:**266, 1959.

Carpenter, S., et al.: The childhood type of dermatomyositis, Neurology **26:**952, 1976.

Carpenter, S., et al.: Inclusion body myositis: a distinct variety of idiopathic inflammatory myopathy, Neurology **28:**8, 1978.

Chou, S. M.: Myxovirus-like structures in a case of human chronic polymyositis, Science **158:**1453, 1967.

Chou, S. M., and Gutmann, L.: Picornavirus-like crystals in subacute polymyositis, Neurology **20:**205, 1970.

Clawson, B. J., Noble, J. F., and Lufkin, N. H.: Nodular inflammatory and degenerative lesions of muscles from 450 autopsies, Arch. Pathol. **43:**579, 1947.

Cook, C. D., Rosen, F. S., and Banker, B. Q.: Dermatomyositis and focal scleroderma, Pediatr. Clin. North Am. **10:**979, 1963.

Currie, S., and Walton, J. N.: Immunosuppressive therapy in polymyositis, J. Neurol. Neurosurg. Psychiatry **34:**447, 1971.

Dabich, L., Sullivan, D. B., and Cassidy, J. T.: Scleroderma in the child, J. Pediatr. **85:**770, 1974.

Dawkins, R. L., and Mastaglia, F. L.: Cell-mediated cytotoxicity to muscle in polymyositis, N. Engl. J. Med. **288:**435, 1973.

DeVere, R., and Bradley, W.: Polymyositis: its presentation, morbidity and mortality, Brain **98:**637, 1975.

Dietzman, D. E., et al.: Acute myositis associated with influenza-B infection, Pediatrics **57:**255, 1976.

Dowben, R. M., et al.: Polymyositis and other diseases resembling muscular dystrophy, Arch. Intern. Med. **115:**584, 1965.

Drachman, D., et al.: Experimental arthrogryposis caused by viral myopathy, Arch. Neurol. **33:**362, 1976.

Dubowitz, V.: Treatment of dermatomyositis in childhood, Arch. Dis. Child. **51:**494, 1976.

Everett, M. A., and Curtis, A. C.: Dermatomyositis: a review of nineteen cases in adolescents and children, Arch. Intern. Med. **10:**70, 1957.

Fidziańska, A.: Virus-like structures in muscle in chronic polymyositis, Acta Neuropathol. **23:**23, 1973.

Fischer, R. J., et al.: Childhood dermatomyositis and polymyositis, Am. J. Dis. Child. **133:**386, 1979.

Fraga, A., et al.: Mixed connective tissue disease in childhood: the relationship of Sjögren's syndrome, Am. J. Dis. Child. **132:**263, 1978.

Galton, M. M., et al.: Leptospirosis: epidemiology, clinical manifestations in man and animals, and methods in laboratory diagnosis. Public Health Service Publications No. 951, Washington, D.C., 1962, U.S. Government Printing Office.

Goel, K. M., and Shanks, R. A.: Dermatomyositis in childhood: review of eight cases, Arch. Dis. Child. **51:**501, 1976.

Grose, C.: Staphylococcal polymyositis in South Texas, J. Pediatr. **94:**457, 1978.

Hanson, V., and Kornreich, H.: Systemic rheumatic disorders ("collagen disease") in childhood: lupus erythematosus, anaphylactoid purpura, dermatomyositis, and scleroderma. Part I. Bull. Rheum. Dis. **17:**435, 1967.

Harvey, J. C.: A myopathy of Boeck's sarcoid, Am. J. Med. **26:**356, 1959.

Henrickx, G. F., et al.: Dermatomyositis and toxoplasmosis, Ann. Neurol. **5:**393, 1979.

Horsfall, F. L., Jr., and Tamm, I.: Viral and rickettsial infections of man, ed. 4, Philadelphia, 1965, J. B. Lippincott Co.

Howard, J. M., and Inui, F. K.: Clostridial myositis-gas gangrene: observations of battle casualties in Korea, Surgery **36:**1115, 1954.

Hutchinson, W. F., and Bryan, M. W.: Studies on the hydatid worm echinococcus granulosus: I and II, Am. J. Trop. Med. Hyg. **9:**606, 1960.

Jacobs, J. C.: Methotrexate and azathioprine treatment of childhood dermatomyositis, Pediatrics **59:**212, 1977.

Jennekens, F., et al.: Inflammatory myopathy in scapulo-ilio-peroneal atrophy with cardiopathy, Brain **98:**709, 1975.

Kagan, I. G.: Trichinosis: a review of biologic, serologic and immunologic aspects, J. Infect. Dis. **107:**65, 1960.

Koch, M., Brody, J., and Gillespie, M.: Childhood polymyositis: a case control study, Am. J. Epidemiol. **104:**627, 1976.

Korones, S. B., et al.: Congenital rubella syndrome syndrome: study of 22 infants, Am. J. Dis. Child. **110:**435, 1965.

Lane, S. L., Kutscher, A. H., and Chaves, R.: Oxytetracycline in the treatment of oral cervical facial actinomycosis, J.A.M.A. **151:**968, 1953.

Laranja, F. S., et al.: Chagas' disease, Circulation **14:**1035, 1956.

Machtey, I., et al.: Penicillamine-induced polymyositis, Ann. Int. Med. **86:**832, 1977.

Magyar, T., et al.: Muscle changes in rheumatoid arthritis—review of literature with a study of 100 cases, Virchows Arch. **373:**267, 1977.

Michael, J., and Mitch, W.: Reversible renal failure and myositis caused by phenytoin hypersensitivity, J.A.M.A. **236**:2773, 1976.

Munsat, T. L., and Bradley, W. G.: Serum creatine phosphokinase levels and prednisone treated muscle weakness, Neurology **27**:96, 1977.

Munsat, T. L., et al.: Inflammatory myopathy with facioscapulohumeral distribution, Neurology **22**:335, 1972.

Nahir, A. M., et al.: Gas gangrene following intramuscular injection of aqueous solution, N.Y. State J. Med. **78**:1948, 1978.

Obrador, S.: Clinical aspects of cerebral cysticerosis, Arch. Neurol. Psychiatry **59**:457, 1948.

Pearson, C. M.: Polymyositis: clinical forms, diagnosis and therapy, Postgrad. Med. **31**:450, 1962.

Pearson, C. M., and Bohan, A.: The spectrum of polymyositis and dermatomyositis, Med. Clin. North Am. **61**:439, 1977.

Plummer, W. W., Sanes, S., and Smith, W. S.: Hematogenous tuberculosis of skeletal muscle: report of a case with involvement of the gastrocnemius muscle, J. Bone Joint Surg. **16**:631, 1934.

Rose, A. L.: Childhood polymyositis: follow-up study with special reference to treatment with corticosteroids, Am. J. Dis. Child. **127**:518, 1974.

Rose, A. L., and Walton, J. N.: Polymyositis: a survey of 89 cases with particular reference to treatment and prognosis, Brain **89**:747, 1966.

Rothstein, T. L., Carlson, C. B., and Sumi, S. M.: Polymyositis with facioscapulohumeral distribution, Arch. Neurol. **25**:313, 1971.

Samuels, B., and Rietschel, R.: Polymyositis and toxoplasmosis, J.A.M.A. **235**:60, 1976.

Sato, T., et al.: Chronic polymyositis and myxovirus-like inclusions: electron microscopic and viral studies, Arch. Neurol. **24**:409, 1971.

Sharp, G. C.: Association of antibodies to ribonucleoprotein and Sm antigens with mixed connective-tissue disease, systematic lupus erythematosus and other rheumatic diseases, N. Engl. J. Med. **295**:1149, 1976.

Siim, J. C.: Human toxoplasmosis conference, 1956, Copenhagen. Baltimore, 1960, The Williams & Wilkins Co.

Silverman, A., et al.: Inflammatory myopathy, IgA deficiency, and intestinal malabsorption, J. Pediatr. **89**: 216, 1976.

Singsen, B., et al.: Childhood polymyositis with cardiac conduction defects, Am. J. Dis. Child. **130**:72, 1976.

Singsen, B., et al.: Lymphocytic leukemia, atypical dermatomyositis, and hyperlipidemia in a four-year-old boy, J. Pediatr. **88**:602, 1976.

Singsen, B. H., et al.: Mixed connective tissue disease in childhood—a clinical and serologic survery, J. Pediatr. **90**:893, 1977.

Sokoloff, L., Wilens, J. J., and McEwen, C.: Diagnostic value of histologic lesions of striated muscle in rheumatoid arthritis, Am. J. Med. Sci. **219**:174, 1950.

Sokoloff, M. C., Goldberg, L. S., and Pearson, C. M.: Treatment of corticosteroid-resistant polymyositis with methotrexate, Lancet **1**:14, 1971.

Spiro, A. J., and Rorke, L. B.: Skeletal muscle lesions in congenital rubella syndrome, Am. J. Dis. Child. **112**:427, 1966.

Sullivan, D. B., et al.: Prognosis in childhood dermatomyositis, J. Pediatr. **80**:555, 1972.

Thompson, C. E.: Polymyositis in children, Clin. Pediatr. **7**:24, 1968.

Unverricht, H.: Polymyositis acuta progressiva, Z. Klin. Med. **12**:533, 1887.

Walton, J. N., and Adams, R. D.: Polymyositis. Edinburgh, 1958. E & S Livingstone.

Wedgwood, R. J. P., Cook, C. D., and Cohen, J.: Dermatomyositis: report of 26 cases in children with a discussion of endocrine therapy in 13, Pediatrics **12**: 447, 1953.

Weed, L. A., et al.: Nocardiosis: clinical, bacteriologic and pathologic aspects, N. Engl. J. Med. **253**: 1137, 1955.

Whitaker, J. N., and Engel, W. K.: Vascular deposits of immunoglobulin and complement in idiopathic inflammatory myopathy, N. Engl. J. Med. **286**:333, 1972.

Whitaker, J. N., and Engel, W. K.: Mechanisms of muscular injury in idiopathic inflammatory myopathy, N. Engl. J. Med. **289**:107, 1973.

# Index